Plant Tissue Culture as a Source of Biochemicals

Editor

E. John Staba, Ph.D.

Professor of Pharmacognosy
College of Pharmacy
University of Minnesota
Minneapolis, Minnesota

CRC Press, Inc.
Boca Raton, Florida

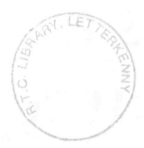

Library of Congress Cataloging in Publication Data

Main entry under title:

Plant tissue culture as a source of biochemicals.

   Bibliography: p.
   Includes index.
   1. Plant tissue culture. 2. Plant products.
I. Staba, E. John.
SB123.6.P52   631.5'8   79-12074
ISBN 0-8493-5557-5

PREFACE

Plant tissue culture techniques are profitably used today throughout the world. The technique is used to rapidly and uniformly propagate many horticultural plants, occasionally important food plants — for example, potato and sugar cane, and economically valuable plants containing steroids and pyrethrins. Academic, government, and industrial laboratories are also developing tissue culture techniques to rapidly propagate trees; to develop plants which will resist specific pathogens or will grow better in unfavorable environments; to be used for bio-assays; or to introduce desirable nuclear- or epi-genetic factors into plants. Aseptic plant cells, tissues, and organs are also used to better understand the biochemical processes of a plant. Although some microbial procedures are applied to plant tissue culture systems, plant cells are dramatically larger, and genetically and physiologically more complex than microorganisms. The major objectives of this book are to inform the reader of these significant differences, and of the scientific progress made in growing aseptic plant cell suspension cultures for biochemical production.

After approximately two decades of study it has been demonstrated that serially propagated plant tissue culture systems will produce many unusual secondary compounds; that cell strains can be selected for high production of some alkaloids and pigments; that some plant tissue cultures can be stored for long periods; and that plant cells can be grown in fermentors containing thousands of gallons of medium. However, several problems remain to be solved. For example, some compounds of interest are not produced in detectable or adequate amounts; selected strains are not always stable; and growth may be undesirably long and costly. Regardless of these important considerations, plant biochemical systems are *now* available for use in a controlled environment of our choosing. It should be remembered that single plant cells are totipotent in that they can be regenerated into whole plants. These cells are probably also biochemically equivalent to the plant at selected stages of cell, tissue, organ, or plant growth. Today, the art of plant tissue culture has become a science that is very much in an active developmental phase.

Although the obvious use of plant tissue culture systems to produce biochemicals industrially is not yet realized, one should not ignore the advantages of being able to produce plant substances independently of weather, geography, or even the confines of the surface of the earth. Indeed, the use of plant tissue culture may in the foreseeable future become greatest in space colonies!

I wish to thank the many contributors to this book, some of whom are easily identifiable as they have authored chapters. Others are not as easily identified to the reader, as they contributed by their correspondence and their personal suggestions to the authors. Lastly, I wish to thank some of the dedicated scientists to this research specialty whose works continue to inspire us — G. Morel, H. E. Street, and P. R. White.

E. John Staba

THE EDITOR

E. John Staba, Ph.D., Professor of Pharmacognosy, College of Pharmacy, University of Minnesota, was born May 16, 1928 in New York City, New York. He received his B.S. (Pharm.) (1952) from St. John's University; M. S. (1954) from Duquesne University; and Ph.D. (1957) from the University of Connecticut. He is married to Joyce E. Staba and has five children, three girls and two boys. He was Assistant Professor of Pharmacognosy (1957) and Professor and Chairman of the Pharmacognosy Department (1965) at the University of Nebraska. In 1968 he assumed the position of Professor and Chairman, Department of Pharmacognosy at the University of Minnesota.

He served as a consultant for the U.S. Army Quartermaster Corp., National Aeronautics and Space Administration (NASA) and various pharmaceutical and industrial concerns. His publications (60 +) and patents (2) have been in the area of medicinal plant tissue culture, aquatic plant phytochemistry, and pharmacy education. He received the Lunsford-Richardson Honorary Research Award (1957), and was a Gustavus and Louise Pfeiffer Visiting Professor, University of Connecticut (1966). In 1969 he was a National Academy of Sciences Visiting Scientist to Poland, Czechoslovakia, and Hungary. In 1970 he was a recipient of a Fulbright Hays Research Fellowship to Germany, and in 1973 a Council of Scientific and Industrial Research (CSIR) Visiting Scientist appointment to India. In 1974 he was an invited participant in a U.S.-Republic of China Cooperative Science Program Seminar on Plant Cell Tissue and Cell Culture, and a Vice President and participant in the 3rd International Congress of Plant Tissue and Cell Culture, Leicester, England. He has participated as a member of the visitation team for the American Foundation for Pharmaceutical Education (1976); presided over the Pharmaceutical section of a special NASA Colloquium on Bioprocessing in Space—March, 1976; and was invited by the German Ministry of Science and Technology to participate in an International Congress on Plant Cell Cultures and their Biotechnological Applications (Munich, September, 1976). He is listed in Who's Who in America, and American Men of Science.

He has served on many committees of the Academy of Pharmaceutical Sciences (Section of Pharmacognosy and Natural Products), the American Society of Pharmacognosy, the American Association of College of Pharmacy, and the Tissue Culture Association. He was President of the American Society of Pharmacognosy (1971—72), Chairman of the AACP Conference of Teachers (1972—73), and Chairman of the Plant Division, Tissue Culture Association (1972—74). He was a member of the In-Vitro Editorial Board, Tissue Culture Association (1974—76).

He served as Vice Chairman (1975—76) and Chairman-elect (1976—77) of the Academy of Pharmaceutical Sciences Section on Pharmacognosy and Natural Products. He also served as the AACP Council of Sections representative to the AACP Board of Directors' (1976—78).

CONTRIBUTORS

Donald K. Dougall, D. Phil.
Senior Scientist
W. Alton Jones Cell Science Center
Lake Placid, New York

Walter E. Goldstein, Ph.D.
Director
Chemical Engineering Research and
 Pilot Services
Research and Development
Industrial Products Group
Miles Laboratories
Elkhart, Indiana

M. B. Ingle, Ph.D.
Vice President
Research and Development
Industrial Products Group
Miles Laboratories
Elkhart, Indiana

P. G. Kadkade, Ph.D.
Staff Scientist
GTE Laboratories, Inc.
Waltham, Massachusetts

Linda Lasure, Ph.D.
Senior Research Scientist
Biosynthesis Research
Industrial Products Group
Miles Laboratories
Elkhart, Indiana

S. M. Martin, Ph.D.
Senior Research Officer
Division of Biological Sciences
National Research Council of Canada
Ottawa, Ontario
Canada

Masanaru Misawa, Ph.D.
Manager of Research
Tokyo Research Laboratory
Kyowa Hakko Kogyo Co. Ltd.
Tokyo, Japan

Louis G. Nickell, Ph.D.
Vice President
Research and Development
Velsicol Chemical Corporation
Chicago, Illinois

Janet E. A. Seabrook, Ph.D.
Department of Biology
University of New Brunswick
Fredericton, New Brunswick
Canada

Michael Seibert, Ph.D.
Senior Scientist
Solar Energy Research Institute
Golden, Colorado

J. M. Widholm, Ph.D.
Professor of Plant Physiology
Department of Agronomy
University of Illinois
Urbana, Illinois

for Joyce

TABLE OF CONTENTS

Chapter 1

LABORATORY CULTURE

Janet E. A. Seabrook

TABLE OF CONTENTS

I. INTRODUCTION

Plant tissue culture is the technique of growing plant cells, tissues, and organs in a prepared nutrient medium and in the absence of microorganisms. There are two main applications of plant tissue culture. As a unique and valuable research tool, growing plant tissues in vitro can help minimize variables such as environmental factors. Better control can be attained of light, temperature, gas mixtures, and nutrition. Correlative influences, which are working relationships between two or more organs within a plant, can be reduced. Plant tissues can be grown in the absence of artifacts attributable to bacteria, fungi, algae, small organisms, and possibly, viruses. Plant tissue culture can also be employed to preserve valuable germ plasma and as a tool for the plant breeder.

A recent application of plant tissue culture is the use of this technique for the production of economically valuable chemicals. Plant cells and tissues in culture can be manipulated so that specific chemicals can be extracted from the cultured tissues or from the medium in which the tissues have grown. In addition, the principle of totipotency, which states that every cell within the plant has the potential to regenerate into a whole plant, can be applied to regenerate plants from cultured cells and tissues. The propagation of valuable economic plants through tissue culture is based on the principle of totipotency.

A general feature of plant tissue culture is the disinfestation of the tissue to be cultured. A suitable nutrient medium has to be selected and, then, appropriate environmental conditions chosen for the kind of tissue to be cultured and for the type of culture desired.

For both research and economic purposes, most plant tissue culture involves the growth of callus on a semisolid medium. Liquid-suspension cultures of cells are not as widespread, probably due to the cost of equipment. Commercial plant propagators use cultures started from shoot tips or lateral buds, sometimes erroneously referred to as "meri-cloning" or "meristem cultures." Plant pathologists culture meristems in an attempt to obtain virus-free plants. Because of the potential for possible dramatic strides in genetic modification and crop improvement, the fusion protoplasts have also become a popular field of research in recent years.

This chapter will attempt to consider the parameters associated with the establishment of callus from explants, factors required for the growth of callus in culture, and the subsequent regeneration of plants from callus. Appendix I provides a sample methodology for the induction of callus and for the regeneration of shoots.

The information we have at present on the culture of plant tissues in vitro may not be applicable to all plants. Techniques of regenerating plants by auxillary branching, adventitious shoots, etc. have been discussed in a recent review by Murashige[1] and will not be repeated here.

II. THE SOURCE PLANT

The successful production of callus and subsequent plant regeneration is dependent, in part, upon the qualities associated with the explants used. These, in turn, are related to the condition of the source plant.

Often, there is considerable variability associated with the genotype of the plants used as explants.[1] While it has been convenient to categorize success in vitro with taxonomic grouping, this classification has not been entirely valid. There is as much variability in vitro between cultivars of the same species as there is between families. The ease of organ regeneration, e.g., root regeneration, in vitro is usually related to the ease of vegetative propagation by traditional nursery methods. Conversely, plants which are difficult to propagate vegetatively are also often difficult to regenerate in vitro.

Tissue culture should normally be viewed as a situation that allows for the enhancement of a process which can be observed in nature, i.e., as a means to enhance an ability already present. Tissue culture is not the miracle which will allow for the expression of genetically nonexistent characters.

A. Organ Source

The tissue or organ used as a source of explants can also be a determinant of the success, or degree of success, of a plant tissue culture. It is advisable to compare the culture of various organs and tissues systematically for each plant before selecting any given tissue or organ.

Even though totipotentiality may be a universal characteristic of plant cells, its expression has been limited to certain types of cells, identified as meristemoids by Torrey.[2] Meristemoid cells are apparently cells that respond to organogenetic stimuli, such as auxin/cytokinin balances. They can be distinguished among cultured cells by their relatively small size, dense cytoplasm, isodiametric shape, thin cell walls, minimal vacuolation, and large nuclei. They usually occur as clusters within the cultured tissues and sometimes appear as nodules or proembryonic masses.

If whole-plant regeneration is desired, the presence of meristemoids, or cells which can readily develop into meristemoids, are necessary. Such cells have been found in shoot tips of *Asparagus*,[3] immature leaf bases of *Narcissus*,[4] *Osmunda* leaf tips,[5] *Pseudotsuge menziesii* cotyledons,[6] *Citrus* nucellus,[7] *Citrus* ovary,[8] *Daucus carota* root,[9] *Nicotiana* stem internode,[10] and *Datura* microspores.[11]

B. Developmental Phase

Juvenile plants or growths usually provide more regeneration explants than adult plants. The juvenile and adult phases are reversible to varying degrees, the ease of reversibility being dependent on the plant species. Both juvenile and adult growth can be found on the same plant at the same time. The juvenile phase is characterized by vigorous vegetative development and the absence of reproductive-structure formation. The adult material usually grows more slowly and is sexually reproductive. The two phases can sometimes be distinguished by different leaf shapes and other morphological characteristics.

C. Ontogenetic Age

Even among materials in the juvenile development phase, tissue and organ regeneration is more likely to be accomplished with the younger tissues. Young plants provide the best explants. Older plants may have accumulated more pathogens in their tissues and, therefore, not be as healthy. Furthermore, older plants probably contain less meristematic tissue and may have the additional problem of being physiologically mature. Unfortunately, one often does not know if plants have characteristics which are desirable (e.g., superior blooms, higher fruit yields, production of a biochemical) until they are physiologically mature. This is a particular problem with woody perennials. Murashige[12] has illustrated the relationship between ontogenetic age and the organogenetic behavior of tissues in vitro.

D. Preculture Treatment of the Source Plant

Preculture treatment of source plants can make the difference between the success and failure of a culture. Standard greenhouse conditions such as soil mixtures and fertilizer applications should be maintained with as much uniformity as possible.

1. Seasonal Requirements

The position of the explant on the source plant[12] and the season of the year can make a difference to the regeneration of *de novo*-formed bulbils on *Lillium* bulb scales.[13,14,15] Fellenberg[16] noted that organogenesis in *Solanum tuberosum* tissue cultures was seasonally mediated. Thus, climatic requirements such as photoperiod[17] and temperature (cold treatment) may have to be satisfied prior to culture.[15]

2. Nutritional Requirements

The nutritional status of the source plant probably affects the successful establishment of explants in tissue culture. Heavy applications of fertilizer to the source plants prior to their use as explants for tissue culture can drastically change the response of the explants to the cultural conditions.

3. Etiolation

Changes in the light intensity to which source plants are subjected can alter the response of tissues to experimental conditions.[18]

4. Pretreatment with Growth Regulators

Pretreatment of the source plants with growth regulators can enhance or change the response of the explants to cultural conditions. Pretreatment with gibberellic acid can, in some plants, produce juvenile tissue which is easier to culture.[19]

The application of the growth retardant CCC (β-chloroethyltrimethyl ammonium chloride) as a foliar spray on tomato plants before using them as a source of culture material altered the response of the resultant callus to the application of exogenous auxin and cytokinin.[20]

5. Reduction of Microorganisms by Pretreatment of Source Plant

Explants which are free of microorganisms, especially pathogens, can be obtained by pretreating the source plant with antibiotics or with fungicides. Treatment of source plants with antiviral agents such as "virozol", heat-treatment, and drying out can all reduce the microorganism content of the explant in culture.

Plants established in growth chambers usually provide the cleanest explants for culture, whereas green-house-grown and field-grown plants provide explants which are successively more difficult to rid of microorganisms.

E. Explant Size

The larger the explant, the greater the danger of the inclusion of microbial contaminants in the tissues. There is, however, a minimum effective size for explants, as very small explants such as meristems do not grow as fast or respond as effectively to cultural conditions as do larger explants. This dilemma can be partly solved by culturing several small explants together in one culture vessel. In this way, shock due to dissection and transfer are also reduced. There appears to be a "population effect" in vitro. When several small explants are cultured in the same vessel they grow faster than small explants cultured singly.

F. Disinfestation of Tissue to be Used for Culture

It is always necessary to remove all microorganisms from tissue to be cultured because they will outgrow the tissues and destroy them. Secondly, the presence of microorganisms changes the environment by removing nutrients from the medium and by releasing metabolic by-products into it. Results obtained from contaminated cultures may not be reproducible. Surface sterilization is particularly difficult with hairy or unevenly surfaced materials as they harbor pockets of microorganisms. Occasionally a combination of more than one kind of disinfesting agent is effective. A compromise has to be achieved between adequate disinfestation and causing as little damage as possible to the tissues to be cultured.

Plants to be used as a source of explants should be removed from the field or greenhouse and all soil washed from the roots. If only small sections of a large plant are required, the tissue can be removed with a sharp scalpel and the cut surface dipped in hot wax before transport to the laboratory. All necrotic, old, or obviously unclean tissue should be removed before applying sterilizing agents. Sharp scalpel blades should be used to prevent unnecessary damage to the explants. When suitable, outer tissues such as bud scales and older leaves can be left on until after surface-sterilization. They can then be removed under sterile conditions.

A mild soap and running tap water can be used to remove much of the surface dirt from tissue to be cultured. Placing the tissue in 70% ethylalcohol for 5 to 20 sec removes some contaminants. The most common method of surface-sterilizing plant material is the use of a chlorine solution, Purex® sodium hypochlorite, or calcium hypochlorite for 5 to 30 min (15 min is usually sufficient).

Penetration of the disinfesting agent into uneven or hairy surfaces can be promoted by the addition of a wetting agent such as Tween 20® (1 to 2 drops per 100 mℓ disinfestant, ca. 0.05%). Placing the explant and surface sterilant together in an erlenmeyer flask on a rotary shaker (50 to 150 rpm) for 15 to 30 min enhances disinfestation.[21] The use of a vacuum can further increase penetration of the disinfestant into the surface crevices of the tissue.

After disinfestation, all manipulations should be performed in a sterile environment. Utilizing a laminar-flow transfer hood is the most effective way to ensure sterility of material to be cultured. All equipment placed in a transfer hood should be sterile or swabbed with alcohol or Purex®. Sterilized tissue should be rinsed at least three times with sterile, distilled water. This is best done in the transfer hood.

All damaged or dead material should be removed from the disinfested explant which is now ready to be planted on a suitable nutrient medium.

III. ESTABLISHING A CALLUS CULTURE

The most commonly cultured plant tissue is callus, which is wound tissue composed of differentiated, highly vacuolated, unorganized cells.

Callus and cell-suspension cultures of most plant species have been easier to culture than shoot cultures. Callus is usually obtained by culturing explants on a semisolid medium containing a high concentration of salts, high auxin, and casein hydrolysate. Once friable callus has been obtained, the tissue can be transferred to a liquid medium. If vigorous agitation and aeration is applied, a suspension of free cells and aggregates of cells can be obtained. Callus cultures are usually maintained in darkness, and 2,4-D is frequently added to suppress organogenesis.

A. Media Formulations

Although whole plants have simple requirements for growth, plant-tissue cultures have more complex needs and are seldom autotrophic. That is, plant tissue in vitro requires the usual macro- and microelements supplied in hydroponic culture. In addition, other nutrients, such as a source of bound carbon and vitamins, are necessary. Isolated plant cells and tissues frequently require the addition of vitamins and plant-growth regulators that in vivo are synthesized by one part or organ of a plant and transported to another part where they are metabolized. Little is known of the effect of many of the individual constituents on the production of secondary metabolites because the chemical composition of most plant-tissue-culture formulations have been devised with the aim of improving cell growth and organogenesis. Media composition for suspension cultures is discussed in Chapter 2. Thus, only generalities will be noted here.

1. Salt Requirement for Cultured Plant Tissues

Although early tissue-culture formulations[22,23] were suitable for the culture of callus cells, later formulations, such as those of Murashige and Skoog[24] and Gamborg, Miller and Ojima,[25] are more suitable for a wider range of plants and for the promotion of organogenesis in cultures. A formulation has to be determined which supports the growth of cultured cells for each species, and sometimes each variety within a species. Generally, the Murashige and Skoog (MS)[24] salt solution will support the growth of most plant cells in culture, and this is in part due to its high salt concentration. Some ions, the NH_4 ion in particular, may be in too high a concentration for all plants and tissue at all stages of development in vitro. The addition of $NaH_2PO_4 \cdot H_2O$ to the MS salt solution has been beneficial for some tissue. Huang and Murashige[26] have listed the major constituents of plant tissue culture media and have indicated how they can be prepared.

Even though there are trace impurities of minor elements in supplies of major elements such as N, K, and P, additional quantities of these microelements are almost always necessary. The MS salt solution is particularly high in microelements when compared to other media formulations.[26] The addition of chelating agents such as Fe-EDTA* ensures that iron is available over a wide range of pH.

---

*   EDTA, ethylenediaminetetraacetic acid.

2. Osmolarity and Ion Concentration

Embryogenesis is more likely to occur when tissue is grown in a salt solution of high osmolarity such as the MS formulation.[27] The concentration of N and K ions appear to be important for somatic embryogenesis. Reinert[28] proposed an interaction between nitrogen and auxin which enhanced embryogenesis.

3. Organic Constituents
a. Vitamins

The use of vitamins in plant tissue culture media has been a matter of custom rather than proven necessity. Thiamine·HCl is the only vitamin for which there seems to be a consistent requirement for growth of plant tissues in vitro. Other vitamins should be added to media formulations where enhancement of growth or morphogenesis indicate they are necessary.[26]

b. Carbon Source

The addition of an organic carbon source, such as sucrose, to plant tissue culture media, is absolutely necessary for nearly all tissue, as very few plant cells in vitro are autotrophic. Sucrose, in concentrations of 2 to 3%, is the most commonly used carbon source. There is evidence that the production of some metabolites by plant tissue may be affected by the concentration of sucrose.[29]

c. Growth Regulators

Hormones, in intact plants, act to regulate and coordinate processes which lead to normal development. Growth, as well as differentiation of tissue and cells and secondary metabolism, is affected by these hormones. The addition of plant-growth regulators to tissue-culture media, is not always necessary for callus cultures. However, supplementation with growth regulators is usually obligate for callus cultures in which an increase in the growth rates or organogenesis is required.

Very few plant tissues in vitro will produce extensive callus in the absence of growth regulators.[30] *Helianthus tuberosus* callus from dormant tubers and callus from the root of *Cichorium* are autotrophic for cytokinin, but require auxin.[30]

Indole-3-acetic acid (IAA) is the most generally used auxin for plant tissue culture because it has fewer adverse effects on organogenesis than other auxins. IAA is weaker than naphthaleneacetic acid (NAA). NAA can sometimes be used in higher concentrations than IAA, which is usually used on concentrations of 10^{-5} to 10^{-10} M.[30] Media containing IAA deteriorates faster than media containing NAA, especially if not refrigerated.

The most potent of the commonly used auxins is 2,4-dichlorophenoxyacetic acid (2,4-D). It strongly suppresses organogenesis and is particularly useful for the maintenance of callus cultures. 2,4-D is generally active in plant tissue cultures at concentrations from 10^{-5} to 10^{-7} M.[30] It should be recalled that 2,4-D is a commonly used herbicide for the control of broadleaved weeds, and therefore, its use in cultures of dicotyledonous plants may be restricted.

A second class of commonly used growth regulators in tissue culture are the cytokinins. The most active of the common synthetic cytokinins is N_6-isopentenyladenine (2iP). N_6-Benzyladenine (BA) has a particularly enhancing effect on the release from apical dominance of axillary shoots and on the proliferation of shoots induced in vitro. Tobacco pith callus requires a concentration of 10^{-6} to 10^{-7} M kinetin for growth, whereas organogensis in tobacco pith callus needs a concentration of 10^{-5} to 10^{-7} M kinetin.[30] As there is some evidence that kinetin, which is a synthetic cytokinin, can be degraded by light (300 to 800 nm), care should be taken to store stock solutions in darkness.[31]

Skoog and Miller[32] reported that the balance of auxin to cytokinin levels had an effect on organ formation. Their concept states that both auxin and cytokinin are necessary for the control of growth and of organogenesis in vitro. The kind of development, i.e., callus, roots or shoots, is determined by the relative amounts of these two growth regulators. This concept should be applied when trying to obtain organ formation in cultures. Phenolic compounds[33] and excess gibberellins[20] can mask the effect of a balance of auxins to cytokinins and, therefore, suppress organ formation.

Gibberellins have been used in tissue culture, but they generally have the effect of suppressing organ formation.[10] The proporion of various growth regulators and the concentrations that are required for plant tissues varies with the stage of development of the cultured tissue.[1] Organ initiation is generally enhanced by higher levels of growth regulators than is required for the growth of callus.[1]

d. Amino Acids and Amides

The requirement for amino acids by a plant-tissue culture can be estimated by adding varying amounts of a protein hydrolysate (e.g., enzymatic casein hydrolysate). Any enhancement of growth or morphogenesis can be explored further by testing a mixture of amino acids and amides.[26] The use of amino acids in plant-tissue culture media should take into account possible antagonisms between them.

The amino acids and amides which commonly give beneficial effects are L-argenine, L-aspartic acid, L-asparagine, L-glutamic acid and L-glutamine.[26]

e. Nitrogen Bases

The nitrogen bases, cytidylic and guanylic acids, have been reported to enhance growth in callus cultures.[26]

f. Natural Complexes

Natural complexes, such as coconut milk, yeast extract, and protein hydrolysates (hydrolysates of casein, lactalbumin, peptone, and tryptone) which have been used in the past for plant tissue cultures, should be avoided. Quality control with these products is nearly impossible. Use can result in nonreproducible results.

A more effective way of supplementing media with organic constituents is to add various known chemicals when it has been determined that they improve growth or morphogenesis of cultures.

g. Materials which Enhance the Quality of the Medium by Physical Means
(1) Semisolid Media

In early plant tissue culture techniques, agar was used to solidify the medium. Only simple laboratory equipment is required for a semisolid medium, but the yields of biomedicals may not be as high as can be obtained from liquid cultures. Agar is still the most commonly used material for gelling media, however the quality should be very carefully monitored. Unless one is reasonably sure that the agar is pure, it should be washed at least three times with distilled water. Romberger and Tabor[34] found that the best growth of *Picea abies* was with a nutrient medium solidified with Difco®, "Purified" agar, and that Difco,® "Noble" agar, which is more refined, gave poorer growth. High concentrations of agar can inhibit the growth of plant tissue in culture. The precise concentration of agar suitable for each medium and plant tissue should be determined for each situation. However, a concentration of 0.8% is usually sufficient for most purposes.

Gelatin and silica gel have been used to support plant tissue, and recently acrylamide gels have been developed. Starch co-polymers have been suggested as agar substitutes.[35] They have the advantage that they do not require boiling to dissolve in water. There are problems at present with adjusting the pH, and these will have to be solved before starch co-polymers can be widely used.

Charcoal is frequently added to media formulations. It enhances growth by adsorbing toxic metabolites of tissue cultures.[36]

(2) Liquid-Media Formulations

Liquid formulations are also common. Tissue can be continuously immersed in the liquid medium or suspended on small filter-paper bridges. Glass wool can also be used to support cultured tissue. Cheng and Voqui[6] have used a fabric support (100% polyester) saturated with a liquid medium for the growth and organogenesis of Douglas fir cotyledon explants. Immersed cultures can be agitated at 1 rpm to 150 rpm to improve aeration. Some cultures, e.g., domestic carrot callus, proliferate faster when only periodically immersed in the medium. This is achieved by the use of a roll-a-drum apparatus which holds test tubes at a 10 to 12° angle as they are rotated.

The quantity of medium used for a particular-sized inoculum of plant tissue may be important. There appears to be a critical cell population of minimum effective density for each tissue.[30] Small quantities of cells in culture often have to be supplied with substances such as amino acids, which are not required by a large mass of cells. This "population effect" may be similar to that reported in pollen germination studies[37,38] in which there appears to be a critical concentration of boron or calcium required. It is possible that cells not only take up nutrients from the culture medium, but also release metabolites into the medium which affect other cells.

h. pH of Nutrient Media

Both the growth-promoting effect and the selectivity of plant tissue culture media are pH dependent. Tissue culture media are usually adjusted to a pH of 5.0 to 6.0 prior to the addition of agar and to autoclaving. In time, the pH of a medium will drift to a neutral pH. Extremes of pH should be avoided as this will block the availability of some nutrients to the tissue. For instance, at both an alkaline pH and at a pH below 3.0, gibberellic acid is activated.[39]

The incorporation of EDTA into media may be important as it maintains the availability of iron and other metal ions as the pH drifts during culture.[30] In sycamore cell suspension cultures, the minimum effective cell density can be reduced by adjusting the pH to 6.4.[30]

B. Optimum Volume of Medium per Culture Vessel

The correct amount of medium for each tissue and vessel type should be tested carefully. Too much medium can adversely affect tissue growth. Conversely, an inadequate quantity of medium can slow growth rates of tissue.

C. Sterilization of Medium

Plant tissue culture media are sterilized by autoclaving or by filter sterilization. The most common technique is to sterilize the media, which has previously been dispensed into culture vessels, at 121°C for 15 min in an autoclave. The use of pressure allows a high temperature to be used without the liquid overboiling. When autoclaved, sucrose in combination with other media constituents can cause a nonenzymatic browning which can be toxic to cultured plant cells.[40]

Media constituents which are heat labile (e.g., gibberellin),[39] can be filter sterilized and added to the remainder of the constituents which have been autoclaved and maintained at 40°C to prevent agar solidification. The heat-sterilized and filter-sterilized components are combined under aseptic conditions in a laminar-flow transfer hood. Filter sterilization can be accomplished by using a membrane filter (millipore), which is a two-dimensional screen made of homogenous polymers with a uniform pore size. Bacteria and fungi are normally removed with a pore size of 0.45 μm. This technique is particularly useful for the sterilization of heat-labile components.

If desired, all media components can be filter sterilized and the medium dispensed into sterile culture vessels under aseptic conditions. This tends to be time-consuming for large quantities of media, but may be necessary if degradation of media components by heat is suspected.

D. The Culture Environment for Callus
1. Light
Plant-tissue cultures are not photosynthetically efficient and therefore, generally are not autotrophic. Nevertheless, the influence of light on morphogenetic processes within the cultured tissue should not be discounted. When maintaining callus cultures, the tissue should be maintained in darkness to avoid morphogenesis.

2. Temperature
A temperature of 25-27°C is normally employed for in vitro culture. The optimum temperature for the growth of callus cultures may have to be investigated individually for each species.

3. Humidity
The climatic conditions of each area dictate the treatment required by cultures. In tropical, humid regions, dehumidifiers may have to be used in the culture area if high rates of fungal contamination are experienced. When dry atmosphere is encountered, enclosures such as "Kaputs" may have to be used to reduce loss of moisture from both cultures and the medium.

E. Removal or Suppression of Microbial Contaminants from Cultures
Contamination of cultures is a serious problem and can be disastrous when working with valuable material. Attempts to resterilize contaminated tissue by the use of the aforementioned surface sterilants are not usually successful, as the tissue is often damaged. Antibiotics, such as gentamycin, partially suppress bacterial contaminants, but may also reduce growth rates.

IV. REGENERATION OF PLANTS FROM CALLUS CULTURES

Some valuable biochemicals are only synthesized (or synthesized in greater quantity) by differentiated tissue or are only accumulated in specialized organs or tissues. For instance, the total alkaloid content of callus cultures is often low, but is increased with morphogenesis and plant growth.[41] Therefore, it may be necessary to obtain and maintain differentiated and organized tissue for the purpose of extracting drugs. Ideally, one would prefer to obtain chemical diffentiation in suspension cultures, which are easier to grow, without having to resort to morphological specialization. Further, the clonal propagation of a high-yield plant, and its subsequent multiplication by modern nursery techniques, may be at present the most efficient method for the commercial production of a drug. In any event, the principles of regeneration of shoots and plantlets for the two above purposes are similar.

If plant cells are totipotent, that is, capable of regenerating a whole plant from a single cell or small group of cells, then their ability to undergo organogenesis depends on their differentiation to meristematic cells and then their further differentiation to specialized cells.

There are two ways to regenerate plants from callus, through the initiation of shoots or by somatic embryos.[12] The removal of suppressive influences, such as 2,4-D, and a salt solution of high osmolarity are required for the formation of shoots and somatic embryos in vitro. The presence of light is required for the normal germination of somatic embryos and for the growth of shoots.[12]

The nutrient requirements for organogenetic cultures are generally the same as for callus cultures. The growth-regulator levels may have to be adjusted.[1]

A. Regeneration of Shoots From Callus Cultures

Regeneration of shoots is generally accomplished in the presence of light and in a culture medium of high osmolarity containing chelating agents.[12] An exogenous supply of carbohydrates is usually necessary for shoot initiation.[42] The maintenance of shoot cultures usually requires the presence of exogenous cytokinin as well as auxin.[12] In some plants, continued proliferation of shoots can be maintained for several months,[20] although organ formation declines with time.[12]

1. Growth Regulators

The single most important factor determining organ formation in tissue culture is the relative quantities of auxin and cytokinin.[32] There appears to be a universal control, by the relative levels of auxin and cytokinin, of a regulatory mechanism which leads to organogenesis within the cells and tissues of plants. Tobacco stem segments produce callus when supplied exogenously with auxin and cytokinin of approximately the same molar concentration. If the auxin level is raised relative to the cytokinin concentration, roots are induced. Conversely, when the auxin concentration is lower than that of the cytokinin, shoots are formed on the tobacco tissue.

The synergism between coconut milk and auxin which was reported by Steward and Shantz[43] has been found to be, in part, due to an auxin/cytokinin synergism. When tissues in vitro do not appear to require a balance in the levels of exogenously applied auxin and cytokinin in the above manner, it may be that sufficient endogenous levels exist for organogenesis.

2. Amino Acids

Skoog and Miller[32] reported that L-tyrosine could replace casein hydrolysate for the enhancement of root and shoot formation in tobacco callus cultures.

3. Adenine

Increased shoot initiation in tobacco callus cultures was noted by Skoog and Tsu[44] when adenine was added to the nutrient medium.

4. Other Factors

Phenolic substances can enhance shoot formation in tobacco callus cultures.[33] Increased levels of inorganic phosphate (e.g., $NaH_2PO_4 \cdot H_2O$) can increase shoot production in plant-tissue cultures.[12]

B. Regeneration of Plants by Somatic Embryogenesis

Regeneration of plants from cultured cells can occur through somatic embryogenesis and has been reported for over 300 plants in vitro.[45] Somatic embryos, which often lack a suspensor, are morphologically indistinguishable from sexual embryos.

1. Removal of Auxin

When callus from certain plants is transferred from a medium containing an auxin (2,4-D or NAA) to a medium lacking auxin, somatic embryos are formed.[46,47] The addition of the antiauxin, 2,4,6-trichlorophenoxyacetic acid, to the culture medium increases the number of embryos formed in wild-carrot cultures.[48] The precise mechanism by which 2,4-D and other embryogenic suppressants act is, as yet, unclear.[44] Wochok and Wetherell[49] reported that ethylene suppressed embryogenesis, but other studies[50] indicate that additional chemicals may be involved. Supplementing the medium with charcoal increases embryogenesis by apparently adsorbing inhibitory substances from the medium.[36]

2. Nitrogen and Potassium Ions

Enriching the nutrient medium with nitrogen enhances somatic embryogenesis.[47] The potassium ion also positively affects the number of somatic embryos formed in cultured tissues.[51]

C. The Culture Environment for Regenerating Shoots and Somatic Embryos
1. Light

Although light is not required for the initiation of asexual embryos in carrot, Murashige[1] has noted that light is essential for shoot initiation in tobacco cultures. Light intensity, photoperiod, and spectral quality are all factors which should be considered when attempting to initiate shoots in vitro.

The optimum light intensity for shoot initiation in *Gerbera* is 1000 lux,[1] and many cultures respond favorably to this level of intensity.[12] A photo-period of 16 hr daily is commonly used for tissue culture. When working with obligate long- or short-day plants, it would be wise to test the photo-period required by tissue in vitro. Continuous illumination has generally been found to be unsuitable for optimal rates of organogenesis.[12]

Seibert[52] has reported that the significant wavelength of light for the induction of shoots in tobacco callus was 467 nm. Daily 16-hr exposure to 1000-lux Gro Lux® light should provide adequate light for most tissue culture.[12]

2. Temperature

Skoog[53] noted that there was increased bud formation in tobacco pith callus when the tissue was incubated at 18°C as compared with cultures maintained at 12 and 33°C.

Although one might expect plants which experienced diurnal fluctuation in their native habitat to exhibit a positive response to similar changes in vitro, this does not always seem to be the case. Hasegawa, Murashige, T., and Takatori,[54] reported no advantage to lowering the night (dark period) temperature of *Asparagus* tissue cultures. In addition, a lowering of the night temperature to which cultures of *Narcissus* were subjected, did not increase the fresh weight of the tissue or the number of shoots induced.[67] The rooting of *Helianthus* tuber sections in vitro was increased when the temperature was 26°C in the daytime and lowered to 15°C at night.[55]

In contrast, Kefford and Caso[56] noted that the maximum yield of adventitious shoots in *Chondrilla juncea* root cultures occurred when the night temperature was 16 to 22°C and the day temperature was 21 to 27°C.

Temperature pretreatment of source plants prior to their use as tissue-culture explants may increase the yields of shoots produced in vitro. *Lillium* bulbs of some cultivars, which have had a cold treatment, produced more propagules,[12,13,15] and the number of shoots and plantlets obtained from prechilled *Narcissus* is greater than that for untreated bulbs.[4]

3. Oxygen Tension

When plant tissues are placed in a liquid or on an agar-gell medium containing the same constituents, different morphogenetic effects are observed. White[57] and Skoog[53] observed that *Nicotiana* cultures produced more shoots in a liquid medium in contrast to an agar-gelled medium. Generally, relatively anaerobic conditions favor embryogenesis and shoot initiation in carrot callus cultures, and more aerobic conditions favor the production of roots.[58]

V. GENERAL DISCUSSION

A. Regeneration of Plants from Long-Term Callus Cultures

Cell and callus cultures, when maintained over a long period of time, tend to lose their morphogenetic potential.[59,60] That is, the ability of the cultures to regenerate shoots, roots, and somatic embryos, which was previously exhibited by the culture, is progressively lost with time. This may be partly due to karyotypic and ploidy changes in the cultured cells in response to auxin.[59,60] In addition, epigenetic changes can occur in cultured tissues such that there is a change in the response of the cultured cells to the cultural conditions.

One way of reducing the hazard of genetic changes in cultured cells is to preserve desirable cells lines by freezing. This will be discussed in Chapter 5.

B. Rooting of In Vitro-Produced Plants

Rooting of plants produced by means of tissue culture is an important step in the clonal multiplication of a desirable plant. Propagules have to have an adequate root system before they can be reestablished satisfactorily.

A reduction in the concentration of both sucrose and salt generally enhances the induction of adventitious roots on shoots grown in vitro. Lowering the sucrose concentration from 3 to 1 and reducing the concentration of a MS salt solution by 50% is usually satisfactory.[4,25] Auxin has also been beneficial in inducing rooting.[61] The rooting of shoots should be distinguished from the induction of roots on callus or on explants *de novo* via the manipulation of the relative levels of auxin and cytokinin.

Amemiya[62] noted that a high osmotic pressure was inhibitory to root growth of rice embryos. Kartha, Gamborg, and Constabel[63] produced roots on over 50% of cultured shoots of *Pisum* by transferring them to one-half-strength B5 medium with the addition of NAA (1.0 μM).[25]

An increase in light intensity may be advantageous for rooting plantlets. Hasegawa et al.[54] noted an optimum light intensity (10,000 lux) for rooting of *Asparagus* shoot cultures (stage III) which was higher than that required for the multiplication of propagula in stage II (1,000 lux).

C. Hardening-Off Propagules for Reestablishment in Soil

Many valuable propagules can be lost if care is not taken when transferring them to soil. The change from the heterotrophic to the autotrophic state has to be somewhat gentle. A good root system should help propagules to withstand some moisture stress. Placing the small plants in a shaded greenhouse and under an intermittent mist spray can reduce excessive transpiration.

Sterilizing soil in an autoclave or by the use of steam rods can reduce pathogens, particularly those which cause damping off. Soil sterilized in an autoclave should be allowed to remain, covered, at room temperature, for 1 to 2 weeks prior to use.

D. Production of Biochemicals by Organized Cultured Tissues

The production of drugs or other biochemicals by plant tissues may, in some instances, be more efficient when organized tissues are employed. Although we can presently culture the organs and tissues in which specialized cells occur, we cannot culture higly specialized cells such as glandular hair or lactifers.

If the efficient production of a specific biochemical is not technically feasible at present, the most economical way of producing the compound could be by clonal multiplication through the tissue culture of superior genotypes.

ACKNOWLEDGMENT

I wish to express my deep appreciation to Dr. Toshio Murashige, University of California, Riverside, for the generous use of facilities. Dr. Murashige's discussions and comments on this manuscript have been invaluable and are gratefully acknowledged.

APPENDIX I

SAMPLE METHODOLOGY FOR THE CULTURE OF *NARCISSUS* SCAPE CALLUS AND FOR THE REGENERATION OF SHOOTS.

APPENDIX I

SAMPLE METHODOLOGY FOR THE CULTURE OF *NARCISSUS* CALLUS AND FOR THE REGENERATION OF SHOOTS.

I.   Equipment

    1.   Autoclave
    2.   Laminar-flow cabinet
    3.   Distilled-water apparatus
    4.   Gyratory shaker
    5.   Refrigerator and freezer
    6.   Balance
    7.   Glassware:

        •   Delong flasks (50 mℓ)
        •   Stoppers or caps (kaputs) for flasks
        •   Erlenmeyer flasks (200 mℓ)
        •   Pipettes
        •   Pasteur pipettes

8. Reagents:

- Water should be demineralized or double distilled.
- Chemicals as in Table 1.
- Reagent-grade chemicals should be used.
- Growth regulators and other organic constituents may require further purification.

II. Preparation of Media for the Induction of Callus on Scape Tissue of *Narcissus* (Daffodil)[4,64]

1. Prepare stock salt solutions (modified Murashige and Skoog (MS) salt solution)[24] as follows:*

TABLE 1

Stock Solutions for Modified MS Salt Solution

Constituent	g/ℓ
1. NH_4NO_3	165.0
2. KNO_3	190.0
3. $CaCl_2 \cdot 2H_2O$	37.0
4. $MgSO_4 \cdot 7H_2O$	37.0
5. $NaH_2PO_4 \cdot H_2O$	30.0
6. H_3BO_3	0.62
7. $MnSO_4 \cdot 4H_2O$	2.23
8. $ZnSO_4 \cdot 7H_2O$	0.86
9. KI	0.083
10. $Na_2MoO_4 \cdot 2H_2O$	0.025
11. $CuSO_4 \cdot 5H_2O$	0.0025
12. $CoCL \cdot 6H_2O$	0.0025
13. $FeNa_2EDTA$	
$\quad FeSO_4 \cdot 7H_2O$	28.00
$\quad Na\ EDTA$	37.25

2. Place 400 mℓ double-distilled water in a 2000 mℓ Erlenmeyer flask.
3. Add 10 mℓ each of above 12 stock solutions.
4. Add 10 mℓ of organics stock solution prepared as follows:

Constituent	mg/ℓ
Thiamine $\cdot$ HCl	50.0
Pyridoxine	100.0
Nicotinic acid	500.0
Glycine	200.0

5. Add

Constituent	amount
i-inositol	100.0 mg
Adenine sulfate	160.0 mg
Casein hydrolysate	1000.0 mg
Sucrose	30.0g

* Note: 4.33 g/ℓ of GIBCO premixed MS salts + 3.0 g/ℓ $NaH_2PO_4 \cdot H_2O$ may be used in place of the above 12 stock solutions.

6. Add 10 mℓ of a 100 mg/ℓ NAA stock solution and 100 mℓ of a 100.0 mg/ℓ BAP stock solution.
7. Dilute to 800 mℓ with double-distilled water.
8. Adjust pH to 5.4 ± 0.1 with 1 *N* NaOH.
9. Add 8.0 g agar which has been washed 3 times with double-distilled water. Use good quality agar such as Difco Bactoagar®.
10. Bring up to final volume of 1000 mℓ with double-distilled water.
11. Dissolve agar by heating or by placing in an autoclave at 121°C for 5 min.
12. Make sure that the medium is well mixed. Dispense 20 mℓ into each 50 mℓ delong flask and stopper with foam plugs covered with aluminum foil or Bellco® "kaputs".
13. Sterilize by placing the culture vessels in an autoclave at 121°C for 15 min.

III. Preparation and Surface Disinfestation of Explant Source (*Narcissus* [Daffodil] Bulbs).
1. Remove the brown outer scales and lower half of the basal plate from a healthy, prechilled daffodil bulb which has not been replanted in soil.
2. Working very carefully with a clean, sharp scalpel, remove the white, inner bulb scales so that the shoot covered with protective sheaths remains with a small amount of basal plate. There are usually 2 to 3 shoots per double-nosed daffodil bulb.
3. Dip the shoots in 70% ethyl alcohol for 10 to 15 sec.
4. Place the shoots in a surface disinfestant (9% filtered calcium hypochlorite solution, to which 2 to 3 drops of Tween 20® wetting agent have been added) for 10 to 15 min.
5. Remove the shoots from the disinfestant and rinse three times with sterile double-distilled water.
6. In a laminar-flow transfer hood, dissect the daffodil shoots in a sterile petri dish. Using surgical instruments which have been sterilized by dipping in 95% ethyl alcohol and flaming, carefully dissect out the immature leaves and floral parts.
7. Dissect out the scape (floral stem) so that the top and bottom of each section can be identified.* This can be accomplished by cutting the scape with a straight transverse cut for the lower portion of each section and an angled cut for the upper portion of the explant. The small, wedge-shaped section remaining when each explant is dissected can be discarded.
8. Plant all scape sections in an *inverted* position, ca. one third into the medium, 2 per delong flask.

IV. Transfer of Ovary Callus to Liquid Medium for Maintenance of Callus
  A. Preparation of Medium for Maintenance of Callus
1. Prepare medium as in section B.1 to 4 (above).
2. Add 10 mℓ of a 100 mg/ℓ 2,4-D stock solution and 10 mℓ of a 100 mg/ℓ BAP stock solution.
3. Dilute to 800 g with double-distilled water.

---

* Note: The base of the immature leaves can be cultured in the same way as the scape (above). Cultured leaf bases do not usually produce callus. Ovaries produce callus on a medium (II 1-13) containing 25 mg/ℓ NAA and 4 mg/ℓ BAP.

4. Adjust pH to 5.4 ± 0.1 with 1 *N* NaOH.

5. Bring up to final volume of 1000 m*l* with double-distilled water. Do not add agar.

6. Dispense 20 m*l* into each 50-m*l* delong flask, and sterilize as above.

B. Transfer of Scape Callus Tissue to Callus-Maintenance Medium

1. In a laminar-flow transfer hood, dissect the callus off the top portion of the scape.

2. Place 2 to 3 0.5 × 0.5 cm pieces in each flask of liquid callus maintenance medium.

3. Place flask on a rotary shaker (100 rpm) in darkness at 25°C for 2 to 6 weeks.

V. Transfer of Scape Callus from Callus Maintenance Medium to Shoot-Inducing Medium.

1. Prepare medium as in II.1 to 13 (above).

2. Transfer 0.5 × 0.5 cm sections of scape callus tissue on medium as prepared in 1.

3. Place at 25°C in a growth cabinet with a 300 fc cool-white fluorescent 16 hr daily photoperiod for 4 to 8 weeks or until small unrooted plants 4 to 8 cm are formed.

VI. Rooting of In Vitro-Induced Shoots

1. Prepare a modified Hellers[65] and Knudson[66] media as follows:

TABLE 2

Salt	gm/l	mg/l
$Ca(NO_3)_2 \cdot 4H_2O$	1.0	—
KH_2PO_4	0.25	—
$MgSO_4 \cdot 7H_2O$	0.25	—
$(NH_4) \cdot 7H_2O$	0.25	—
$(NH_4)_2SO_4$	0.5	—
Na_2EDTA	0.018625	—
$FeSO_4 \cdot 7H_2O$	0.013925	—
$MnSO_4 \cdot 4H_2O$	—	0.1
$ZnSO_4 \cdot 7H_2O$	—	1.0
H_3BO_3	—	1.0
KI	—	0.01
$CuSO_4 \cdot 5H_2O$	—	0.03
$AlCl_3$	—	0.03
$NiCL_2 \cdot 6H_2O$	—	0.03
Sucrose	1.5%	—
Agar	0.6%	—
pH	5.5 (± 0.1)	—

2. Transfer shoots 4-8 cm in length to medium prepared in 1.

3. Place in environmental cabinet as in V.3.

REFERENCES

1. **Murashige, T.**, Clonal crops through tissue culture, in *Plant Tissue Culture and Its Bio-technological Application*, Barz, N., Reinhard, E., and Zenk, M. H., Eds., Springer-Verlag, Berlin, 1977, 392.
2. **Torrey, J. G.**, The initiation of organized development in plants, *Adv. Morphog.*, 5, 39, 1966.
3. **Murashige, T., Shabde, M. N., Hasegawa, P. M., Takatori, F. H., and Jones, J. B.**, Propagation of asparagus through shoot apex culture. I. Nutrient medium for formation of plantlets, *J. Am. Soc. Hortic. Sci.*, 97, 158, 1972.
4. **Seabrook, J. E. A., Cumming, B. G., and Dionne, L. A.**, The *in vitro* induction of adventitious shoot and root apices on *Narcissus* (daffodil and narcissus) cultivar tissue, *Can. J. Bot.*, 54, 814, 1976.
5. **Steeves, T. A. and Sussex, I. M.**, Studies on the development of excised leaves in sterile culture, *Am. J. Bot.*, 44, 665, 1957.
6. **Cheng, T.-Y. and Voqui, T. H.**, Regeneration of douglas fir plantlets through tissue culture, *Science*, 198, 306, 1977.
7. **Esan, E. B.**, A Detailed Study of Adventive Embryogenesis in the Rutaceae, Ph.D. thesis, University of California, Riverside, 1973.
8. **Mitra, G. C. and Chaturvedi, H. C.**, Embryoids and complete plants from unpollinated ovaries and from ovules of *in vitro*-grown emasculated flower buds from *Citrus* spp., *Bull. Torrey Bot. Club*, 99, 184, 1972.
9. **Levine, M.**, Differentiation of carrot root tissue grown *in vitro*, *Bull. Torrey Bot. Club*, 74, 321, 1947.
10. **Murashige, T.**, Suppression of shoot formation in cultured tobacco cells by gibberellic acid, *Science*, 134, 280, 1961.
11. **Guha, S. and Maheshwari, S. C.**, *In vitro* production of embryos from anthers of *Datura*, *Nature (London)*, 204, 497, 1964.
12. **Murashige, T.**, Manipulation of organ initiation in plant tissue cultures, *Bot. Bull. Acad. Sin.*, 18, 1, 1977.
13. **Robb, S. M.**, The culture of excised tissue from bulb scales of *Lilium speciosum* Thun., *J. Exp. Bot.*, 8, 348, 1957.
14. **Hackett, W. P.**, Control of bulbet formation of bulb scales of *Lilium longiflorum*, *Hortic. Sci.*, 4, 171, 1969.
15. **Simmonds, J. A. and Cumming, B. G.**, Propagation of *Lillium* hybrids. I. Dependence of bulblet production on time of scale removal and growth substances, *Scientia Hortic.*, 5, 77, 1976.
16. **Fellenberg, G.**, Über die Organibildung au in vitro kultviertem Knollengewebe von *Solanum tuberosum*, *Z. Bot.*, 51, 113, 1963.
17. **Alleweldt, G. and Radler, F.**, Interrelationship between photoperiodic behavior of grapes and growth of plant tissue cultures, *Plant Physiol.*, 37, 376, 1962.
18. **Aloni, R. and Jacobs, W. P.**, Polarity of tracheary regeneration in young internodes of *Coleus* (Labiatae), *Am. J. Bot.*, 64, 395, 1977.
19. **Schwabb, W. W.**, Applied aspects of juvenility and some theoretical considerations, in Symp. on Juvenility in Woody Perennials, Zimmerman, R. H., Ed., International Society of Horticulture Science, The Hague, 1975, 45.
20. **deLanghe, E. and de Bruijne, E.**, Continuous propagation of tomato plants by means of callus cultures, *Scientia Hortic.*, 4, 221, 1976.
21. **Gamborg, O. L.**, Callus and cell culture, in *Plant Tissue Culture Methods*, Gamborg, O. L. and Wetter, L. R., Eds., National Research Council of Canada, Saskatoon, Saskatchewan, 1975, 1.
22. **White, P. R.**, Potentially unlimited growth of excised tomato root tips in a liquid medium, *Plant Physiol.*, 9, 585, 1934.
23. **Gautheret, R.**, Sur la possibilite dé réaliser la culture indefinié des tissues du tubercules de carotte, *C. R. Acad. Sci. Ser. D*, 208, 118, 1939.
24. **Murashige, T. and Skoog, F.**, A revised medium for rapid growth and bio-assays with tobacco tissue cultures, *Physiol. Plant.*, 15, 473, 1962.
25. **Gamborg, O. L, Miller, R. A., and Ojima, K.**, Nutrient requirements of suspension cultures of soybean root cells, *Exp. Cell Res.*, 50, 151, 1968.
26. **Huang, L.-C. and Murashige, T.**, Plant tissue culture media: major constituents, their preparation and some applications, *Tissue Culture Assoc. Man.*, 3, 539, 1977.
27. **Ammirato, P. V. and Steward, F. C.**, Some effects of environment on the development of embryos from cultured free cells, *Bot. Gaz. (Chicago)*, 132, 149, 1971.
28. **Reinert, J.**, Control of morphogenesis in plant tissue cultures by hormones and nitrogen compounds, in *Plant Growth Substances 1970*, Carr, D. J., Ed., Springer-Verlag, New York, 1972, 686.

29. Tabata, M., Recent advances in the production of medicinal substances by plant cell cultures, in *Plant Tissue Culture and Its Bio-technological Application*, Barz, W., Reinhard, E. and Zenk, M. H., Eds., Springer-Verlag, Berlin, 1977, 3.

30. Street, H. E., Ed., *Plant Tissue and Cell Culture*, Blackwell Scientific, Oxford, 1973, 503.

31. Bezemer-Sybrandy, S. M., Tasseron-de Jong, J. G., and Veldstra, H., Effect of visable light on kinetin solutions, *Biochim. Biophys. Acta*, 161, 568, 1968.

32. Skoog, F. and Miller, C. O., Chemical regulation of growth and organ formation in plant tissues cultured *in vitro*, *Symp. Soc. Exp. Biol.*, 11, 118, 1957.

33. Lee, T. T. and Skoog, F., Effects of substituted phenols on bud formation and growth of tobacco tissue cultures, *Physiol. Plant*, 18, 386, 1965.

34. Romberger, J. A. and Tabor, C. A., The *Picae abies* shoot apical meristem in culture. I. Agar and autoclaving effects, *Am. J. Bot.*, 5, 131, 1971.

35. Cooke, R. C., The use of an agar substitute in the initial growth of Boston Ferns *in vitro*, *Hortic. Sci.*, 12, 339, 1977.

36. Fridborg, G. and Eriksson, T., Effect of activated charcoal on growth and morphogenesis in cell cultures, *Physiol. Plant.*, 34, 306, 1975.

37. Mariani Colombo, P., Analisi dell'effetto del boro sulla germinazione del polline, *Acad. Patavinia Sci.*, 72, 103, 1960.

38. Brewbaker, J. L. and Majumder, S. K., Cultural studies on the pollen population effect and the self-incompatibility inhibition, *Am. J. Bot.*, 48, 457, 1961.

39. Van Bragt, J. and Pierik, R. L. M., The effect of autoclaving on the gibberellin activity of aqueous solutions containing gibberellin A_3. in, *Effects of Sterilization on Components in Nutrient Media*, van Bragt, J., Mossel, D. A. A., Pierik, R. L. M., and Veldstra, H., Eds., H. Veenman and Zonen N. V., Wageningen, 1971, 133.

40. Peer, H. G., Degradation of sugars and their reaction with amino acids, in *Effects of Sterilization on Components in Nutrient Media*, van Bragt, J., Mossel, D. A. A., Pierik, R. L. M., and Veldstra, H., Eds., H. Veenman and Zonen N. V., Wageningen, 1971, 105.

41. Hiraoka, N. and Tabata, M., Alkaloid production by plants regenerated from cultured cells of *Datura innoxia*, *Phytochemistry*, 13, 1671, 1974.

42. Thorpe, T. A. and Murashige, T., Starch accumulation in shoot-forming tobacco callus cultures, *Science*, 160, 421, 1968.

43. Steward, F. C. and Shantz, E. M., The growth of carrot tissue explants and its relation to the growth factors in coconut milk. II. The growth-promoting properties of coconut milk for plant tissue cultures. *Ann. Biol.*, 30, 139, 1954.

44. Skoot, F. and Tsui, C., Chemical control of growth and bud formation in tobacco and stem segments and callus cultures, *in vitro*, *Am. J. Bot.*, 35, 782, 1948.

45. Tisserat, B. H., A Factor in Citron That Represses Asexual Embryogenesis in *Citrus* and *Daucus* Tissues *In Vitro*, Ph.D. thesis, University of California, Riverside, 1976.

46. Halperin, W. and Wetherell, D. F., Ammonium requirement for embryogenesis *in vitro*, *Nature (London)*, 395, 519, 1965.

47. Reinert, J., Tazawa, M., and Semenoff, S., Nitrogen compounds as factors of embryogenesis *in vitro*, *Nature (London)*, 216, 1215, 1967.

48. Newcomb, W. and Wetherell, D. F., The effects of 2,4,6-trichlorophenoxyacetic acid on embryogenesis in wild carrot tissue cultures, *Bot. Gaz. (Chicago)*, 131, 242, 1970.

49. Wochok, Z. S. and Wetherell, D. F., Suppression of organized growth in cultured wild carrot tissue by 2-chloroethylphosphonic acid, *Plant Cell Physiol.*, 12, 771, 1971.

50. Tisserat, B. and Murashige, T., Probable identity of substances in citrus that repress asexual embryogenesis, *In Vitro*, 13, 785, 1977.

51. Tazawa, M. and Reinert, J., Extracellular and intracellular chemical environments in relation to embryogenesis *in vitro*, *Protoplasma*, 68, 157, 1969.

52. Seibert, M., Light — The effects of wave length and intensity on growth and shoot initiation in tobacco callus, *In Vitro*, 8, 435, 1973.

53. Skoog, F., Growth and organ formation in tobacco tissue cultures, *Am. J. Bot.*, 31, 19, 1944.

54. Hasegawa, P. M., Murashige, T., and Takatori, F. H., Propagation of *Asparagus* through shoot apex culture. II. Light and temperature requirements, transplantability of plants, and cyto-histological characteristics, *J. Am. Soc. Hortic. Sci.*, 98, 143, 1973.

55. Gautheret, R. J., Investigations on the root formation in the tissues of *Helianthus tuberosus* cultured *in vitro*, *Am. J. Bot.*, 56, 702, 1969.

56. Kefford, N. P. and Caso, O. H., Organ regeneration on excised roots of *Chondrilla juncea* and its chemical regulation, *Aust. J. Biol. Sci.*, 25, 691, 1972.

57. White, P. R., Controlled differentiation in a plant tissue culture. *Bull. Torrey, Bot. Club*, 66, 507, 1939.

58. **Kessell, R. H. J. and Carr, A. H.**, The effect of dissolved oxygen concentration on growth and differentiation of carrot (*Daucus carota*) tissue, *J. Exp. Bot.,* 23, 996, 1972.
59. **Torrey, J. G.**, Morphogenesis in relation to chromosomal constitution in long-germ plant tissue cultures, *Physiol. Plant.,* 20, 265, 1967.
60. **Murashige, T., Nakano, R., and Tucker, D. P. H.**, Histogenesis and rate of nuclear change in *Citrus limon* tissue *in vitro, Phytomorphology,* 17, 469, 1968.
61. **Kartha, K. K.**, Organogenesis and embryogenesis, in *Plant Tissue Culture Methods,* Gamborg, O. L. and Wetter, L. R., Eds., National Research Council of Canada, Saskatoon, Saskatchewan, 1975, 44.
62. **Amemiya, A.**, Effect of peptone on growth of rice embryos (studies on the embryo culture in rice plant. IV. *Bull. Natl. Instit. Agric. Sci. Ser. D,* 11, 151, 1964.
63. **Kartha, K. K., Gamborg, O. L., and Constabel, F.**, Regeneration of pea (*Pisum sativum* L.) plants from shoot apical meristems. *Z. Pflanzenphysiol.,* 72, 172, 1974.
64. **Seabrook, J. E. A. and Cumming, B. G.**, Vegetative propagation of *Narcissus* using tissue culture, *Daffodils 1976,* Royal Horticultural Society, London, 1976, 16.
65. **Heller, R.**, Recherches sur la nutrition numerale des tissues vegetaux cultives, *in vitro, Ann. Sci. Nat. Bot. Biol. Veg.,* 14, 1, 1953.
66. **Knudson, L.**, A new nutrient solution for the germination of orchid seed. *Am. Orchid Soc. Bull.,* 15, 214, 1946.
67. **Seabrook, J. E. A.**, unpublished data.

Chapter 2

NUTRITION AND METABOLISM

Donald K. Dougall

TABLE OF CONTENTS

I. INTRODUCTION

The objective in this chapter is to outline the available information on nutrition and metabolism related to nutrition in plant cell cultures. It will also serve to identify areas of deficiency of information. The information on nutrition is beginning to change in character. In the past, it has been concerned with simply achieving growth of cell cultures. The information becoming available is beginning to answer questions concerned with growth yield from specific nutrients, effects of concentrations of nutrients on growth rate, and effects of concentrations of nutrients on secondary product synthesis. In terms of metabolism, the area is also at a transition point. In the past, the validity and relevance of studies of metabolism in cell cultures have been doubted. This opinion appears now to have changed. We can anticipate further developments in the understanding of metabolism in plant cell cultures which should lead to the ability of investigators to approach questions of yield on a rational basis.

In the following discussion, the highest priority will be given to data obtained using suspension cultures of plant cells. There are two reasons for this. First, experience shows that the limiting growth rates in suspension culture are higher than those obtained on semisolid media. This may be the result of diffusion being a rate-limiting process in such media. Second, there appears to be little economic incentive in growing many thousands of cultures per week when a single stirred fermentor can be used to produce the same biomass.

A. Media and Culture pH

An examination of the major ions in media used for suspension cultures over the last 20 years, i.e., compare the media of White,[1] Gamborg,[2] Gamborg et al.,[3] Murashige and Skoog,[4] Schenk and Hildebrandt,[5] and Kato et al.,[6] shows a progressive increase in the concentrations of nitrate, potassium, ammonium, and phosphate.

Media for suspension culture of plant cells are prepared with an initial pH of 5 to 6. The component of the medium which is capable of buffering in this range is phosphate. The usual concentration of phosphate in media is 1 to 5 mM. The media, therefore, have very low buffering capacities. During the course of growth of plant cells in media which are in general use, the pH of the medium changes; thus, it may drop as low as pH 4 and rise to pH 7.[7-12] Such changes can be expected to have an impact on the metabolism of the cells. The available information on the behavior of plant cell cultures when the pH is controlled is very limited.[8,9,13,14]

B. Establishment and Development of Suspension Cultures

In the past, suspension cultures have been mainly established from callus cultures. Suspension cultures can be established directly from primary explants. The limitation on the direct initiation of suspension cultures is probably the availability of equipment for agitation of the cultures and the long time required to initiate the cultures. Some of these limitations may be minimized in the future if primary explants are disaggregated, e.g., with pectinase prior to initiation of cultures. This would be analogous to the first step of a two-step protoplast preparation.[15,16]

The ease of establishment of suspension cultures from callus tissue is influenced by the friability of the callus tissue.[17] In those cases where the callus is very friable, suspension cultures of cells and small aggregates may form with a simple shaking in culture media.[18,19] The friability of callus may be increased by increasing the auxin concentration in the medium. Friable variants sometimes appear as sectors in callus cultures.[20] Even with increased friability of the callus tissue, suspension cultures may not form readily and require a period of adaptation in liquid medium to give suitable suspension cultures[21-23] or may even require alternating periods of growth in agitated liquid and agar medium[24] to give suitable or improved suspension cultures. The possibility of selecting a variant which has improved characteristics for suspension culture clearly exists in these procedures.

In addition to adaptation by prolonged subculture in liquid media, some aspects of media composition influence the degree of dispersion of a suspension culture. Lamport[17] concluded that decreasing the amount of coconut water and increasing the 2,4-D in the medium increased the pipettability of suspension cultures of *Acer pseudoplatanus*. Wallner and Nevins[20] showed that the average clump size in suspension cultures of Paul's Scarlet Rose was decreased by using glucose instead of sucrose as a carbon source, by increased NAA in the medium, by decreased kinetin, and by replacement of nitrate by casein hydrolysate. Eriksson[25] comments that kinetin decreased cell separation in *Haplopappus gracilis* suspension cultures. Matsumoto et al.[26] showed that increased thiamine enhanced the dispersion of tobacco crown gall tumor tissue. Morris and Northcote[27] comment that the degree of dispersion of *A. pseudoplatanus* suspension cultures is increased by increased calcium in the medium. Oswald et al.[28] concluded that increased iron, the presence of vitamin E, and the omission of EDTA increased the degree of dispersion of clover and soybean suspension cultures. Street[29] describes the temporary increase in dispersion of *A. pseudoplatanus* suspension cultures by the presence of macerozyme and cellulase in the culture medium. Lamport[17] has discussed in general terms the basis for the formation of suspensions of cells. He concluded that factors which minimize the mechanical stability of the walls between cells, i.e., rapid cell division and wall extension throughout the cell, are important in the formation of suspensions. When tissue is suspended in liquid and agitated, the shear forces generated by agitation will separate cells if the adhesion between cells has been decreased.

C. Uptake of Nutrients

The mechanism of uptake of a nutrient by plant cells can be anticipated to have some important consequences for growth rate and yield of cells. Two cases may be considered as illustrations. The first is uptake by diffusion, and the second is an active uptake which is energy dependent or against a concentration gradient. For uptake by diffusion, one can anticipate that growth rate and yield will be dependent on relatively high external concentrations and that a considerable proportion of the nutrient initially supplied may be present in the medium at the end of growth. For active uptake, one can anticipate that the growth rate will be independent of concentration at relatively high external concentrations, that the final yield will be dependent on the amount of nutrients supplied, and that very little of the nutrient will remain in the medium after growth. As a consequence, one may anticipate that the mechanism of uptake of a nutrient may have ramifications for metabolism, for the control of processes which occur in cells, e.g., growth vs. secondary product synthesis, and for the economics of growing cells.

An important question then is whether nutrients enter the cells by passive diffusion or whether they are taken into the cells by some selective and active systems. In most cases, data from an examination of the effect of concentration of a nutrient on its uptake rate can be treated by a formalism which is analogous to the Michaelis-Menten treatment of enzyme-catalyzed reactions. This suggests that an analogue of an enzyme, i.e., a carrier, is involved in the uptake of nutrients. However, Harrington and Smith[30] argue that the formalism should be used only to describe the process and should not be taken as implying a mechanism. The effects of inhibitors, such as dinitrophenol, cyanide, etc., has led to the interpretation of the uptake process as being "active" or requiring energy.[31-37] Cases where the measurement of uptake of nutrients by plant cells in culture has been made and the affinity of the transport system estimated are given in Table 1. For the usual nutrients of a medium, the affinities vary from 0.003 to 1500 μM. These transport systems will be operating at 95% of their maximal velocity when the concentration of a compound transported is 19 times the affinity constant. It seems, therefore, that the media formulated by Murashige and Skoog,[4] Gamborg,[2] etc. are adequately supplied to insure that carriers are operating at or near their maximal velocity.

The entries in Table 1 for glucose and for L-alanine have, in common, very small affinity constants when the cells are starved and very large affinity constants when the cells have an excess of the nutrient or an alternative. King and Oleniuk[37] suggest that this might reflect scavenging mechanisms which can come into play when nutrients are depleted. Such scavenging would allow some continuation of growth by the use of materials which were lost from the cells during the early part of growth.

With respect to the entries in general, they cannot be interpreted to very great depth because there are not enough species examined. In the one case where more than one species has been examined for the uptake of a nutrient, i.e., nitrate, the values are from two different methods. Heimer and Filner[31] estimated uptake of nitrate by tobacco cells essentially uncomplicated by utilization. King and Street[38] measured growth

TABLE 1

Affinities of Uptake Systems for Nutrients of Plant Cell Cultures

Nutrient	Affinity (μM)	Condition	Ref.
NO_3^-	130		38
	400		31
PO_4^{--}	32		38
SO_4^{--}	15		40
	20—40		35
Glucose	15	Sucrose grown	33, 34
	1400	Glucose grown	33, 34
L-alanine	2.55	N starved	37
	46	N starved	36
	∞	NO_3^- present during growth	37
	8000	N starved; measured at high alanine concentrations	36
L-arginine	103	Lysine absent	32
	127	Lysine present	32
L-lysine	7900	Arginine absent	32
	2450	Arginine present	32
L-cysteine	17		30
	350		
2,4-Dichloro- phenoxy acetic acid	3×10^{-3} (estimated)		190
Indole acetic acid	1—5		54

of *A. pseudoplatanus* in continuous culture; thus, their value represents the concentration giving a one-half maximal growth rate which includes utilization as well as uptake. King and Hirji[39] have examined amino acid transport in nitrogen-starved soybean cells. They identified at least three transport systems by competition experiments. Hart and Filner[40] showed that L-cysteine and L-homocysteine, but not D-cysteine, would inhibit sulfate uptake by tobacco cells. They also showed that L-cysteine uptake by tobacco cells gave a straight line in a Lineweaver-Burke plot and that the uptake was inhibited by L-leucine, L-arginine, L-tyrosine, and L-phenylalanine. Their observation that there was a lag of approximately 2 hr before the inhibitory effects of amino acids on L-cysteine uptake could be observed, suggested to them that these inhibitors might not be acting on a membrane transport system.

Harrington and Smith[30] did not observe a lag in L-cysteine uptake by tobacco cells. They showed that the effect of the L-cysteine concentration on its transport by tobacco cells was biphasic and describe the transport as consisting of a "high affinity system" having a K_m of $1.7 \pm 0.17 \times 10^{-5}$ M and a "low affinity system" having a K_m of $3.5 \pm 0.13 \times 10^{-4}$ M. They also examined the effects of a number of inhibitors of metabolism and amino acids on L-cysteine transport. Smith[35] showed that selenate was a competitive inhibitor of sulfate transport and that sulfide was a noncompetitive inhibitor. Bellamy and Bieleski[41] measured the rate of phosphate uptake from 10^{-5} M phosphate by tobacco cells and showed that it varied from 17.3 nmol/g/hr in the midexponential phase of growth to 135 nmol/g/hr in the early stationary phase of growth. They also showed the effect of phosphate concentration on the uptake rate of phosphate for exponentially growing cells. Danks et al.[42] measured the ability of Paul's Scarlet Rose cells in suspension culture to abosrb $^{86}Rb^+$ from culture media. They demonstrated the presence of two systems of $^{86}Rb^+$ uptake which operated at different external concentrations. One system was saturated at 0.7 mM; the other was not saturated at 100 mM Rb^+. The rates of uptake at 100 mM Rb^+ was approximately ten times higher than that measured at 0.7 mM Rb^+. The characteristics of these two systems changed with progression through the batch culture cycle.

D. Manipulation of Cultures May Lead to Rapid Changes

It may be necessary to exercise some caution in drawing conclusions from the available data on the uptake of nutrients. The measurements of affinities and uptake rates published have been made over periods of time which vary with the author from 1 min to 20 hr. There have been demonstrations of some extremely rapid changes in plant cell cultures as a result of changing their environment. Wahlstrom and Eriksson[43] showed that glutamic acid uptake by *Daucus carota* suspension cultures were reduced to 60% of the controls by inoculating the cells into fresh medium. The decrease in uptake occurred within 10 min, remained lowered for 20 min, and had reached the capacity of the controls in 80 min. Bellamy and Bieleski[41] showed that the uptake rate of phosphate increased three-fold in 2 hr when early stationary phase cells were transferred into 10^{-4} M $CaCl_2$. Under these conditions, the sulfate uptake rate dropped over the first 2 hr and then rose 20-fold in the next 6 hr.

Thoiron et al.[44] showed, with *A. pseudoplatanus* suspension cultures, that a vigorous agitation of cultures led to a two- to three-fold drop in the sulfate uptake rate over an hour period. The uptake rate began to rise between 1 and 5 hr, reached a maximum at approximately 10 hr, sometimes showed an oscillation between 10 and 25 hr, and thereafter became relatively stable.

Changes in other cellular properties also occur rapidly on changing the environment of cells. Towill and Mazur[45] showed loss of viability of *A. saccharum* cells within 5 min of exposure to increased sucrose levels. Morris and Northcote[27] showed that increasing the calcium concentration in the medium of *A. pseudoplatanus* suspension cultures to 100 mM markedly increased the rate of release of polysaccharides, which reached a maximum within 15 min. Increases in the specific activity of phenylalanine ammonia lyase on dilution of suspension cultures of *Petroselinum hortense* into water or fresh medium, which begins with a lag of 2.5 hr and are maximal after 15 hr, have been shown by Hahlbrock and Wellmann,[46] Hahlbrock and Schroder,[47] and Hahlbrock.[48]. Phenylalanine ammonia lyase reached its maximum value 12 hr after the subculturing of *H. gracilis* suspension cultures.[49] Changes in the polysome/monosome ratio within 3 hr of subculturing soybean cells have been shown.[50] Verma and Marcus[51] showed that the two- to three-fold increase in respiration within a few minutes, the three-fold increase in ATP, and the ten-fold increase in the rate of protein synthesis within 2 hr of dilution of stationary phase *Arachis hypogaea* suspension cultures was due to changes in oxygen availability to cells. The increase in nitrate reductase in *Nicotiana tabacum* suspension cultures in 24 hr[52] and in *Glycine max* suspension cultures beginning at 3 to 5 hr and reaching a maximum at 60 to 80 hr[53] are dependent on the presence of nitrate in the medium. While these latter cases have an explanation, they also point out that rapid changes in the cells occur on changing their environment.

The studies of auxin transport in suspension cultures of *Parthenocissus tricuspidata* crown gall cells show further complexities of transport that may need to be taken into account in interpreting experimental data.[54,55]

Some of the available data on transport may be complicated by the effects of changing cellular environments, which lead to very rapid changes in the cells. Thus, care should be exercised in drawing conclusions from the available data.

E. Osmotic Effects on Plant Cell Cultures

The possibility that culture media may have effects on cells which are due to the osmotic effects of medium components has been explored in three studies in addition to the study of Towill and Mazur[45] which has already been mentioned. These three studies have been performed by supplementing media with nonmetabolized compounds, such as mannitol, Carbowax®-1000, and NaCl. Maretzki et al.,[56] using sugarcane suspension cultures, showed alterations in growth and metabolism resulting from an increased osmotic pressure of media. Withers and Street[57] showed changes in cell size and increased resistance to chilling injury in suspension cultures of *Acer pseudoplatanus* and *Capsicum annuum* by growing these cells in media supplemented with mannitol. The fresh and dry weights of soybean callus were increased and the cell size decreased by growing the tissue on media containing increased mannitol, sorbitol, sucrose, or glucose.[58] In general practice, osmotic effects of media composition on cell performance are ignored. As quantitative studies become important in plant tissue culture, osmotic effects may turn out to be of greater importance than currently realized.

II. CARBOHYDRATES

A. Growth

The ability of various carbohydrates to support growth of callus and suspension cultures of plant cells was reviewed by Maretzki et al.[59] Their conclusion was that sucrose or its component monosaccharides, glucose or fructose, were the carbon sources giving the best growth of most plant cell cultures. They go on to say: "Other carbohydrates can, however, be substituted for sucrose, glucose, or fructose. Growth responses differ, depending on the species or clone, but generally not the tissue, from which the explant was isolated." Their conclusions are still valid.

Concentrations of sucrose giving maximal growth have been given as 60 g/ℓ for *A. pseudoplatanus*,[60] not less than 50 g/ℓ for *Populus* hybrids, *N. glutinosa*, and *N. tabacum* var. Xanthi by Matsumoto et al.[61] and *N. tabacum* L. cv. BY-2 by Ikeda et al.,[62] 30 to 40 g/ℓ for *H. gracilis*,[25] 60 g/ℓ for *Phytolacca americana*,[63] 40 g/ℓ for *Morinda citrifolia*,[64] and 30 g/ℓ for *Scopolia japonica*,[65] and for *Camptotheca acuminata*.[278]

Yasuda et al.,[66] in describing the effects of sucrose concentration on the growth of *N. tabacum* var. Xanthi, concluded that the concentration of sucrose giving a one-half maximal growth rate was 6.9 mM (2.35 g/ℓ). They also comment that high concentrations of sucrose lead to a decrease in the specific growth rate. This effect can also be seen in the studies with *A. psuedoplatanus*.[60] Using callus cultures of *N. rustica*, Hunt and Loomis[67] concluded that the concentration of sucrose giving a one-half maximum growth rate was 3.7 mM (1.26 g/ℓ).

The abilities of suspension cultures to grow on large numbers of different carbohydrates has been examined for *D. carota*,[68] *Saccharum* species,[69] a *Populus* hybrid,[70] *Rosa* species,[20] *Papaver bracteatum*,[71] *N. tabacum* var. Xanthi,[66] and *M. citrifolia*.[64] In all of these cases, growth was apparent only on hexoses and hexose di, tri, etc. saccharides. Pentoses, uronic acids, or inositol as the sole carbon and energy source would not support growth. Stuart and Street[72] concluded that for the growth of cultures of *A. pseudoplatanus* at low inoculum densities, sucrose could not be replaced by glucose and/or fructose. Scala and Semersky[73] and Grout et al.[74] have described some aspects of the growth of *A. pseudoplatanus* cells on glycerol as a sole carbon source. This is the only example of glycerol as a sole carbon source for plant cell cultures.

The limited available data support the conclusions of Maretzki et al.[59] with respect to growth. The data is, however, limited not only in quantity but in quality. In several studies, growth on different carbohydrates was measured at only one point in time. With measurement at one point in time, an observed decrease in growth relative to that obtained on sucrose may be due to an increased lag, with the growth rate achieved being equal to that on sucrose. An example of such behavior is the growth of suspension cultures of *D. carota* on galactose.[68]

B. Inositol

There are some reports in the literature that supplementing media with inositol, which will not serve as a sole carbon source, can enhance growth or, in some cases, is essential for growth. Cases where *myo*-inositol is essential for growth are suspension cultures of *M. citrifolia*,[64] Iaul's Scarlet Rose,[75] and probably callus cultures of *Haworthia* sp.[76] *myo*-Inositol (10 to 100 mg/ℓ) enhanced the plating efficiency and colony growth of *Convolvulus arvensis*[18] and promoted the growth of tobacco pith explants and callus.[4, 77] Matsumoto et al.,[26] showed a small stimulation of growth of suspension cultures of tobacco crown gall tissue by *myo*-inositol. Suspension cultures of maize endosperm,[78] soybean root cells,[3] *Catharanthus roseus*,[79] *D. carota*,[80] and rice[81] showed no effect on growth with inositol in the medium.

C. Effects of Carbohydrates on Secondary Products

The effects of the sucrose concentration on the yield of secondary products in plant cell cultures has been examined by several groups. Increasing sucrose from 2 to 4% increased the polyphenols per culture in *Rosa* sp. suspension cultures[82] and in *A. pseudoplatanus* suspension cultures.[83] Increasing sucrose from 2 to 5% decreased the ubiquinone per gram of dry cells in *N. tabacum* L. cv. BY-2,[62] but increased the total dry weight, thus, there is probably little systematic effect on the total ubiquinone per flask. The yield of shikonin derivatives per gram fresh weight of callus cultures of *Lithospermum erythrorhizon* increased with increasing sucrose from 1 to 5% and then remained fairly constant at 7 and 10% sucrose. However, at a higher sucrose concentration, the fresh weight of callus per flask declined. Total anthocyanin in callus cultures from a *Populus* hybrid increased with the increasing sucrose from 0.3 to 5%, while growth was not affected. The total anthraquinones produced by a culture of *M. citrifolia* was maximal at 7% sucrose.[64] Increasing glucose from 0.05 to 0.2 M increased the total phenols and the total leucoanthocyanins produced by *Rosa* sp. suspension cultures.[84]

The response of secondary products to different carbohydrates supplied in the medium appears to indicate that sucrose may be the best general carbon source. The extent of data available is limited, and this conclusion should be regarded with caution. Davies[82] describes differences in phenol production in *Rosa* sp. cultures grown on sucrose or glucose and an interaction between carbohydrates and auxin concentration leading to particular conditions where higher yields are obtained on glucose. The yield of ubiquinone (μg/g dry weight) in *N. tabacum* var. BY-2 is comparable at equal concentrations of sucrose and glucose.[62] Sucrose is clearly superior to glucose, fructose, or an equal mixture of both in the level of shikonin derivatives achieved by *L. erythrorhizon* callus cultures.[85] Sucrose and glucose gave essentially identical anthocyanin per culture in *Populus* cultures and were higher than fructose and eight other carbohydrates.[70] Of 14 carbohydrates tested at 2%, sucrose gave the highest yield of anthraquinones in *M. citrifolia* cultures.[64] Zenk et al.[64] also showed that, at the optimal concentration of glucose for anthraquinone production per culture (7.5%), the yield was 75% of that obtained at the optimal concentration of sucrose (7%).

D. Metabolism of Carbohydrates

The metabolism of carbohydrates can be conveniently considered as having two parts. The first is metabolism via glycolysis, the tricarboxylic acid cycle, and the pentose phosphate pathway leading to energy and intermediates in biosynthesis. The second is metabolism leading polysaccharides, such as starch or components of cell walls.

1. Carbohydrate Breakdown

Much information available to support the view that glycolysis, the tricarboxylic acid cycle, and the pentose phosphate pathway are operating in tissue cultures is reviewed by Maretzki et al.[59] Recent evidence includes the measurement of the activities of some enzymes of glycolysis and the pentose phosphate pathway in suspension cultures of *A. pseudoplatanus* growing under the conditions of a constant dilution rate,[86] measurement of the levels of metabolites in batch cultures of *A. pseudoplatanus* leading to the conclusion that phosphofructokinase and pyruvickinase are points of regulation,[87] studies of two isozymes of glucose-6-phosphate dehydrogenase from suspension cultures of *N. tabacum* L. var. Xanthi,[88] and a study of the subcellular location of hexokinase in *A. pseudoplatanus* cells grown in batch culture.[89] Hunt and Fletcher[90] have concluded that during rapid protein synthesis the amount of carbon removed from the tricarboxylic acid cycle for amino acid synthesis equals one quarter of that evolved as CO_2. The replenishment of the acids of the tricarboxylic acid requires dark fixation of CO_2. Dark fixation of CO_2 by suspension cultures of *Rosa* sp. has been examined by Nesius and Fletcher.[99] Gathercole et al.[100] have shown that CO_2 is required for the growth of suspension cultures of *A. pseudoplatanus*, especially when grown at low cell densities. This requirement is presumably met by CO_2 produced by metabolism in cultures at higher densities.

2. Cell Wall Synthesis

The synthesis of cell wall monosaccharides of *A. pseudoplatanus* from glucose has recently been documented by Morris and Northcote[27] and from galactose by Verma et al.[91] The enzymes for the conversion of glucose into *myo*-inositol have been isolated from *A. pseudoplatanus* cells and studied by Loewus and Loewus.[92,93] The synthesis of *myo*-inositol from glucose and galactose by *D. carota* cultures has been established.[80] The conversion of inositol into pentoses and uronic acids has been shown in *A. pseudoplatanus*[91] and in *D. carota*.[80]

E. Photoheterotrophic Growth

Bergmann[94] has discussed work by his group and from other laboratories which leads to the conclusion that chlorophyll-containing cells, when grown heterotrophically in light, can provide for some of their nutritional requirements by photosynthesis. Light increases both plating efficiency in low density cultures and growth of higher-density cultures. The paper of Nato et al.,[95] provides an excellent description of photoheterotrophic growth of tobacco suspension cultures including photosynthetic oxygen evolution and CO_2 fixation, CO_2 metabolism, and the relationships of these to the phases of the growth cycle. They observed substantial (25 to 50%) CO_2 fixation into C_4 compounds during the lag and early exponential phases of growth, which declined to 10% of the total CO_2 fixed in the stationary phase. One can calculate from their data that, in the period between 8 and 18 days when the dry weight of their cultures doubles, the total CO_2 fixed is equivalent to 720 mg of carbohydrate per gram dry weight of cells. Thus, the photosynthetic activity can provide for a significant proportion of the cellular dry weight accumulated.

F. Photoautotrohpic Growth

While achieving photoautotrophic growth of plant cells in culture has been of interest to investigators, little success has been achieved until recently when Husemann and Barz[96] described photoautotrohpic growth of suspension cultures of *Chenopodium rubrum.* They noted that at least four passages, each of 18 days, were required to improve the growth rate of the cells. Following this adaptation, an 80% increase in fresh weight was achieved at each passage. Factors which increased the growth rate of their cultures were lowered 2,4-D levels in the medium and increased CO_2 levels, with 1% giving as much as double the growth of tissue compared to 0.5%. They also measured the chlorophyll content, the total $^{14}CO_2$ fixed in the light and dark, and the amount of $^{14}C_2$ going into ethanol-insoluble components of the cells. Limited photoautotrophic growth of tobacco suspension cultures had been previously described by Chandler et al.[97] Photoautotrophic growth of tobacco callus cultures has been described by Berlyn and Zelitch.[98]

III. LIPIDS

There is no evidence in the literature to suggest that plant cell cultures need lipid like materials provided in the culture medium. The one published report which comes anywhere near such a demonstration is that of McChesney[101] in which the stimulation of growth of nine plant cell cultures by the addition of mevalonic acid to the culture medium was demonstrated.

The composition of lipids in plant cell cultures and the state of knowledge of effects of environmental conditions and medium components on lipid composition and of the biosynthesis and interconversion of lipids in plant cell cultures is reviewed by Mangold.[102]

IV. NITROGEN

A. Nitrogen Sources

An examination of the composition of media generally used for the culture of plant cells reveals that they contain NO_3^- and NH_4^+, which are the sources of nitrogen for growth. An examination of media for the growth of cells from particular species or specific cell lines reveals that there are quite large differences in the ability to grow with these two ions as nitrogen sources.

1. Nitrate as a Sole Nitrogen Source

Nitrate is an adequate sole nitrogen source for tobacco,[1,103-105] Paul's Scarlet Rose,[106-108] *A. pseudoplatanus,*[109] carrot,[103,110] tomato and soybean,[103] wheat, flax, horseradish and *Reseda luteoli,*[2] and sweet clover, *Ammi visnaga* and *H. gracilis.*[104]

2. Nitrate Plus Ammonium as a Nitrogen Source

The presence of NH_4^+ in the medium inhibits the growth of *H. gracilis* with NO_3^-.[104] The addition of NH_4^+, to medium containing NO_3^- as a sole nitrogen source enhances the growth of soybean,[2,11,104] azuki bean, wax bean, mung bean, and rice,[104] onion,[111] and flax, horseradish, and *R. luteoli*[2] and is required for the growth of carrot.[9] Bayley et al.[112] found that the requirement for NH_4^+ for the growth of soybean cells had been lost after 18 to 48 hr of growth in the presence of NH_4^+ and that the cells could then be grown on a medium containing NO^{-3} as a sole nitrogen source. Sargent and King[104,113] have shown that within this period much of the NH_4^+ is converted into glutamine.

In addition to enhancing or allowing growth, the presence of NH_4^+ in the culture medium enhances or allows the formation of somatic embryos in carrot[9,110,114,276] and *Atropa belladonna*,[115] suggesting that there are qualitative differences in tissue grown on NO_3^- and NO_3^- + NH_4^+ as nitrogen sources. Quantitative differences in tissue grown in the presence and absence of NH_4^+ as a supplement to NO_3^- have also been demonstrated. Craven et al.[116] have shown differences in free organic acids, amino acids, sugars, and K^+ in carrot explants grown on KNO_3 or NH_4NO_3. Bergmann et al.[105] and Bergmann[94] have shown differences in glutamine, alanine, malate, and the level of malic enzyme in tobacco cells grown on NO_3^- and NO_3^- + NH_4^+. They also showed that, while the doubling times for dry weight were the same on both nitrogen sources, in the presence of NH_4^+ the doubling time for protein was 48 hr and in the absence the doubling time for protein was 70 hr. Rose and Martin[117,118] have concluded that when suspension cultures of *Ipomoea* sp. and *D. carota* are grown with NH_4^+ available, the ratio of total nitrogen to the dry weight in cells is increased compared to cultures grown on NO_3^- alone. The available data consistently shows major differences in tissue grown on NO_3^- in the presence or absence of NH_4^+, but the metabolic basis of this difference is not understood.

3. Ammonium as a Sole Nitrogen Source

The growth of plant cells with NH_4^+ as a sole nitrogen source was first reported by Gamborg and Shyluk.[10] They showed that soybean, wheat, and flax suspension cultures would grow on NH_4^+ as a sole nitrogen source provided a Krebs' cycle acid was also supplied. Since that report, others have reported the growth of soybean,[53,119] carrot,[9,103,120] tobacco, and tomato.[103] Behrend and Mateles[121] explored the role of succinate in allowing tobacco cells to grow with NH_4^+ as a sole nitrogen source, but were not able to identify the significant effects of succinate. Dougall and Verma[14] were able, by continuous titration of cultures, to grow carrot suspension cultures on NH_4Cl as a sole nitrogen source to give yields of embryos and biomass comparable to that achieved on NH_4^+, + NO_3^- as a nitrogen source. Martin et al.[13] similarly have shown the growth of *Ipomoea* and soybean suspension cultures on ammonia as a sole nitrogen source. These demonstrations suggest that the failure of plant cell cultures to grow on NH_4Cl or $(NH_4)_2SO_4$ as sole nitrogen sources was due to an excessive decrease in pH in weakly buffered culture media. It is not clear, however, whether the only function of the Krebs' cycle acids in allowing growth on NH_4^+ is to control the pH of the media within tolerable limits.

4. Effects of Nitrate and Ammonium on Medium pH During Growth

In addition to decreases in the medium pH associated with growth of plant cells on NH_4^+ as a sole nitrogen source,[9,10,11,14] increases in the medium pH occur when plant cells are grown on NO_3^- as a sole nitrogen source.[112] Increases in the pH of culture media are also observed when NH_4^+ has been used and NO_3^- remains in the medium of growing cultures.[7,118] Furthermore, the pH of cultures near the end of growth is increased with increased NO_3^- and decreasd with increased NH_4^+ initially in the culture medium.[7,9] In addition to the utilization of NH_4^+ and NO_3^- leading to changes in culture media pH, the rate of utilization of NH_4^+ and NO_3^- is different at different pHs. Rose and Martin[118] showed with suspension cultures of *Ipomoea* that the utilization rate of NO_3^- increased with decreased pH and that the utilization rate of NH_4^+ increased with increased pH. Similar data was obtained by Sheat et al.[122] during studies of tomato root cultures. The effects of uptake of NH_4^+ and NO_3^- on culture pH and the effects of culture pH on the assimilation of these ions suggests an explanation for the pH changes observed during the growth of many cell cultures and suggests the outline of a mechanism by which cells are able to maintain the medium pH within limits which allow growth.

5. Other Sole Nitrogen Sources

In addition to NO_3^- and NH_4^+ as nitrogen sources for growth, other sole nitrogen sources have been used. Soybean suspension cultures have been grown on urea, if Ni^{2+} is provided in the medium,[119,123] and on glutamine.[53] Paul's Scarlet Rose,[107] *Acer pseudoplatanus*,[285] tobacco, tomato, and carrot cells[103] have also been grown on urea. Tobacco cells have been grown on casein hydrolysate, urea, or γ-amino butyric acid as sole nitrogen sources.[52,125] Carrot cultures have been grown on glutamine, casein hydrolysate, or alanine as sole nitrogen sources.[9] Meins[126,127] has shown that tobacco teratoma tissue can grow on glutamate as a sole nitrogen source provided auxin is also supplied.

6. Amino Acids

Single amino acids have been used to supplement other nitrogen sources in many studies. Glutamine is widely used, and arginine is used with nitrate for the growth of sugarcane cells.[128] Filner[52] showed that when single amino acids were added to tobacco cells growing with nitrate as a sole nitrogen source their effects fell into two classes: those which inhibited both growth and induction of nitrate reductase in the cells were alanine, asparagine, glycine, methionine, proline, threonine, valine, aspartic acid, glutamic acid, histidine, and leucine, and those which did not inhibit growth or induction of nitrate reductase were arginine and lysine. When added with an inhibitory amino acid, arginine or lysine always allowed growth and induction of nitrate reductase. Cysteine or isoleucine could prevent inhibition by all amino acids except alanine and methionine. Most of the effects of amino acids on growth of *M. citrifolia* cultures obtained by Zenk et al.[64] are consistent with the pattern obtained in tobacco by Filner.[52] Salonen and Simola[129] examined the effects of eight amino acids on the growth of callus cultures of *Atropa belladonna* in the presence and absence of nitrate. In the presence of nitrate, alanine and proline gave no inhibition of growth, but arginine did inhibit growth.

Behrend and Mateles[103] showed that single amino acids added to tobacco, tomato, carrot, or soybean cells growing on nitrate as a sole nitrogen source inhibited both the growth and the induction of nitrate reductase in a pattern similar, but not identical, to that shown by Filner[52] for tobacco. Arginine reversed the inhibition of growth by other amino acids in each of the tissues tested. When grown on urea as a sole nitrogen source, many of the amino acids again inhibited the growth of tobacco, tomato, and carrot. When grown on NH_4^+ and succinate, an inhibition of growth was not observed. As the authors point out, the amino acid inhibition of growth on urea is difficult to explain only on the basis of prevention of induction of nitrate reductase.

The available data on the effects of single amino acids added to media with nitrate as a sole nitrogen source did not appear to be completely reproducible between investigators. Whether this is due to differences in experimental conditions, changes in cultures with increased passaging, differences between species of origin, or differences in the mechanism of action of amino acids is not clear.

7. Utilization of Nitrogen Sources When Several Are Present in Media

There are several studies of nitrogen utilization when several sources of nitrogen are simultaneously available to the cells. The data of Sargent and King[104] show that NH_4^+ is removed from medium by soybean cells in less than 2 days and suggests that NH_4^+ is predominantly converted into glutamine, while Bayley et al.[11] showed that little or no nitrate is utilized in this period. Veliky and Genest[130] showed the preferential utilization of amino acids over NH_4^+ by cultures of *Cannabis sativa*. Their data further show a preferential utilization of NH_4^+ over NO_3^-. Cultures of *Ipomoea* show a preferential utilization of amino acids over NO_3^-.[131] Veliky and Rose[7] show a preferential utilization of NH_4^+ over NO_3^- by carrot cell cultures. Rose and Martin[118] show the same for *Ipomoea*. In these cases, the utilization of the more-reduced nitrogen source was preferential, but not exclusive, over other available nitrogen sources. In all these cases, the pH of the cultures were not controlled. This generalization appears not to hold when the pH of *Ipomoea* cultures is held at 4.8 or 5.6. Here, the initial rate of NO_3^- disappearance from the medium is higher than the initial rate of NH_4^+ disappearance.[8]

B. Metabolism of Nitrogen

The largest portion of the nitrogen assimilated by cells is used for the synthesis of proteins or amino acids. Proteins and amino acids, together with nucleic acids, account for most of the cellular nitrogen. The assimilation of nitrogen can be dealt with in three parts; the reduction of NO_3^- to NH_4^+, the incorporation of NH_4^+ into organic compounds, and the interconversions of the nitrogen-containing organic compounds.

The reduction of NO_3^- to NH_4^+ can be further subdivided into two parts. The first is the reduction of NO_3^- to NO_2^- catalyzed by nitrate reductase. The second is the reduction of NO_2^- to NH_4^+ catalyzed by nitrate reductase.

1. Nitrate Reductase

Nitrate reductase has been demonstrated in soybean,[11,53,132] Ipomoea,[133] wheat,[11] Paul's Scarlet Rose,[107,108] tobacco,[31,52,103,125,134] tomato,[103] *Acer psuedoplatanus*,[135] and *Convolvulus arvensis*.[136] The induction of nitrate reductase and the nitrate uptake system by nitrate have been studied extensively in tobacco cells by Filner and co-workers.[31,52,125] The synthesis and turnover of the enzyme has been studied by Zielke and Filner.[137] Evidence has been obtained for two distinct pools of nitrate and for their roles within cells by Ferrari et al.[138] The induction of the nitrate uptake system and nitrate reductase by nitrite was demonstrated by Heimer[134] and of nitrate reductase by nitrite by Chroboczek-Kelker and Filner.[139] A requirement for molybdenum for active nitrate reductase has been demonstrated in tobacco by Heimer and Filner[31] and in Paul's Scarlet Rose by Jones et al.[107] In addition to amino acids preventing the induction of nitrate reductase in cell cultures,[52,103] NH_4^+ or glutamine prevents its induction in soybean,[53] and NH_4^+ appears to repress nitrate reductase in *Ipomoea*.[133]

2. Nitrite Reductase

Nitrite reductase has been measured in tobacco cells[139,140] and *Ipomoea* cells.[133] The regulation of nitrite reductase levels by several nitrogen sources was examined by Chroboczek-Kelker and Filner.[139] The addition of NH_4^+ to *Ipomoea* cultures reduced the levels of nitrite reductase.[133] Evidence for the localization of nitrite reductase in proplastids from tobacco cells has been described by Washitani and Sato.[140] Jessup and Fowler[141] have discussed evidence which points to the pentose phosphate pathway as the source of NADPH for the reduction of nitrate.

3. Incorporation of Ammonia into Glutamic Acid

The assimilation of NH_4^+ into organic compounds has long been known to give glutamic acid as an early and the major compound. Some NH_4^+ also appears early in the amide nitrogen atom of glutamine. The assimilation of NH_4^+ was assumed to be by the reaction,

$$NH_4^+ + \alpha\text{-ketoglutarate} + \text{reduced pyridine nucleotide} \rightleftharpoons \text{glutamic acid} + \text{oxidized}$$
$$\text{pyridine nucleotide}$$

which is catalyzed by glutamic dehydrogenase. The reaction catalyzed by glutamic dehydrogenase was the only reaction known by which NH_4^+ could be assimilated until 1974 when Dougall,[120] as a result of studies with carrot cell cultures, provided evidence for a second route of assimilation. The enzymatic activity demonstrated in that study was

$$\text{glutamine} + \alpha\text{-ketoglutarate} + \text{reduced pyridine nucleotide} \rightarrow 2 \text{ glutamic acid} + \text{oxidized pyridine}$$
$$\text{nucleotide}$$

The enzyme catalyzing this reaction is often referred to by the acronym, GOGAT, or the trivial name, glutamate synthase. Its systematic name is L-glutamate: NADP$^+$ oxido reductase (Transaminating) (EC 1.4.1.13). This enzyme has been demonstrated in tissue cultures from six species,[142] *A. pseudoplatanus* cell cultures, pea roots,[143] pea cotyledons,[144] and maize endosperm.[145] A second GOGAT, initially described by Lea and Miflin[146] from pea leaves, has been found in a number of higher plants.[147] This enzyme uses ferredoxin as a reductant. The enzyme from the leaves of *Vicia faba* has been partly purified by Wallsgrove et al.[148] The ferredoxin-dependent enzyme has been demonstrated in proplastids from tobacco cell cultures.[149]

This second route for the assimilation of NH_4^+ into glutamic acid requires the activities of GOGAT together with glutamine synthetase. Glutamine synthetase catalyses the synthesis of glutamine as follows:

$$NH_4^+ + \text{glutamic acid} + ATP \xrightarrow{\text{Mg}^{++}} \text{glutamine} + ADP + Pi$$

combined with GOGAT catalyzing the reaction,

$$\text{glutamine} + \alpha\text{-ketoglutarate} + \text{reductant} \rightarrow 2 \text{ glutamic acid} + \text{oxidized reductant}$$

gives the net reaction,

$$NH_4^+ + \alpha\text{-ketoglutarate} + ATP + \text{reductant} \rightarrow \text{glutamic acid} + ADP + Pi + \text{oxidized reductant}$$

The advantages of these two reactions and their characteristics have been discussed by Dougall[150] and Miflin and Lea.[147] The current conclusion is that, at least at low levels of NH_4^+, these two enzymes constitute the pathway of NH_4^+ assimilation in plant cells.

The metabolism of urea when it is used as a nitrogen source for plant cell cultures requires the presence of urease in the cells to convert the urea into $NH_4^+ + CO_2$. The fornation of urease in rice, tobacco, and soybean cell cultures and the requirement for Ni^{++} for urease formation have been described by Polacco.[119,123,151]

4. Biosynthesis of Other Nitrogen-Containing Compounds

The current state of information on the pathways of the biosynthesis of amino acids from glutamic acid and glutamine has been reviewed by Miflin and Lea.[147] In addition, Smith[152] has provided evidence for the presence of *o*-acetylserine, the immediate precursor of cysteine, in tobacco suspension cultures. Glenn and Maretzki[153] have described the properties and subcellular distribution of two ornithine transcarbamoylases in sugarcane suspension cultures. Aspartate kinase from carrot cell suspension cultures has been partly purified by Davies and Miflin,[154] who describe some properties of the enzyme and show that it is inhibited additively by lysine and threonine (end products of aspartate metabolism). Sakano and Komamine[155] have shown that carrot root tissue contains predominantly an aspartyl kinase which is inhibited by threonine (70%). A second aspartyl kinase which is inhibited by lysine (16%) is also present. When carrot root slices are incubated for 3 days under conditions where cultures would be initiated, the threonine-sensitive aspartyl kinase increases 1.5- to two-fold, while the lysine-sensitive aspartyl kinase increases 700-fold and becomes the predominate form of the enzyme.

C. Effects of Nitrogen Nutrition on Secondary Product Formation

The accumulation of phenolic compounds in *A. pseudoplatanus* cell cultures is decreased by increased nitrate or urea in the medium and is decreased by the delayed addition of urea to the culture medium.[156,157] Phillips and Henshaw[157] have shown that the labeling of protein by phenylalanine decreases, while the labeling of phenols increases over the period of increasing total phenols in these cultures, showing that phenylalanine is preferentially used for protein synthesis and that, as this use declines, the phenylalanine is metabolized to phenolic compounds. Davies[82] showed that the levels of polyphenols produced in suspension cultures of *Rosa* sp. was decreased at 20 mM NO$_3^-$ when compared with 10 mM NO$_3^-$. Amorim et al.[84] showed that, in suspension cultures of *Rosa* sp., increased nitrate decreased the total phenols when 0.2 M glucose, but not when 0.1 M glucose, had been provided to the cultures and only between 8 and 12 days of growth. Leucoanthocyanin accumulation in these cultures, which occurred between 8 to 12 days of growth, was substantially decreased by increased nitrate in the culture medium.[84] Mizukami et al.[85] showed that the formation of shikonin derivatives (1:4-naphthoquinones) by callus cultures of *Lithospermum erythrorhizon* was increased when total nitrogen in the medium was raised from 67 to 104 mM. Further increases in the total nitrogen decreased the formation of these compounds. The addition of 0.3% peptone or casein hydrolysate to their medium containing 67 mM nitrogen decreased the amount of shikonin derivatives formed. The delayed addition of urea to cultures also decreased the yield of shikonin derivatives. Anthraquinone production by suspension cultures of *M. citrifolia* was not inhibited, and growth was not stimulated when KNO$_3$ was increased from 2.0 to 4.5 g/ℓ. Both growth and anthraquinone production declined rapidly above and below this range.[64] Zenk et al.,[64] also showed that when their medium was supplemented with casein hydrolysate at levels greater than 4 g/ℓ, anthraquinone production, but not growth, was strongly inhibited. The total ubiquinone per culture of tobacco was not altered by altering the NH$_4^+$:NO$_3^-$ ratio in the medium from 3:1 to 1:3, with total nitrogen held constant.[158] The production of glutamine by suspension cultures of *Symphytum officinale* was maximal with 4.95 g of NH$_4$NO$_3$ per liter + 5.7 g of KNO$_3$ per liter. Both growth and glutamine declined when both nitrogen sources were increased proportionately. When both nitrogen sources were decreased proportionately, the accumulation of glutamine fell, while growth was not affected. The production of plasmin inhibitor by suspension cultures of *Scopolia japonica* was markedly increased, while growth was little affected, by decreasing the NH$_4$NO$_3$ from 1.66 to 0.83 g/ℓ and increasing the KNO$_3$ from 1.9 to 7.6 g/ℓ in the culture medium.[65] The synthesis of tryptophan-derived alkaloids by callus cultures of *Peganum harmala* was decreased by substituting NH$_4^+$ or glutamine for nitrate, but not by substituting alanine for nitrate.[160] The growth of the tissue was not affected by these changes in the medium.

V. SULFUR

A. Sulfur Sources

Sulfate is the usual source of sulfur provided in media used for plant tissue culture. Murashige and Skoog[4] concluded that for tobacco callus tissue 1.65 mM of sulfate was suitable, although it may be slightly higher than optimal. Kato et al.[6] modified sulfate levels for growth of tobacco suspension cultures to 1.20 mM as a result of measuring sulfate uptake during growth. Ohira et al.[81] showed that sulfate from 0.5 to 10 mM had no effect on the growth of rice suspension cultures. For suspension cultures of *N. tabacum* var. Xanthi, the 2.5 mM of NO_3^- + 0.1 mM of SO_4^{2-} provided in the medium were both used up when growth was complete.[161] Hart and Filner[40] concluded that thiosulfate, L-cyst(e)ine, L-methionine, and gluthathione give growth of tobacco cells equal to that obtained on sulfate and that D-cyst(e)ine, D-methionine, and DL-homocyst(e)ine would support the growth, but at a slower rate than on sulfate. Reuveny and Filner[161] confirmed the growth of tobacco cells on L-cyst(e)ine and/or L-methionine and showed that glutathione or djenkolate would allow a reduced growth of the cells. Bergmann and Rennenberg[162] showed that glutathione inhibited growth of soybean callus cultures.

B. Metabolism of Sulfate

The uptake of sulfate has been discussed earlier under *Uptake of Nutrients*. The first metabolic alteration in sulfate is a reaction with ATP in which pyrophosphate and adenosine-5'-phosphosulfate (APS) are the products. ATP sulfurylase (EC 2.7.7.4, ATP:sulfate adenylyl transferase), the enzyme catalyzing this reaction, has been measured in the direction of APS synthesis in extracts of tobacco cells by Reuveny and Filner.[163] ATP sulfurylase is derepressed in tobacco cells under conditions of sulfur starvation or limited sulfur availability[161] and in the presence of sulfate analogues (molybdate and selenate).[164] In tissue grown on sulfate or cysteine (the end product of sulfate assimilation), the enzyme is detectable, and its specific activity is identical in both culture conditions, showing that the fully repressed level is sufficient to allow maximum growth on sulfate as a sulfur source.[161] The dependence of derepression of ATP sulfurylase on the availability of nitrogen to tobacco cells has been demonstrated directly.[279]

A correlation between sulfate transport capacity and ATP sulfurylase in developing maize roots has been demonstrated.[165] Rennenberg[166] has demonstrated the presence of glutathione in conditioned medium from tobacco suspension cultures.

VI. POTASSIUM

Murashige and Skoog[4] chose 20 mM of K^+ as suitable for tobacco callus cultures. Lavee and Hoffman[167] concluded that 3.6 mM K^+ is optimal for apple callus tissue growth. Kato et al.[6] showed that when 21.3 mM K^+ is provided to tobacco cells growing in suspension culture approximately 50% of the K^+ is present in the medium at the end of growth. Ohira et al.[81] show a small (30%) stimulation of the growth of rice suspension cultures as K^+ was varied from 0 to 100 mM. In contrast, the measurements of conductivity and nitrate levels during the growth of soybean and parsley cells[12,132,168] and *M. citrifolia*[64] in media containing KNO_3 as the major ionic component suggests that the K^+ is largely taken up by the cells. Suspension cultures of *Pogostenum cablin* also removed the majority of K^+ from the medium.[169] The K^+ may serve as an essential nutrient as well as a counter ion to preserve electrical neutrality. The effects of K^+ on growth and embryogenesis in carrot suspension cultures using a variety of nitrogen sources was examined by Brown et al.[170] They showed that K^+ at 1 mM gave maximal growth but that 10 to 50 mM of K$^+$ was optimal for embryogenesis. Veliky and Rose[7] comment that they made no attempt to replace the K$^+$ when KNO$_3$ was removed from their media and saw no indication of a K$^+$ requirement. Dobberstein and Staba[171] concluded that a reduction of K$^+$ from 784 to 49 mg/ℓ had little discernible effect on the growth of *Ipomoea*, *Rivea* or *Argyreia* tissue cultures. Alkaloids in the culture were higher on low-K$^+$ medium only for the Argyreia cultures.

VII. PHOSPHORUS

Murashige and Skoog[4] concluded that, despite a variability in tissue response to PO$_4^{3-}$ and an interaction with K$^+$ and perhaps also with sucrose and iron, 1.25 mM of PO$_4^{3-}$ was close to the optimal level for tobacco pith explants and callus cultures. Bellamy and Bieleski,[41] Ueki and Sato,[172] and Kato et al.[6] showed that tobacco suspension cultures depleted PO$_4^{3-}$ very rapidly when the initial concentration was 1.25 mM. Kato et al.[6] showed with tobacco suspension cultures that increased KH$_2$PO$_4$ in the medium increased the growth rate of the cultures, and they raised the concentration of PO$_4^{3-}$ to 4.41 mM in their modified medium. Eriksson[25] showed that increased PO$_4^{3-}$ from 1.25 to 10 or 20 mM gave a 50% increase in the final yield of *H. gracilis*. Gamborg et al.[3] comment that a variation in the PO$_4^{3-}$ concentration near 1 mM resulted in minor changes in the growth rate for soybean. Misawa et al.[63] showed with *P. americana* suspension cultures that raising the PO$_4^{3-}$ from 1.25 to 1.9 mM or greater increased the dry weight achieved by more than 50%. Wilson[173] showed that *Acer pseudoplatanus* cells in a batch culture with an initial 1.1 mM of PO$_4^{3-}$ depleted the medium PO$_4^{3-}$ very rapidly, and that below 0.55 mM PO$_4^{3-}$, the final yield of cells achieved was approximately proportional to the amount of PO$_4^{3-}$ supplied. Zenk et al.[64] comment that the growth of *M. citrifolia* was not affected by changing phosphate in the range of 10^2 to 10^4 ppm. Dobberstein and Staba[171] concluded that a four-fold increase in the PO$_4^{3-}$ concentration to 593 mg/ℓ decreased the growth of *Ipomoea* and Argyreia suspension cultures and stimulated *Rivea* suspension cultures. Ohira et al[81] showed that growth of rice suspension cultures was stimulated (20%) by increasing phosphate from 1 to 20 mM. Carew and Krueger[79] showed that the growth rate of suspension cultures of *C. roseus* was higher with 2.2 and 5.45 mM of PO$_4^{3-}$ than with 1.1 mM of PO$_4^{3-}$ and that, when 10.9 mM of PO$_4^{3-}$ was present in the medium, the growth rate declined again. Bayliss[174,175] showed that, in medium containing 1.25 mM of PO$_4^{3-}$, suspension cultures of carrot were phosphate limited. He further showed that the competitive advantage of a subtetraploid line of carrot over a diploid cell line was associated with the ability of the former to maintain its exponential growth at a lower PO$_4^{3-}$ concentration than could the diploid line. The growth index of *P. harmala* callus cultures was not altered over one passage by omitting PO$_4^{3-}$ from the medium or by increasing it from 4 to 20 mM.[160]

Ueki and Sato[172] showed that acid phosphatase appeared in the culture medium of tobacco cells as the phosphate was taken up by the cells and that delayed phosphate addition to the medium caused a rapid decrease in the specific activity of the medium acid phosphatase. Igaue et al.[176] showed the presence of an acid phosphatase repressible by PO$_4^{3-}$ in rice cells and that this acid phosphatase can be separated into six isoenzymes.[177] Ninomiya et al.[178] have examined the phosphatase activity produced by tobacco cells by chromatography. They showed the presence of three phosphatases, one of which, a nonspecific acid phosphatase, is markedly increased under conditions of phosphate deprivation. Suzuki and Sato[179] have provided some evidence for a particular acid phosphatase being associated with the walls of tobacco cells from suspension culture.

There are three interesting papers on phosphodiesterases from tobacco cells grown in suspension culture. Shinshi et al.[180] described the purification and some properties of phosphodiesterases from tobacco cells and later[181] showed that the enzyme would preferentially cleave the pyrophosphate linkages by which methylated guanosine residues are attached to the 5′ end of many messenger RNAs without cleavage of the polynucleotide chain of the RNA. These observations were confirmed by Efstratiadis et al.[182] and extended to provide a method for the ^{32}P-end labeling of messenger RNA for further studies.

The effects of the PO_4^{3-} supply on secondary products produced by plant cell cultures have been examined in only a few cases. Nettleship and Slaytor[160] showed that removal of phosphate from the medium increased the content of harmalol and harmine in *P. harmala* callus cultures. Carew and Krueger[79] showed that increased phosphate in the medium increased the indole compounds in the medium of *C. roseus* suspension cultures. Dobberstein and Staba[171] found that, for *Ipomoea* suspension cultures, increased phosphate increased the alkaloids, whereas the alkaloids in *Argyreia* and in *Rivea* cultures were not altered by increased phosphate. Zenk et al.[64] obtained a 50% increase in anthraquinones in *M. citrifolia* when phosphate was increased to 5 g/ℓ.

VIII. CALCIUM

The fresh weight increase of tobacco pith explants was unaffected by a Ca^{++} concentration in the range of 1.5 to 6 mM.[4] The dry weight achieved by soybean suspension cultures was not altered by Ca^{++} from 1 to 4 mM.[3] Calcium was absolutely required for growth and pigment production in *M. citrifolia*.[64] For *H. gracilis*, 3 mM of Ca^{++} seemed to be near optimal.[25] Ohira et al.[81] obtained the maximum growth of rice suspension cultures when Ca^{++} was 0.2 to 1 mM and a decreased growth with a further increase in Ca^{++}. Kato et al.[6] selected 1.5 mM of Ca^{++} for the growth of suspension cultures of tobacco cells and showed that in excess of 50% of the Ca^{++} provided remained in the medium after growth was completed. Morris and Northcote[27] have shown that increased Ca^{++} (100 mM) in the culture medium of sycamore suspension cultures had no effect on the O_2 uptake, gave similar growth rates to that observed in 1 mM of Ca^{++}, increased the degree of dispersion of the tissue, and increased the secretion into the medium of polysaccharides, precursors of cell walls. The growth of *L. erythrorhizon* callus cultures and the yield of shikinon derivatives was decreased by increasing the Ca^{++} above 3 mM.[85]

IX. MAGNESIUM

For tobacco pith cultures, Murashige and Skoog[4] chose 1.5 mM of Mg^{++} as a suitable concentration. For suspension cultures of tobacco, Kato et al.[6] reduced the concentration to 1.05 mM, but here the level of sulfate and not the level of Mg^{++} being supplied was the important factor. The dry weight achieved by soybean suspension cultures was not affected in the range of 0.5 to 3.0 mM of Mg^{++}.[3] For *H. gracilis*,[25] 1.5 mM was near optimal, and 0.5 to 5 mM of Mg^{++} had no effect on the growth of rice suspension cultures.[81] Growth and embryogenesis in wild carrot suspension cultures is not affected by an alteration in the Mg^{++} supplied from 2.25 to 0.25 mM. Veliky et al.[183] concluded that 0.3 mM of Mg^{++} was sufficient to support a full growth of *Ipomoea* cells in batch culture. They studied the effect of controlled pH on Mg^{++} uptake and concluded that as the pH of the medium was increased, an increased uptake of Mg^{++} occurred. With increased Mg^{++} availability (up to 10 mM), the uptake was increased, and there was little effect on growth, indicating a minimal toxicity of Mg^{++}.

X. IRON

The optimal level of iron supplied with an equimolar amount of Na_2EDTA was 0.1

mM for tobacco pith and callus cultures[4] and *H. gracilis.*[25] Neumann and Steward[184] examined the effects of iron on the growth of carrot root explants and concluded that a minimum level of iron for good growth and at which toxicity is not displayed was 0.05 mM. Oswald et al.[28,185] have described some effects of altered iron and EDTA levels in the medium on the growth and degree of dispersion of clover, soybean, and maize tissues in culture. The effects described are in the range of concentration of $FeSO_4$ from 0.07 to 0.36 mM with EDTA from 0 to 0.46 mM. In these studies, the $FeSO_4$, and EDTA were not always used in equimolar proportions, suggesting that the Fe^{++} concentrations may have significant effects. Growth of *L. erythrorhizon* callus was increased by raising Fe^{++} from 0.1 to 0.2 mM and decreased at 1 mM, while the production of shikonin derivatives was decreased with both increases in Fe^{++}.[85] Neither growth or anthraquinone production occurred in *M. citrifolia* when iron was omitted from the medium.[64] Ojima et al.[186] showed that, in suspension culture of *Ruta graveolens*, the chlorophyll content of the tissue decreased in the first passage in the absence of iron and growth decreased to 20% of the controls in the second passage in the absence of iron. Rice suspension cultures were very dependent on iron in the medium.[187] Growth and respiration was decreased to 50%, protein per gram of fresh weight was elevated by 20%, and the soluble amino acids were increased four-fold in the first passage in an iron-free medium.

XI. TRACE ELEMENTS

A. Requirements for Trace Elements

Trace amounts of iodine, boron, zinc, manganese, molybdenum, copper, cobalt, aluminum, and nickel are added to plant tissue culture media.

R. graveolens suspension cultures have been shown to require manganese, zinc, copper, and perhaps molybdenum.[186] Rice suspension cultures ceased to grow at the end of three passages in medium free of zinc or copper. In contrast, the growth in the absence of manganese, molybdenum, iodine, or boron was little affected over six passages.[187] Stimulation of growth of *D. carota* explants by manganese and molybdenum in combination has been shown by Neumann and Steward.[184] Stimulation of growth of *P. americana* suspension cultures by a five-fold increase in $CuSO_4 \cdot 5H_2O$ to 0.125 mg/ℓ was shown by Misawa et al.[63] They also showed that doubling the levels of trace elements did not lead to toxicity. A dependence of growth of *A. pseudoplatanus* on copper at concentrations below 2 μg/ℓ has been shown.[188] Eriksson[25] showed a toxicity of trace elements to *H. gracilis* suspension cultures, particularly with small inocula, and reduced the concentrations used to 10% of those recommended by Murashige and Skoog[4] for tobacco. Murashige and Skoog[4] included 0.1 mM of H_3BO_3, 0.1 mM of Mn^{++}, 0.03 mM of Zn^{++}, 0.005 mM of I^-, 0.001 mM of Na_2MoO_4, 0.0001 mM of Cu^{++}, and 0.0001 mM of Co^{++} in their medium for tobacco pith explants because, although these additions did not stimulate growth, they did not show toxicity and there are other reasons for expecting that these ions are essential. Zenk et al.[64] concluded that KI could be omitted from the medium for the growth of *M. citrifolia* and that the trace elements, Mn, B, Zn, Mo, Cu, and Co, could be omitted for at least one passage without affecting the growth, but with a 30% reduction in anthraquinone production.

B. Roles of Trace Elements

The role of zinc in the growth of normal and crown gall callus tissue of *Parthenocissus tricuspidata* was examined by Klein et al.,[189] who showed that the effects of zinc deficiency on the growth of crown gall tissue could be reversed by auxin or tryptophan and in the normal tissue by tryptophan.

Molybdenum is required for the synthesis of active nitrate reductase.[31,107] Nickel,

TABLE 2

Growth Yields for Plant Cell Cultures

Nutrient	Growth yield (g dry wt per gram of nutrient)	Cell type	Ref.
Sucrose	0.53	Tobacco suspension culture	6
	0.43	Tobacco suspension culture	273
	0.36—0.50	Tobacco suspension culture	274
	0.50	Carrot cells growing exponentially	275
	0.20	Carrot cells growing with limited O_2	275
	0.61	Tobacco callus tissue	67
NO_3^-	10.4	Tobacco suspension cultures	6
	11.1	Carrot cells growing exponentially	275
	4.0	Carrot cells growing with limited O_2	275
SO_4^{--}	107	Tobacco suspension cultures	6
NH_4^+	50	Carrot cells growing exponentially	275
	16.6	Carrot cells growing with limited O_2	275
K^+	30.1	Tobacco suspension cultures	6
	25.0	Carrot cells growing exponentially	275
	3.57	Carrot cells growing with limited O_2	275
Ca^{++}	414	Tobacco suspension cultures	6
PO_4^{3-}	50	Carrot cells growing exponentially	275
	33.3	Carrot cells growing with limited O_2	275

which is not added to many plant tissue culture media, is part of the active site of urease, an enzyme which is required for the growth of cell cultures on urea as a sole nitrogen source.[119,123,151] Bligny and Douce[188] examined the effects of Cu^{++} deficiency on mitochondria of *A. pseudoplatanus*. They found that oxygen uptake was very similar to that of normal mitochondria, but was much more sensitive to KCN inhibition. The levels of cytochrome aa_3 were reduced in Cu^{++} deficiency. They conclude that in Cu^{++} deficiency, it is not the rate of respiration which limits growth.

Whether or not Na^+ and Cl^- are essential elements is not known. If they are required, they are provided as contaminants of other chemicals, as counter ions, or during an adjustment of the pH of culture media.

XII. GROWTH YIELDS FROM NUTRIENTS

A limited amount of information of growth yields is available in the literature. Some of this is shown in Table 2. Additional data from which growth yields can be estimated is available.[7,11,13,106,118,169] Leguay and Guern[190] have estimated that the growth yield

TABLE 3

Demonstrated Vitamin Requirements in Plant Tissue Cultures

Tissue	Thiamine	Nicotinic acid	Pyridoxine	Pantothenic acid	Ref.
Tobacco[a]	+[b]	0	0	0	77
Tobacco[c]	+	NT	NT	NT	191
	+	0	0	0	62
Morinda citrifolia[c]	+	+	±	0	64
Soybean[c]	+	0	0	0	3
	+	NT	NT	NT	191
Haplopappus gracilis	±	±	±	0	25
Convolvulus arvensis (plating single cells)	±	0	0	0	18, 19
Rice[c]	+	0	0	0	191
Ruta graveolens[c]	0	NT	NT	NT	191
Peanut[c]	0	NT	NT	NT	191
Paul's Scarlet Rose[c]	0	0	0	0	5, 99
Tobacco crown gall[c]	±[d]	±	0	0	26
Tobacco crown gall[c]	+	0	NT	NT	23
Phytolacca americana[c]	0	0	0	0	63
Catharanthus roseus[c]	0	0	0	0	79
Ephedra gerardiana[a]	0	0	0	0	200
Corn endosperm[c]	+	0	0	0	78

Note: NT denotes not tested.

[a]   Callus or pith cultures.
[b]   + denotes an absolute requirement, ± denotes that the compound was promotive of growth, and 0 denotes no requirement demonstrated.
[c]   Suspension cultures.
[d]   Promoted dispersion of the tissue.

of *A. pseudoplatanus* cells in suspension culture is 2.5×10^6 cells per nanomole of 2,4-D.

XIII. VITAMINS

Plant tissue culture media in general use contain members of the water-soluble or B group of vitamins, e.g., thiamine, nicotinic acid, pyridoxine, and pantothenic acid. In many cases, these vitamins are added to insure that a deficiency does not occur rather than on the basis of demonstrated need. Listed in Table 3 are cases where the requirements for vitamins have been examined. There appears to be a requirement for thiamine for many, but not all, of the cultures examined. In several cultures, a requirement for or a stimulation by nicotinic acid and pyridoxine also appears. Ohira et al.[191] point out that, in their study, it was cultures showing some low level of differentiation, i.e., *R. graveolens* and peanut, that did not need exogenous thiamine, while those showing no capacity for differentiation, i.e., soybean, tobacco, and rice, required exogenous thiamine. In the case of *C. arvensis*, where growth is promoted by added thiamine, the cells clearly underwent an extensive division in the absence of thiamine. With *H. gracilis*, Eriksson[25] showed that the cultures would grow to the extent of 30 to 50% of the control in the absence of thiamine, nicotinic acid, or pantothenic acid, Matsumoto et al.[26] showed that, in the absence of any vitamin, their tobacco crown gall tissue would grow to approximately one half the settled volume of their best medium, but required twice the time period to do so. Of the vitamins, nicotinic acid gave the greatest stimulation of growth on the first passage. Noguchi et al.[23] showed that the doubling time of this tobacco crown gall suspension culture decreased from 3 to 1.5 days over ten passages in the absence of nicotinic acid. They show similar decreases in doubling time for these cells subsequent to a change from medium containing yeast extract to one with yeast extract replaced by thiamine plus nicotinic acid plus inositol, suggesting that these adaptations to growth in the absence of organic compounds may be a general phenomenon rather than one specifically associated with nicotinic acid. For many cell cultures, there is good evidence for a thiamine requirement in at least one passage. However, it is not known whether the cultures could be adapted to growth in media not containing thiamine or other vitamins. In *Ephedra* callus cultures, which grew only very slowly in the first passage in the absence of thiamine or inositol, growth was as rapid as in the presence of these compounds in the second passage.[192]

In many ways, the lack of requirement for vitamins in plant cell cultures is not surprising because whole plants are autotrophic for vitamins. This presumably means that they have the genetic information for the synthesis of these compounds. The correlation of Ohira et al.[191] between a lack of a thiamine requirement and a capacity for differentiation in cell cultures might be a reflection of such an idea.

The advantage of providing these compounds in plant tissue culture media may lie in minimizing stress on explants or cultures. The stress may result from a low-expressed capacity to synthesize vitamins, leakage of vitamins into the medium, or general stress due to a transfer to fresh medium which has not been conditioned. Examples which can be interpreted as stressful situations are available. One of these is the plating experiments of Earle and Torrey[18,19] with *C. arvensis* where thiamine stimulated growth. Another is the culturing of *A. pseudoplatanus* cells at low density,[72] where the omission of thiamine, pantothenic acid, cysteine, choline, and inositol from the medium led to a significant reduction in growth, but the omission of one of these had no significant effect on growth. Linsmaier-Bednar and Skoog[193] showed that increased cytokinin in the medium of tobacco pith and callus cultures removed the requirement for thiamine. Dravnieks et al.[194] showed that thiamine synthesis in tobacco callus tissue was stimulated by elevated cytokinin levels.

There are a series of effects of vitamins which may be effects at much more subtle level than growth. Matsumoto et al.[26] illustrated that the degree of dispersion of tobacco crown gall suspension cultures was increased by the presence of thiamine. Wilson, Edwards, and Street (cited by Stuart and Street[72]) observed an abnormal "clumping" of *A. pseudoplatanus* cultures grown in the absence of thiamine, pantothenic acid, cysteine, choline, and inositol. The addition of 10^{-4} *M* of ascorbic acid to callus cultures of *L. erythrorhizon* stimulated the production of shikonin (napthoquinone) derivatives,[85] and the addition of up to 0.05 mg/ℓ of riboflavin stimulated anthocyanin accumulation by *Populus* cells in suspension culture grown in the light.[70]

In the context of the effects of exogenously supplied vitamins on plant cell cultures, the observations of Oswald et al.[185] are of interest. Their results appear to show that the addition of vitamin E (*dl*-alpha-tocopherol acetate) to the media, along with other modifications, allows the growth of callus tissue and the establishment of suspension cultures from maize somatic tissue and white clover. The vitamin E also promoted the dispersion of soybean suspension cultures. This is the first time to the author's knowledge that vitamin E has had a promotive effect in plant tissue cultures. An independent verification of these effects would greatly strengthen the documentation of the effects of vitamin E.

XIV. OTHER ORGANIC COMPOUNDS

The requirement for inositol by a number of cultures has been discussed under *Carbohydrates*. The addition of Krebs' cycle acids in culture media when NH_4^+ is a sole nitrogen source has been discussed. There are, in addition, sporadic observations of the stimulation of cell cultures by other organic compounds. Kamimura and Akutsu[71] showed a stimulation of the growth of *Papaver bracteatum* suspension cultures by malic and malonic acids when 200 mg/l were added. Streptomycin sulfate in the range of 1 to 50 mg/l inhibited growth and increased the yield of shikonin derivatives in *L. erythrorhizon* callus cultures.[85] The addition of 1.32 mM of sodium acetate substantially increased the viability of corn suspension cultures.[185] Mevalonate stimulated the growth of a number of callus cultures.[101] Citric acid stimulated the growth of Shamouti orange albedo callus cultures.[195] Adenosine stimulated the increase in cell number in carrot and oil palm cultures and increased the number of adventive embryos formed in carrot cultures.[196]

Wood and Braun[197] showed with normal tissue of *Vinca rosea* that progressively increased growth was obtained when White's medium containing auxin and cytokinin was supplemented with

1. Inositol
2. Inositol plus glutamine
3. Inositol plus glutamine plus cytidyllic acid
4. Inositol plus glutamine plus cytidyllic acid plus asparagine plus guanylic acid

In similar experiments, Sogeke and Butcher[198] showed a stimulation of growth of normal *V. rosea* tissue and an inhibition of growth of normal *Helianthus annuus* tissue by these organic compounds. Note that inositol was not included in any of the media, and not all combinations were tested. Wood and Braun[197] further showed that if White's medium containing auxin, cytokinin, inositol, and glutamine, i.e., medium containing supplement 2, was further supplemented with 845 mg/l of KCl, 1800 mg/l of $NaNO_3$, and 300 mg/l of $Na_2HPO_4H_2O$, then growth was greater than that obtained on the medium containing supplement 4. Thus, for the achievement of growth of normal *V. rosea* cells, auxin and cytokinin appeared to be necessary, and growth was improved by either supplementing White's medium containing auxin and cytokinin with inorganic salts or with organic compounds. Sogeke and Butcher[198] showed that the combination of $NaNO_3$ + $NaH_2PO_4 \cdot 2H_2O$ was the most effective for the stimulation of growth of both normal and crown gall tissue of *H. annuus*, i.e., that the extra KCl was not needed. They further showed with normal *H. annuus* tissue that, while the concentration of auxin required for maximum growth was not altered by supplementing White's medium with KCl, $NaNO_3$, and $NaH_2PO_4 \cdot 2H_2O$, the concentration of kinetin for maximal growth was altered from 0.1 mg/l on White's medium to 1.0 mg/l on White's medium supplemented with inorganic salts. They also showed with an auxin-habituated subline of *H. annuus* that the growth on White's medium occurred in the presence of auxin, but not cytokinin, while on White's medium supplemented with inorganic salts either kinetin or auxin allowed growth. An auxin-habituated tissue of *V. rosea* behaved in the same way,[198] although in this tissue the presence of both auxin and cytokinin in either media gave a stimulation of growth over that achieved with either growth substance. They showed that supplementing White's medium with inorganic salts leads to "increased growth rates throughout the growth period and not a prolongation of the exponential growth phase."

These two papers[197,198] both contained valuable data. They show that growth can be improved by adding either inorganic or organic components to some media. Sogeke and Butcher[206] further show interrelationships between growth regulator requirements and inorganic nutrition. They also showed differences in growth regulator requirements of normal and crown gall tissues of *H. annuus* which are comparable to those demonstrated for *V. rosea*.[197] However, a reader of these papers is cautioned to examine the data presented and draw his or her own conclusions. Much of the discussion in Sogeke and Butcher's paper appears to indicate major differences between their results and those of Wood and Braun.[197] These differences do not appear on a close examination of the data presented.

XV. GROWTH REGULATORS

There are several classes of compounds and several individual compounds which are known to have different regulatory effects on growth and development in whole plants. These are auxins, cytokinins, gibberellins, abscisic acids, and ethylene. In each of the classes of regulatory compounds, there is at least one compound which is produced in growing plants and which is involved in the growth and coordinated development of the plant. In addition, there are other compounds (synthetic) which are not found in plants which mimic part or all of the physiological effects of the naturally occurring compounds.

Of these compounds or classes of compounds, the auxins and cytokinins are clearly those of the greatest significance in plant tissue culture. This is the result of a number of observations, which were initially developed into a coherent picture by Skoog and Miller.[199] Skoog and Miller[199] showed that, by varying the concentrations of these two factors in the culture medium of tobacco pith or callus tissue, they could achieve either unorganized growth, growth plus shoot formation, or growth plus root formation. Thus, organogenesis is achieved in plant cells when a suitable balance between auxin and cytokinin is presented to the cells. These phenomena, initially observed with tobacco, have been shown to occur in cells of a very large number of plant species and have now been recognized as general in plant cells.[200]

While specific cells or tissue in plants produce auxins and cytokinins[201] which are then transported to their sites of action to control growth and development, not all cells appear to produce these compounds. That is, the cells of a plant have the genetic information for the synthesis of auxins and/or cytokinins, but they do not express the information and synthesize these compounds. Thus, the majority of plant cell parts, when excised and placed in tissue culture, require an exogenous supply of auxin and/or cytokinin for growth and cell division. It is to be noted that there are exceptions to this generalization. If the cells placed in culture are actively synthesizing sufficient auxin or cytokinin, then it will not need to be provided in the culture medium. The synthesis of auxin or cytokinin may be initiated in plant cells either spontaneously or as a result of treatment, e.g., the initiation of crown gall by *Agrobacterium tumefaciens*; the cells become autonomous for auxin or cytokinin. Where this happens spontaneously, the terms "habituation" or "habituated" are applied.

The greatest difference between tissues from different species in terms of their behavior in tissue culture lies in the levels of auxins and/or cytokinins required for growth. This aspect of medium composition is the first to be examined in the initiation of cultures. As a consequence, there is very extensive descriptive literature of the effects of these compounds on growth, organogenesis, and secondary product formation. Their effects on secondary product formation will not be discussed.

A. Auxins

The natural auxin is indole-3-acetic acid (IAA). Evidence suggesting that phenylacetic acid may also be a natural auxin is accumulating.[202] Synthetic compounds which have auxin activity and which are most widely used in plant tissue culture are α-na-phthalene acetic acid (NAA) and 2,4-D. Other compounds with auxin activity which are used in plant tissue culture include indole-3-butyric acid (IBA) and p-chlorophen-oxyacetic acid (CPA). In addition to these five compounds, there are many others with auxin activity and a number of compounds which behave as antiauxins.[203] The auxins may be generally ordered in increasing activity as IAA, IBA, NAA, CPA, and 2,4-D, as a general summation of experience. In tests of the effects on primary explants, these compounds are usually initially tested at concentrations from 0.01 to 10 mg/ℓ and occasionally as high as 100 mg/ℓ. 2,4-D is noteworthy in that, when it is provided to tobacco or soybean cell cultures or pea root segments, systems which classically require both an auxin and cytokinin, the addition of exogenous cytokinin is not required,[204-207] although added cytokinin may be stimulatory.[207] Some possibilities for this apparent cytokinin-like activity of 2,4-D are discussed by Witham.[207] The requirements for auxin of some cytokinin-independent tobacco strains is altered by the presence of cytokinin in the medium.[208,209]

Tryptophan, the precursor of IAA, accumulates in a number of 5-methyl trypto-phan-resistant lines of plant cell cultures, but tryptophan accumulation does not automatically confer independence of growth from auxin.[210] IAA is thought to be the least active auxin in the series because it is degraded in tissue. The catabolism of IAA was reviewed by Schneider and Wightman.[202] The metabolism of a large portion of the 2,4-D to an amide of glutamic acid which has auxin activity by soybean callus tissue is described by Feung et al.,[211-214] by N. tabacum and P. hortense by Leguay and Guern.[215] The metabolism of 2,4-D to a compound which, upon treatment with β-glucosidase, yields 2,4-D, by Acer pseudoplatanus cells and not to glutamic acid or asparatic acid conjugates is described by King[124] and Leguay and Guern.[215] Leguay and Guern[215] concluded that the presumed glucose conjugate was no involved in the cell division of A. pseudoplatanus. They also provided evidence for the conclusion that the difference in pH between the medium and the inside of the cells controlled the internal level of 2,4-D and that, if the internal level of 2,4-D exceeded a threshold, then cell division occurred. This is consistent with the data and conclusions of Rubery[55] and Rubery and Sheldrake.[54]

The role of auxins in cell division seems to be at some point in the G_1 phase of the cell cycle because, in the absence of auxin, DNA synthesis is inhibited.[216-218]

B. Cytokinins

The term, cytokinin, is used to encompass compounds which promote cell division in callus cultures of plant tissues. The archetype is N^6-furfuryl adenine, known by the trivial name, kinetin. These compounds have additional physiological effects in plants and plant cells. Their structures, activities, etc. have been reviewed by Skoog and Schmitz,[219] Fox,[220] Hall,[221] and Szweykowska.[222] The naturally occurring cytokinins are N^6-substituted adenine derivatives. The substituents of the naturally occurring cytokinins include Δ^2-isopentenyl (γγ dimethyl allyl) and trans-γ-hydroxymethyl-γ-methyl allyl groups. These compounds are also known by the acronym, 2iP (or DMAAP), and the trivial name, zeatin, respectively.

Cytokinins that are used in plant tissue culture are the naturally occurring compounds 2iP and zeatin together with N^6-benzyl adenine (BA or BAP) and kinetin. In the tobacco callus tissue assay, 2iP gave 50% or more of the maximum tissue yield at concentrations from 3×10^{-9} to $10^{-5} M$. For kinetin and for BA, this range was 3×10^{-7} to $10^{-6} M$.[223] Zeatin appears to be active at slightly lower concentrations that 2iP.[219] From the studies with tobacco callus cultures, zeatin and 2iP appear to have an advantage over BA and kinetin in that they are effective over a wider range of concentrations. This is also observed in A. pseudoplatanus cultures.[224,225] However, Smith et al.[226] and Price et al.[227] concluded that kinetin at 1mg/ℓ was preferred for callus initiation on cotton hypocotyl tissue, but that 0.5 to 1 mg/ℓ of BA or 5 to 10 mg/ℓ of 2iP were preferred for subculture of the callus. In tests involving organ initiation, 2iP was not as effective as BA[228] or kinetin.[229] Thus, different cytokinins give different responses in different tests. It is possible also that different cytokinins may give different responses, at least quantitatively, in the same test.

In evaluating the requirement for cytokinin by a specific cell line, concentrations in the range of 0.01 to 10 mg/ℓ and perhaps as high as 100 mg/ℓ are often tested.

The requirements for cytokinins by cell lines may be different under different conditions or after different treatments. Syono and Furaya[230] showed that a cytokinin-independent (habituated) subline of tobacco isolated from a cytokinin-dependent line was cytokinin dependent when grown at 16°C, but not when grown at 25°C. Meins[231] showed that tobacco pith explants cultured at 35°C for 21 days were cytokinin independent, while those cultured at 25°C were cytokinin dependent. Meins and Binns[232] have shown that the degree of cytokinin independence of a culture can change progressively with time and that all the cells of the population shifted in their degree of cytokinin independence. Binns and Meins[233] have shown that, when plants were regenerated from cytokinin-independent clones of tobacco, the tissue from these plants gave cytokinin-dependent cultures. Evidence that the difference between cytokinin-dependent lines and cytokinin-independent lines is a heritable alteration in phenotype, i.e., epigenetic, but not an alteration in the genotype, i.e., mutation is becoming strong.[234] The production of cytokinin by cytokinin-independent tissue cultures has been demonstrated by Tegley et al.,[235] Linstedt and Reinert,[236] Miller,[237] Wood et al.,[238] Short and Torrey,[239] Dyson and Hall,[240] and Sargent and King.[113]

Cytokinin has been shown to be required for mitosis to occur in tobacco cells.[216,217,241,242] Hagen and Marcus[243] concluded that an important function of cytokinins is the inhibition of cell enlargement, thereby facilitating a balance between cell division and cell expansion. The data on which they concluded that cytokinins do not function directly to stimulate cytokinesis may be the result of the choice of experimental material. It would be of value to know if their observation that kinetin does not stimulate cell division can be repeated in tissue other than that of the *N. glauca* × *N. langsdorffi* hybrid. Jouanneau[242] concluded that the presence of cytokinin and the ability of tissue to synthesize protein are simultaneously required for cytokinin activation of mitosis in tobacco cells. Fosket et al.[50] have shown that specific polypeptides are synthesized by soybean cells treated with cytokinin which are not synthesized in the absence of cytokinin. Note there is also a polypeptide whose synthesis is inhibited by the presence of cytokinin. They further proposed that these polypeptides are specifically involved in cell division. Cytokinins also stimulate the rate of protein synthesis in soybean[244-246] and tobacco.[247,248]

The metabolism of cytokinins is reviewed by Hall,[221] and their presence in transfer RNA is discussed by Hall[221] and Skoog and Schmitz.[219] In addition to the conversion to adenine and to nucleosides and nucleotides, cytokinins are also converted into 3-, 7-, or 9-glucosyl derivatives.[249-251] Studies of the formation of 7-glucosides of cytokinins has led to the conclusion that they are formed from the bases, not the ribosides, and that they are biologically inactive storage forms of cytokinin.[252-254]

Evidence has been presented to show that cyclic AMP derivatives can substitute for cytokinins in tobacco and lettuce pith explants.[255-257]

C. Other Growth Regulators

Included in this group are gibberellins, abscisic acid, and ethylene. Their effects on plant cell and tissue cultures appears to be limited. This may be the result of a very limited exploration of their effects.

Abscisic acid decreased the growth of carraway suspension cultures and promoted the development of normal embryos, while gibberellin had the opposite effects.[258,259] Fujimura and Komamine[260] concluded that gibberellins and abscisic acid did not influence the number of embryos produced by carrot cell cultures, but decreased the progress of embryos to advanced stages of development. Gibberellins enhanced the development of potato meristems into plants.[261,262] Westcott et al.[83] have shown stimulation of shoot tip growth of several *Solanum* species by gibberellins. Meristems of *Opuntia polyacantha* are directed to spine formation by gibberellin.[263] Gibberellins stimulated callus growth and inhibited organogenesis in tobacco.[264,265] Gibberellin and abscisic acid suppressed the development of carnation meristems.[201] Gibberellin and abscisic acid did not alter the growth of bean callus, but did have effects on differentiation.[266] Abscisic acid at 0.01 mg/ℓ stimulated the growth and cell division in callus cultures of *Spinacia oleracea* and inhibited at 1.0 mg/ℓ.[267] Abscisic acid inhibited the growth and production of phenolic compounds by tobacco callus cultures.[265]

Ethylene, a known regulator of the physiology of whole plants,[268] is produced in tissue cultures[269-271] and inhibited the development of chlorophyll in *Spinacia oleracea* suspension cultures.[271] 2-(Chloroethyl) phosphonic acid, which releases ethylene, decreased the production of tannis and the extractable phenylalanine ammonia lyase from *A. pseudoplatanus* suspension cultures, but had no effect on growth.[272]

ADDENDUM

Since this chapter was written, several important papers on the subject have appeared and the Fourth International Congress of Plant Tissue and Cell Culture has been held. At the Congress, the status of many aspects of nutrition and metabolism were covered. The published proceedings of the Congress will appear shortly and should be consulted for articles mentioned here for which no literature citation is given.

The current status of the transport of ions and molecules was reviewed by Maretzki and Thom. Aspects of the regulation of carbohydrate metabolism were reviewed by Fowler. The characteristics of a galactose-adapted line of sugarcane cells have been described (Maretzki and Thom, *Plant Physiol.*, 61, 544, 1978.). The mitochondrial location of isocitrate lyase in cells of Paul's Scarlet Rose has been documented by Hunt et al. (*Plant Physiol.*, 61, 1010, 1978.), who speculate that this enzyme is involved in providing for the synthesis of glycine and serine. Photoautotrohpic growth in tissue culture of two additional species was discussed by Yamada et al. A paper on the photosynthetic characteristics of photoautotrophically grown tobacco cells has appeared (Berlyn et al., *Plant Physiol.*, 61, 606, 1978.). Filner discussed the current information on the regulation of nitrogen and sulphur assimilation in plant cells, including the studies of Skokut and Filner (*Plant Physiol.*, 61, 66, 1978.) on the mechanism of the slow adaptation of tobacco cells to growth on urea as a sole nitrogen source. In addition, Skokut et al. (*Plant Physiol.*, 62, 299, 1978.) have shown that, in tobacco cells, glutamine is the first product of nitrate and ammonium ion assimilation and that glutamine synthetase and glutamate synthase are involved in the assimilation of ammonium ion. There is evidence also to suggest that glutamic dehydrogenase may have a role in nitrogen assimilation in higher plant cells under some circumstances. Some aspects of nitrogen nutrition, especially organic acids which allow growth on ammonium ion as a sole nitrogen source, were discussed by Ojima and Ohira. This area of nutrition has also been the subject of a paper by Fukunaga et al.(*Planta*, 139, 199, 1978.) Iron sources and nutrition were also discussed by Ojima and Ohira.

The effects of extremely low concentrations of ethylene on the growth and tracheid formation in primary explants of lettuce have been described by Zobel and Roberts (*Can. J. Bot.*, 56, 987, 1978). A thorough documentation of the presence of cyclic adenosine 3′:5′-monophosphate in rye grass endosperm cultures has been provided by Ashton and Polya (*Plant Physiol.*, 61, 718, 1978.).

APPENDIX I

ESTABLISHING AND GROWING SUSPENSION CULTURES FROM CALLUS CULTURES

The general condition for the initiation of suspension cultures from callus are as follows:

1. Use the medium used for callus growth with the agar omitted in 25 m*l* batches.
2. Add 2 to 5 g fresh weight of actively growing friable callus broken up into pieces approximately 3 mm on a side or less to each flask.
3. Agitate on a rotary shaker at 100 to 140 r/min in an incubator between 25° and 30°C until a visual observation shows that extensive growth has occurred (2 to 6 weeks).
4. Transfer the suspension to fresh medium using a wide mouth pipette such that it is diluted five- to sixfold.
5. Repeat step 3 above.
6. Repeat step 4 above.
7. Continue to alternate steps 3 and 4 decreasing the intervals between subcultures and increasing the dilution at each subculture as is possible until a suitable suspension culture has been established.

NOTES
Step 1

If the callus does not fragment easily in steps 2 and 3, grow the callus on a medium with increased auxin or decreased kinetin to increase its friability. If callus is grown on a medium containing IAA, then the replacement of IAA by NAA or 2,4-D in step 1 may be advantageous. The amount of NAA or 2,4-D to be used is likely to be about 1 mg/*l* but will need to be examined. Even in cases where the callus is grown of NAA or 2,4-D, the level in liquid medium may need to be changed. If the callus is grown with a cytokinin, this may need to be decreased.

The medium may be supplemented with 250 mg/*l* of casein hydrolysate or 250 mg/*l* of yeast extract in cases where growth in liquid medium appears to be slow.

Step 3

Visual observation can be replaced by a determination of culture density, e.g., by measurement of the settled tissue volume or the fresh weight of aliquots removed aseptically from the cultures. However, this destroys part of the culture being initiated, and reproducible sampling is very difficult to achieve.

REFERENCES

1. **Filner, P.**, Semi-conservative replication of DNA in a higher plant cell, *Exp. Cell Res.*, 39, 33, 1965.
2. **Gamborg, O. L.**, The effects of amino acids and ammonium on the growth of plant cells in suspension culture, *Plant Physiol.*, 45, 372, 1970.
3. **Gamborg, O. L., Miller, R. A., and Ojima, K.**, Nutrient requirements of suspension cultures of soybean root cells, *Exp. Cell Res.*, 50, 151, 1968.

4. **Murashige, T. and Skoog, F.**, A revised medium for rapid growth and bio assays with tobacco tissue cultures, *Physiol. Plant.*, 15, 473, 1962.
5. **Schenk, R. U. and Hildebrandt, A. C.**, Medium and techniques for induction and growth of monocotyledonous and dicotyledonous plant cell cultures, *Can. J. Bot.*, 50, 199, 1972.
6. **Kato, A., Fukasawa, A., Shimizu, Y., Soh, Y., and Nagai, S.**, Requirements of PO_4^{3-}, NO_3^-, SO_4^{2-}, K^+, and Ca^{2+} for the growth of tobaco cells in suspension culture, *J. Ferment. Technol.*, 55, 207, 1977.
7. **Veliky, I. A. and Rose, D.**, Nitrate and ammonium as nitrogen nutrients for plant cell cultures, *Can. J. Bot.*, 51, 1837, 1973.
8. **Martin, S. M. and Rose, D.**, Growth of plant cell (*Ipomoea*) suspension cultures at controlled pH levels, *Can. J. Bot.*, 54, 1264, 1976.
9. **Wetherell, D. F. and Dougall, D. K.**, Sources of nitrogen supporting growth and embryogenesis in cultured wild carrot tissue, *Physiol. Plant.*, 37, 97, 1976.
10. **Gamborg, O. L. and Shyluk, J. P.**, The culture of plant cells with ammonium salts as the sole nitrogen source, *Plant Physiol.*, 45, 598, 1970.
11. **Bayley, J. M., King, J., and Gamborg, O. L.**, The effect of the source of inorganic nitrogen on growth and enzymes of nitrogen assimilation in soybean and wheat cells in suspension cultures, *Planta*, 105, 15, 1972.
12. **Hahlbrock, K. and Kuhlen, E.**, Relationship between growth of parsley and soybean cells in suspension cultures and changes in the conductivity of the culture medium, *Planta*, 108, 271, 1972.
13. **Martin, S. M., Rose, D., and Hui, V.**, Growth of plant cell suspension cultures with ammonium as the sole source of nitrogen, *Can. J. Bot.*, 55, 2838, 1977.
14. **Dougall, D. K. and Verma, D. C.**, Growth and embryo formation in wild carrot suspension cultures with ammonium ion as a sole nitrogen source, *In Vitro*, 14, 180, 1978.
15. **Nagata, T. and Takebe, I.**, Cell wall regeneration and cell division in isolated tobacco mesophyll protoplasts, *Planta*, 92, 301, 1970.
16. **Jensen, R. G., Francki, I. B., and Zaitlin, M.**, Metabolism of separated leaf cells. I. Preparation of photosynthetically active cells from tobacco, *Plant Physiol.*, 48, 9, 1971.
17. **Lamport, D. T. A.**, Cell suspension cultures of higher plants: isolation and growth energetics, *Exp. Cell Res.*, 33, 195, 1964.
18. **Earle, E. D. and Torrey, J. G.**, Morphogenesis in cell colonies grown from *Convolvulus* cell suspensions plated on synthetic media, *Am. J. Bot.*, 52, 891, 1965.
19. **Earle, E. D. and Torrey, J. G.**, Colony formation by isolated *Convolvulus* cells plated on defined media, *Plant Physiol.*, 40, 520, 1965.
20. **Wallner, S. J. and Nevins, D. J.**, Formation and dissociation of cell aggregates in suspension cultures of Paul's Scarlet rose, *Am. J. Bot.*, 60, 255, 1973.
21. **Veliky, I. A. and Martin, S. M.**, A fermenter for plant cell suspension cultures, *Can. J. Microbiol.*, 16, 223, 1970.
22. **Hayashi, T. and Nishinari, N.**, Growth pattern in suspension culture of tobacco cells, *Sci. Pap. Coll. Gen. Educ. Univ. Tokyo*, 23, 45, 1973.
23. **Noguchi, M., Matsumoto, T., Hirata, Y., Yamamota, K., Katsuyama, A., Kato, A., Azechi, S., and Kato, K.**, Improvement of growth rates of plant cell cultures, in *Plant Tissue Culture and Its Bio-technological Application*, Barz, W., Reinhard, E., and Zenk, M. H., Eds., Springer-Verlag, Berlin, 1977.
24. **Wilson, H. M. and Street, H. E.**, The growth, anatomy and morphogenetic potential of callus and cell suspension cultures of *Hevea brasiliensis*, *Ann. Bot. (London)*, 39, 671, 1975.
25. **Eriksson, T.**, Studies on the growth requirements and growth measurements of cell cultures of *Haplopappus gracilis*, *Physiol. Plant.*, 18, 976, 1965.
26. **Matsumoto, T., Okunishi, K., and Noguchi, M.**, Defined medium for crown gall cells of tobacco in suspension culture, *Agric. Biol. Chem.*, 40, 1335, 1976.
27. **Morris, M. R. and Northcote, D. H.**, Influence of cations at the plasma membrane in controlling polysaccharide secretion from sycamore suspension cells, *Biochem. J.*, 166, 603, 1977.
28. **Oswald, T. H., Smith, A. E., and Phillips, D. V.**, Callus and plantlet regeneration from cell cultures of ladino clover and soybean, *Physiol. Plant.*, 39, 129, 1977.
29. **Street, H. E.**, Plant cell cultures: their potential for metabolic studies, in *Biosynthesis and its Control in Plants*, Milborrow, B. V., Ed., Academic Press, London, 1973, 5.
30. **Harrington, H. M. and Smith, I. K.**, Cysteine transport into cultured tobacco cells, *Plant Physiol.*, 60, 807, 1977.
31. **Heimer, Y. M. and Filner, P.**, Regulation of the nitrate assimilation pathway in cultured tobacco cells. III. The nitrate uptake system, *Biochim. Biophys. Acta*, 230, 362, 1971.
32. **Maretzki, A. and Thom, M.**, Arginine and lysine transport in sugarcane cell suspension cultures, *Biochemistry*, 9, 2731, 1970.

33. **Maretzki, A. and Thom, M.**, The existence of two membrane transport systems for glucose in suspensions of sugarcane cells, *Biochem. Biophys. Res. Commun.*, 47, 44, 1972.
34. **Maretzki, A. and Thom, M.**, Membrane transport of sugars in cell suspensions of sugarcane. I. Evidence for sites and specificity, *Plant Physiol.*, 49, 177, 1972.
35. **Smith, I. K.**, Characterization of sulfate transport in cultured tobacco cells, *Plant Physiol.*, 58, 358, 1976.
36. **King, J.**, Uptake by soybean root cells of [^{14}C] alanine over a wide concentration range, *Can. J. Bot.*, 54, 1316, 1976.
37. **King, J. and Oleniuk, F. H.**, The uptake of alanine-^{14}C by soybean root cells grown in sterile suspension cultures, *Can. J. Bot.*, 51, 1109, 1973.
38. **King, P. J. and Street, H. E.**, Growth patterns in cell cultures, in *Plant Tissue and Cell Culture*, Street, H. E., Ed., University of California Press, Berkeley, 1973, 11.
39. **King, J. and Hirji, R.**, Amino acid transport systems of cultured soybean root cells, *Can. J. Bot.*, 53, 2088, 1975.
40. **Hart, J. W. and Filner, P.**, Regulation of sulfate uptake by amino acids in cultured tobacco cells, *Plant Physiol.*, 44, 1253, 1969.
41. **Bellamy, A. R. and Bieleski, R. L.**, Some salt-uptake and tissue-aging phenomena studied with cultured tobacco cells, *Aust. J. Biol. Sci.*, 19, 23, 1966.
42. **Danks, M. L., Fletcher, J. S., and Rice, E. L.**, Influence of ferulic acid on mineral depletion and uptake of ^{86}Rb by Paul's Scarlet rose cell-suspension cultures, *Am. J. Bot.*, 62, 749, 1975.
43. **Wahlström, D. and Eriksson, T.**, Uptake of ^{14}C-L-glutamic acid by *Daucus carota* cell suspension in different shock situations, *Physiol. Plant.*, 38, 138, 1976.
44. **Thoiron, A., Thoiron, B., LeGuiel, J., Guern, J., and Theillier, M.**, A shock effect on the permeability of sulphate of *Acer pseudoplatanus* cell suspension cultures, in *Membrane Transport in Plants*, Zimmermann, U. and Dainty, J., Eds., Springer-Verlag, New York, 1974.
45. **Towill, L. E. and Mazur, P.**, Osmotic shrinkage as a factor in freezing injury in plant tissue cultures, *Plant Physiol.*, 57, 290, 1976.
46. **Hahlbrock, K. and Wellmann, E.**, Light-independent induction of enzymes related to phenylpropanoid metabolism in cell suspension cultures from parsley, *Biochim. Biophys. Acta*, 304, 702, 1973.
47. **Hahlbrock, K. and Schröder, J.**, Specific effects on enzyme activities upon dilution of *Petroselinum hortense* cell cultures into water, *Arch. Biochem. Biophys.*, 171, 500, 1975.
48. **Hahlbrock, K.**, Regulation of phenylalanine ammonia-lyase activity in cell-suspension cultures of *Petroselinum hortense*. Apparent rates of enzyme synthesis and degradation, *Eur. J. Biochem.*, 63, 137, 1976.
49. **Constabel, F., Shyluk, J. P., and Gamborg, O. L.**, The effect of hormones on anthocyanin accumulation in cell cultures of *Haplopappus gracilis*, *Planta*, 96, 306, 1971.
50. **Fosket, D. E., Volk, M. J., and Goldsmith, M. R.**, Polyribosome formation in relation to cytokinin-induced cell division in suspension cultures of *Glycine max* [L.] Merr., *Plant Physiol.*, 60, 554, 1977.
51. **Verma, D. P. S. and Marcus, A.**, Oxygen availability as a control factor in the density-dependent regulation of protein synthesis in cell culture, *J. Cell Sci.*, 14, 331, 1974.
52. **Filner, P.**, Regulation of nitrate reductase in cultured tobacco cells, *Biochim. Biophys. Acta*, 118, 299, 1966.
53. **Oaks, A.**, The regulation of nitrate reductase in suspension cultures of soybean cells, *Biochim. Biophys. Acta*, 372, 122, 1974.
54. **Rubery, P. H. and Sheldrake, A. R.**, Carrier-mediated auxin transport, *Planta*, 118, 101, 1974.
55. **Rubery, P. H.**, The specificity of carrier-mediated auxin transport by suspension cultured crown gall cells, *Planta*, 135, 275, 1977.
56. **Maretzki, A., Thom, M., and Nickell, L. G.**, Infuence of osmotic potentials on the growth and chemical composition of sugarcane cell cultures, *Hawaii. Plant. Rec.*, 58, 183, 1972.
57. **Withers, L. A. and Street, H. E.**, Freeze preservation of cultured plant cells. III. The pregrowth phase, *Physiol. Plant*, 39, 171, 1977.
58. **Kimball, S. L., Beversdorf, D., and Bingham, E. T.**, Influence of osmotic potential on the growth and development of soybean tissue cultures, *Crop Sci.*, 15, 750, 1975.
59. **Maretzki, A., Thom, M., and Nickell, L. G.**, Utilization and metabolism of carbohydrates in cell and callus cultures, in *Tissue Culture and Plant Science 1974*, Street, H. E., Ed., Academic Press, London, 1974, 14.
60. **Carceller, M., Davey, M. R., Fowler, M. W., and Street, H. E.**, The influence of sucrose, 2,4-D, and kinetin on the growth, fine structure, and lignin content of cultured sycamore cells, *Protoplasma*, 73, 24, 1971.
61. **Matsumoto, T., Okunishi, K., Nishida, K., Noguchi, M., and Tamaki, E.**, Studies on the culture conditions of higher plant cells in suspension culture. II. Effect of nutritional factors on the growth, *Agric. Biol. Chem.*, 35, 543, 1971.

62. Ikeda, T., Matsumoto, T., and Noguchi, M., Effects of nutritional factors on the formation of ubiquinone by tobacco plant cells in suspension culture, *Agric. Biol. Chem.*, 40, 1765, 1976.
63. Misawa, M., Hayashi, M., Tanaka, H., Ko, K., and Misato, T., Production of plant virus inhibitor by *Phytolacca americana* suspension culture, *Biotechnol. Bioeng.*, 17, 1335, 1975.
64. Zenk, M. H., El-Shagi, H., and Schulte, U., Anthraquinone production by cell suspension cultures of *Morinda citrifolia*, *Planta Med.*, Suppl., 79, 1975.
65. Misawa, M., Tanaka, H., Chiyo, O., and Mukai, M., Production of a plasmin inhibitory substance by *Scopolia japonica* suspension cultures, *Biotechnol. Bioeng.*, 17, 305, 1975.
66. Yasuda, S., Satoh, K., Ishi, T., and Furuya, T., Studies on the cultural conditions of plant cell suspensions culture, in *Int. Ferment. Symp. 4th, Kyoto, 1972, Proc. Ferment, Technol. Today*, Society of Fermentation Technology, Osaka, 1972, 697.
67. Hunt, W. F. and Loomis, R. S., Carbohydrate-limited growth kinetics of tobacco (*Nicotiana rustica* L.) callus, *Plant Physiol.*, 57, 802, 1976.
68. Verma, D. C. and Dougall, D. K., Influence of carbohydrates on quantitative aspects of growth and embryo formation in wild carrot suspension cultures, *Plant Physiol.*, 59, 81, 1977.
69. Nickell, L. G. and Maretzki, A., The utilization of sugars and starch as carbon sources by sugarcane cell suspension cultures, *Plant Cell Physiol.*, 11, 183, 1970.
70. Matsumoto, T., Nishida, K., Noguchi, M., and Tamaki, E., Some factors affecting the anthocyanin formation by *Populus* cells in suspension culture, *Agric. Biol. Chem.*, 37, 561, 1973.
71. Kamimura, S. and Akutsu, M., Cultural conditions on growth of the cell culture of *Papaver bracteatum*, *Agric. Biol. Chem.*, 40, 899, 1976.
72. Stuart, R. and Street, H. E., Studies on the growth in culture of plant cells. X. Further studies on the conditioning of culture media by suspensions of *Acer pseudoplatanus* L. cells, *J. Exp. Bot.*, 72, 96, 1971.
73. Scala, J. and Semersky, F. E., An induced fructose-1,6-diphosphatase from cultured cells of *Acer pseudoplatanus* (English sycamore), *Phytochemistry*, 10, 567, 1971.
74. Grout, W. W., Chan, K. W., and Simpkins, I., Aspects of growth and metabolism in a suspension culture of *Acer pseudoplatanus* (L.) grown on a glycerol carbon source, *J. Exp. Bot.*, 27, 96, 1976.
75. Nesius, K. K., Uchytil, L. E., and Fletcher, J. S., Minimal organic medium for suspension cultures of Paul's Scarlet rose, *Plants*, 106, 173, 1972.
76. Kaul, K. and Sabharwal, P. S., Morphogenetic studies on *Haworthia*: effects of inositol on growth and differentiation, *Am. J. Bot.*, 62, 655, 1975.
77. Linsmaier, E. M. and Skoog, F., Organic growth factor requirements of tobacco tissue cultures, *Physiol. Plant.*, 18, 100, 1965.
78. Shannon, J. C. and Liu, J.-W., A simplified medium for the growth of maize (*Zea mays*) endosperm tissue in suspension culture, *Physiol. Plant.*, 40, 285, 1977.
79. Carew, D. P. and Krueger, R. J., *Catharanthus roseus* tissue culture: the effects of medium modifications on growth and alkaloid production, *Lloydia*, 40, 326, 1977.
80. Verma, D. C. and Dougall, D. K., *myo*-Inositol biosynthesis and galactose utilization by wild carrot suspension cultures, *Ann. Bot. (London)*, 43, 259, 1979.
81. Ohira, K., Ojima, K., and Fujiwara, A., Studies on the nutrition of rice cell culture. I. A simple, defined medium for rapid growth in suspension culture, *Plant Cell Physiol.*, 14, 1113, 1973.
82. Davies, M. E., Polyphenol synthesis in cell suspension cultures of Paul's Scarlet rose, *Planta*, 104, 50, 1972.
83. Westcott, R. J., Henshaw, G. G., and Roca, W. M., Tissue culture storage of potato germplasm: culture initiation and plant regeneration, *Plant Sci. Lett.*, 9, 309, 1977.
84. Amorim, H. V., Dougall, D. K., and Sharp, W. R., The effect of carbohydrate and nitrogen concentration on phenol synthesis in Paul's Scarlet Rose cells grown in tissue culture, *Physiol. Plant.*, 39, 91, 1977.
85. Mizukami, H., Konoshima, M., and Tabata, M., Effect of nutritional factors on shikonin derivative formation in *Lithospermum* callus cultures, *Phytochemistry*, 16, 1183, 1977.
86. Fowler, M. W. and Clifton, A., Activities of enzymes of carbohydrate metabolism in cells of *Acer psuedoplatanus* L. maintained in continuous (chemostat) culture, *Eur. J. Biochem.*, 45, 445, 1974.
87. Shimizu, T., Clifton, A., Komamine, A., and Fowler, M. W., Changes in metabolite levels during growth of *Acer pseudoplatanus* (sycamore) cells in batch suspension culture, *Physiol. Plant.*, 40, 125, 1977.
88. Hoover, J. D., Wender, S. H., and Smith, E. C., Isoenzymes of glucose-6-phosphate dehydrogenase from tobacco cells, *Phytochemistry*, 16, 195, 1977; Effect of phenolic compounds on glucose-6-phosphate dehydrogenase isoenzymes, *Phytochemistry*, 16, 199, 1977.
89. Fowler, M. W. and Clifton, A., Hexokinase activity in cultured sycamore cells, *New Phytol*, 75, 533, 1975.

90. **Hunt, L. and Fletcher, J. S.,** Estimated drainage of carbon from the tricarboxylic acid cycle for protein synthesis in suspension cultures of Paul's Scarlet rose cells, *Plant Physiol.,* 57, 304, 1976.

91. **Verma, D. C., Tavares, J., and Loewus, F. A.,** Effect of benzyladenine, 2,4-dichlorophenoxyacetic acid, and D-glucose on *myo*-inositol metabolism in *Acer pseudoplatanus* L. cells grown in suspension culture, *Plant Physiol.,* 57, 241, 1976.

92. **Loewus, M. W. and Loewus, F.,** The isolation and characterization of D-glucose 6-phosphate cycloaldolase (NAD-dependent) from *Acer pseudoplatanus* L. cell cultures, its occurrence in plants, *Plant Physiol.,* 48, 255, 1971.

93. **Loewus, M. W. and Loewus, F.,** D-glucose 6-phosphate cycloaldolase: inhibition studies and aldolase function, *Plant Physiol.,* 51, 263, 1973.

94. **Bergmann, L.,** Plating of plant cells, in *Plant Tissue Culture and Its Bio-technological Application,* Barz, W., Reinhard, E., and Zenk, M. H., Eds., Springer-Verlag, Berlin, 1977.

95. **Nato, A., Bazetoux, S., and Mathieu, Y.,** Photosynthetic capacities and growth characteristics of *Nicotiana tabacum* (cv. Xanthi) cell suspension cultures, *Physiol. Plant.,* 41, 116, 1977.

96. **Hüsemann, W. and Barz, W.,** Photoautotrophic growth and photosynthesis in cell suspension cultures of *Chenopodium rubrum, Physiol. Plant.,* 40, 77, 1977.

97. **Chandler, M. T., Tandeau de Marsac, N., and de Kouchkovsky, Y.,** Photosynthetic growth of tobacco cells in liquid suspension, *Can. J. Bot.,* 50, 2265, 1972.

98. **Berlyn, M. B. and Zelitch, I.,** Photoautotrophic growth and photosynthesis in tobacco callus cells., *Plant Physiol.,* 56, 752, 1975.

99. **Nesius, K. K. and Fletcher, J. S.,** Contribution of nonautotrophic carbon dioxide fixation to protein synthesis in suspension cultures of Paul's Scarlet rose, *Plant Physiol.,* 55, 643, 1975.

100. **Gathercole, R. W. E., Mansfield, K. J., and Street, H. E.,** Carbon dioxide as an essential requirement for cultured sycamore cells, *Physiol. Plant.,* 37, 213, 1976.

101. **McChesney, J. D.,** Stimulation of in vitro growth of plant tissues by *dl*-mevalonic acid, *Can. J. Bot.,* 48, 2357, 1970.

102. **Mangold, H. K.,** The common and unusual lipids of plant cell cultures, in *Plant Tissue Culture and Its Bio-technological Application,* Barz, W., Reinhard, E., and Zenk, M. H., Eds., Springer-Verlag, Berlin, 1977.

103. **Behrend, J. and Mateles, R. I.,** Nitrogen metabolism in plant cell suspension cultures. I. Effect of amino acids on growth, *Plant Physiol.,* 56, 584, 1975.

104. **Sargent, P. A. and King, J.,** Investigations of growth-promoting factors in conditioned soybean root cells and in the liquid medium in which they grow: ammonium, glutamine, and amino acids, *Can. J. Bot.,* 7, 1747, 1974.

105. **Bergmann, L., Grosse, W., and Koth, P.,** Influences of ammonium and nitrate on N-metabolism, malate accumulation and malic enzyme activity in suspension cultures of *Nicotiana tabacum, Z. Pflanzenphysiol.,* 80, 60, 1976.

106. **Nash, D. T. and Davies, M. E.,** Some aspects of growth and metabolism of Paul's Scarlet rose cell suspensions, *J. Exp. Bot.,* 23, 75, 1972.

107. **Jones, R. W., Abbott, A. J., Hewitt, E. J., James, D. M., and Best, G. R.,** Nitrate reductase activity and growth in Paul's Scarlet rose suspension cultures in relation to nitrogen source and molybdenum, *Planta,* 133, 27, 1976.

108. **Mohanty, B. and Fletcher, J. S.,** Ammonium influence on the growth and nitrate reductase activity of Paul's Scarlet rose suspension cultures, *Plant Physiol.,* 58, 152, 1976.

109. **Jessup, W. and Fowler, M. W.,** Interrelationships between carbohydrate metabolism and nitrogen assimilation in cultured plant cells. I. Effects of glutamate and nitrate as alternative nitrogen sources on cell growth, *Planta,* 132, 119, 1976.

110. **Halperin, W.,** Alternative morphogenetic events in cell suspension, *Am. J. Bot.,* 53, 443, 1966.

111. **Dunstan, D. I. and Short, K. C.,** Improved growth of tissue cultures of the onion, *Allium cepa, Physiol. Plant.,* 41, 70, 1977.

112. **Bayley, J. M., King, J., and Gamborg, O. L.,** The ability of amino compounds and conditioned medium to alleviate the reduced nitrogen requirement of soybean cells grown in suspension cultures, *Planta,* 105, 25, 1972.

113. **Sargent, P. A. and King, J.,** Investigations of growth-promoting factors in conditioned soybean root cells and in the liquid medium in which they grow: cytokinin-like compounds, *Can. J. Bot.,* 52, 2459, 1974.

114. **Halperin, W. and Wetherell, D. F.,** Ammonium requirement for embryogenesis in vitro, *Nature (London),* 205, 519, 1965.

115. **Thomas, E. and Street, H. E.,** Factors influencing morphogenesis in excised roots and suspension cultures of *Atropa belladonna Ann. Bot. (London),* 36, 239, 1972.

116. **Craven, G. H., Mott, R. L., and Steward, F. C.,** Solute accumulation in plant cells. IV. Effects of ammonium ions on growth and solute content, *Ann. Bot. (London),* 36, 897, 1972.

117. **Rose, D. and Martin, S. M.,** Parameters for growth measurement in suspension cultures of plant cells, *Can. J. Bot.,* 52, 903, 1974.

118. **Rose, D. and Martin, S. M.,** Effect of ammonium on growth of plant cells (*Ipomoea* sp.) in suspension cultures, *Can. J. Bot.,* 53, 1942, 1975.

119. **Polacco, J. C.,** Nitrogen metabolism in soybean tissue culture. I. Assimilation of urea, *Plant Physiol.,* 58, 350, 1976.

120. **Dougall, D. K.,** Evidence for the presence of glutamate synthase in extracts of carrot cell cultures, *Biochem. Biophys. Res. Commun.,* 58, 639, 1974.

121. **Behrend, J. and Mateles, R. I.,** Nitrogen metabolism in plant cell suspension cultures. II. Role of organic acids during growth on ammonia, *Plant Physiol.,* 58, 510, 1976.

122. **Sheat, D. E. G., Fletcher, B. H., and Street, H. E.,** Studies on the growth of excised roots. VIII. The growth of excised tomato roots supplied with various inorganic sources of nitrogen, *New Phytol.,* 58, 128, 1959.

123. **Polacco, J. C.,** Nitrogen metabolism in soybean tissue culture. II. Urea utilization and urease synthesis require Ni^{2+}, *Plant Physiol.,* 59, 827, 1977a.

124. **King, P. J.,** Studies on the growth in culture of plant cells. XX. Utilization of 2,4-dichlorophenoxyacetic acid by steady-state cell cultures of *Acer pseudoplatanus* L., *J. Exp. Bot.,* 27, 1053, 1976.

125. **Heimer, Y. M. and Filner, P.,** Regulation of the nitrate assimilation pathway of cultured tobacco cells. II. Properties of a variant cell line, *Biochim. Biophys. Acta,* 215, 152, 1970.

126. **Meins, F., Jr.,** Auxin-facilitated utilization of glutamic acid by tobacco crown-gall teratoma cells, *Planta,* 92, 240, 1970.

127. **Meins, F., Jr.,** Separate auxin- and cation-dependent mechanisms for glutamate utilization by normal and crown-gall teratoma cells of tobacco in culture, *Planta,* 112, 57, 1973.

128. **Maretzki, A., Nickell, L. G., and Thom, M.,** Arginine in growing cells of sugarcane. Nutritional effects, uptake and incorporation into proteins, *Physiol. Plant.,* 22, 827, 1969.

129. **Salonen, M.-L. and Simola, L. K.,** Dipeptides and amino acids as nitrogen sources for the callus of *Atropa belladonna, Physiol. Plant.,* 41, 55, 1977.

130. **Veliky, I. A. and Genest, K.,** Growth and metabolites of *Cannabis sativa* cell suspension cultures, *Lloydia,* 35, 450, 1972.

131. **Rose, D., Martin, S. M., and Clay, P. P. F.,** Metabolic rates for major nutrients in suspension cultures of plant cells, *Can. J. Bot.,* 50, 1301, 1972.

132. **Hahlbrock, K., Ebel, J., and Oaks, A.,** Determination of specific growth stages of plant cell suspension cultures by monitoring conductivity changes in the medium, *Planta,* 118, 75, 1974.

133. **Zink, M. W. and Veliky, I. A.,** Nitrogen assimilation and regulation of nitrate and nitrite reductases in cultured *Ipomoea* cells, *Can. J. Bot.,* 55, 1557, 1977.

134. **Heimer, Y. M.,** Nitrite-induced development of the nitrate uptake system in plant cells, *Plant Sci. Lett.,* 4, 137, 1975.

135. **Young, M.,** Studies on the growth in culture of plant cells. XVI. Nitrogen assimilation during nitrogen-limited growth of *Acer pseudoplatanus* L. cells in chemostat culture, *J. Exp. Bot.,* 24, 1172, 1973.

136. **Harvey, R. G., Muzik, T. J., and Warner, R. L.,** Differences in nitrogen requirements of two clones of *Convolvulus arvensis* in vitro, *Am. J. Bot.,* 60, 76, 1973.

137. **Zielke, H. R. and Filner, P.,** Synthesis and turnover of nitrate reductase induced by nitrate in cultured tobacco cells., *J. Biol. Chem.,* 246, 1772, 1971.

138. **Ferrari, T. E., Yoder, O. C., and Filner, P.,** Anaerobic nitrite production by plant cells and tissue: Evidence for two nitrate pools, *Plant Physiol.,* 51, 423, 1973.

139. **Chroboczek-Kelker, H. and Filner, P.,** Regulation of nitrite reductase and its relationship to the regulation of nitrate reductase in cultured tobacco cells., *Biochim. Biophys. Acta,* 252, 69, 1971.

140. **Washitani, I. and Sato, S.,** Studies on the function of proplastids in the metabolism of in vitro cultured tobacco cells. I. Localization of nitrite reductase and NADP-dependent glutamate dehydrogenase, *Plant Cell Physiol.,* 18, 117, 1977.

141. **Jessup, W. and Fowler, M. W.,** Interrelationships between carbohydrate metabolism and nitrogen assimilation in cultured plant cells, *Planta,* 133, 71, 1977.

142. **Dougall, D. K. and Bloch, J.,** A survey of the presence of glutamate synthase in plant cell suspension cultures, *Can. J. Bot.,* 54, 2924, 1976.

143. **Fowler, M. W., Jessup, W., and Sarkissian, G. S.,** Glutamate synthetase type activity in higher plants, *FEBS Lett.,* 46, 340, 1974.

144. **Beevers, L. and Storey, R.,** Glutamate synthetase in developing cotyledons of *Pisum sativum, Plant Physiol.,* 57, 862, 1976.

145. **Sodek, L. and da Silva, W. J.,** Glutamate synthase: a possible role in nitrogen metabolism of the developing maize endosperm, *Plant Physiol.,* 60, 602, 1977.

146. **Lea, P. J. and Miflin, B. J.**, An alternative route for nitrogen assimilation in higher plants, *Nature (London),* 251, 614, 1974.
147. **Miflin, B. J. and Lea, P. J.**, Amino acid metabolism, *Annu. Rev. Plant Physiol.,* 28, 299, 1977.
148. **Wallsgrove, R. M., Harel, E., Lea, P. J., and Miflin, B. J.**, Studies on glutamate synthase from the leaves of higher plants, *J. Exp. Bot.,* 28, 104, 1977.
149. **Washitani, I. and Sato, S.**, Studies on the function of proplastids in the metabolism of in vitro cultured tobacco cells. II. Glutamine synthetase/glutamate synthetase pathway, *Plant Cell Physiol.,* 18, 505, 1977.
150. **Dougall, D. K.**, Current problems in the regulation of nitrogen metabolism in plant plant cell cultures, in *Plant Tissue Culture and Its Bio-technological Application,* Barz, W., Reinhard, E., and Zenk, M. H., Eds., Springer-Verlag, Berlin, 1977.
151. **Polacco, J. C.**, Is nickel a universal component of plant ureases?, *Plant Sci. Lett.,* 10, 249, 1977.
152. **Smith, I. K.**, Evidence for *O*-acetylserine in *Nicotiana tabacum, Phytochemistry,* 16, 1293, 1977.
153. **Glenn, E. and Maretzki, A.**, Properties and subcellular distribution of two partially purified ornithine transcarbamoylases in cell suspensions of sugarcane, *Plant Physiol.,* 60, 122, 1977.
154. **Davies, H. M. and Miflin, B. J.**, Aspartate kinase from carrot cell suspension culture, *Plant Sci. Lett.,* 9, 323, 1977.
155. **Sakano, K. and Komamine, A.**, Change in the proportion of two aspartokinases in carrot root tissue in response to in vitro culture, *Plant Physiol.,* 61, 115, 1978.
156. **Westcott, R. J. and Henshaw, G. G.**, Phenolic synthesis and phenylalanine ammonia-lyase activity in suspension cultures of *Acer pseudoplatanus* L., *Planta,* 131, 67, 1976.
157. **Phillips, R. and Henshaw, G. G.**, The regulation of synthesis of phenolics in stationary phase cell cultures of *Acer pseudoplatanus* L., *J. Exp. Bot.,* 28, 785, 1977.
158. **Ikeda, T., Matsumoto, T., and Noguchi, M.**, Effects of inorganic nitrogen sources and physical factors on the formation of ubiquinone by tobacco plant cells in suspension culture, *Agric. Biol. Chem.,* 41, 1197, 1977.
159. **Tanaka, H., Machida, Y., Tanaka, H., Mukai, N., and Misawa, M.**, Accumulation of glutamine by suspension cultures of *Symphytum officinale, Agric. Biol. Chem.,* 38, 987, 1974.
160. **Nettleship, L. and Slaytor, M.**, Adaptation of *Peganum harmala* callus to alkaloid production, *J. Exp. Bot.,* 25, 1114, 1974.
161. **Reuveny, Z. and Filner, P.**, Regulation of adenosine triphosphate sulfurylase in cultured tobacco cells. Effects of sulfur and nitrogen sources on the formation and decay of the enzyme, *J. Biol. Chem.,* 252, 1858, 1977.
162. **Bergmann, L. and Rennenberg, H.**, Growth inhibition of soybean callus tissues by glutathione, *Naturwissenschaften,* 62, 349, 1975.
163. **Reuveny, Z. and Filner, P.**, A new assay for ATP sulfurylase based on differential solubility of the sodium salts of adenosine 5′-phosphosulfate and sulfate, *Ann. Biochem. Exp. Med.,* 75, 410, 1976.
164. **Reuveny, Z.**, Derepression of ATP sulfurylase by the sulfate analogs molybdate and selenate in cultured tobacco cells, *Proc. Natl. Acad. Sci. U.S.A.,* 74, 619, 1977.
165. **Cacco, G., Saccomani, M., and Ferrari, G.**, Development of sulfate uptake capacity and ATP-sulfurylase activity during root elongation in maize, *Plant Physiol.,* 60, 582, 1977.
166. **Rennenberg, H.**, Glutathione in conditioned media of tobacco suspension cultures, *Phytochemistry,* 15, 1433, 1976.
167. **Lavee, S. and Hoffman, M.**, The effect of potassium ions on peroxidase activity and its isozyme composition as related to apple callus growth in vitro, *Bot. Gaz. (Chicago),* 132, 232, 1971.
168. **Hahlbrock, K.**, Further studies on the relationship between the rates of nitrate uptake, growth and conductivity changes in the medium of plant cell suspension cultures, *Planta,* 124, 311, 1975.
169. **Jones, L. H., Barrett, J. N., and Gopal, P. P. S.**, Growth and nutrition of a suspension culture of *Pogostemon cablin* Benth. (Patchouli), *J. Exp. Bot.,* 24, 145, 1973.
170. **Brown, S., Wetherell, D. F., and Dougall, D. K.**, The potassium requirement for growth and embryogenesis in wild carrot suspension cultures, *Physiol. Plant,* 37, 73, 1976.
171. **Dobberstein, R. H. and Staba, E. J.**, *Ipomoea, Rivea* and *Argyeia* tissue cultures: influence of various chemical factors on indole alkaloid production and growth, *Lloydia,* 32, 141, 1969.
172. **Ueki, K. and Sato, S.**, Effect of inorganic phosphate on the extracellular acid phosphatase activity of tobacco cells cultured in vitro, *Physiol. Plant.,* 24, 506, 1971.
173. **Wilson, G.**, A simple and inexpensive design of chemostat enabling steady-state growth of *Acer pseudoplatanus* L. cells under phosphate-limiting conditions, *Ann. Bot. (London),* 40, 919, 1976.
174. **Bayliss, M. W.**, Factors affecting the frequency of tetraploid cells in a predominantly diploid suspension culture of *Daucus carota, Protoplasma,* 92, 109, 1977.
175. **Bayliss, M. W.**, The causes of competition between two cell lines of *Daucus carota* in mixed culture, *Protoplasma,* 92, 117, 1977.

176. Igaue, I., Nishio, M., and Kurasawa, F., Occurrence of acid phosphatase-isozymes repressible by inorganic phosphate in rice plant cell cultures, *Agric. Biol. Chem.,* 37, 941, 1973.

177. Igaue, I., Watabe, H., Takahashi, K., Takekoshi, M., and Morota, A., Violet-colored acid phosphatase isozymes associated with cell wall preparations from rice plant cultured cells, *Agric. Biol. Chem.,* 40, 823, 1976.

178. Ninomiya, Y., Ueki, K., and Sato, S., Chromatographic separation of extracellular acid phosphatase of tobacco cells cultured under Pi-supplied and omitted conditions, *Plant Cell Physiol.,* 18, 413, 1977.

179. Suzuki, T. and Sato, S., Cell-wall column chromatographic identification of the native cell-wall acid phosphatase of cultured tobacco cells, *Plant Cell Physiol.,* 17, 847, 1976.

180. Shinshi, H., Miwa, M., Kato, K., Noguchi, M., Matsushima, T., and Sugimura, T., A novel phosphodiesterase from cultured tobacco cells, *Biochemistry,* 15, 2185, 1976.

181. Shinshi, H., Miwa, M., Sugimura, T., Shimotohno, K., and Miura, K., Enzyme cleaving the 5′-terminal methylated blocked structure of messenger RNA, *FEBS Lett.,* 65, 254, 1976.

182. Efstratiadis, A., Vournakis, J. N., Donis-Keller, H., Chaconas, G., Dougall, D. K., and Kafatos, F. C., End labeling of enzymatically decapped mRNA, *Nucleic Acids,* 4, 4165, 1977.

183. Veliky, I. A., Rose, D., and Zink, M. W., Uptake of magnesium by suspension cultures of plant cells (*Ipomoea* sp.), *Can. J. Bot.,* 55, 1143, 1977.

184. Neumann, K. H. and Steward, F. C., Investigations on the growth and metabolism of cultured explants of *Daucus carota.* I. Effects of iron, molybdenum and manganese on growth, *Planta,* 81, 333, 1968.

185. Oswald, T. H., Nicholson, R. L., and Bauman, L. F., Cell suspension and callus culture from somatic tissue of maize, *Physiol. Plant.,* 41, 45, 1977.

186. Ojima, K., Yamada, M., Yamada, T., and Ohira, K., Studies on the greening of cultured soybean and *Ruta* cells. III. Effects of minorelement deficiency on the growth and photosynthetic activities of *Ruta* cells, *Soil Sci. Plant Nutr. (Tokyo),* 23, 67, 1977.

187. Ohira, K., Ojima, K., Saigusa, M., and Fujiwara, A., Studies on the nutrition of rice cell culture. II. Microelement requirement and the effects of deficiency, *Plant Cell Physiol.,* 16, 73, 1975.

188. Bligny, R. and Douce, R., Mitochondria of isolated plant cells (*Acer pseudoplatanus* L.). II. Copper deficiency effects on cytochrome *C* oxidase and oxygen uptake, *Plant Physiol.,* 60, 675, 1977.

189. Klein, R. M., Caputo, E. M., and Witterholt, B. A., The role of zinc in the growth of plant tissue cultures, *Am. J. Bot.,* 49, 343, 1962.

190. Leguay, J. J. and Guern, J., Quantitative effects of 2,4-dichlorophenoxyacetic acid on growth of suspension-cultured *Acer pseudoplatanus* cells, *Plant Physiol.,* 56, 356, 1975.

191. Ohira, K., Ikeda, M., and Ojima, K., Thiamine requirements of various plant cells, in suspension culture, *Plant Cell Physiol.,* 17, 583, 1976.

192. Nishi, T., Requirement of organic factors for the growth of *Ephedra* tissues cultured in vitro, *Bot. Mag.,* 87, 337, 1974.

193. Linsmaier-Bednar, E. M. and Skoog, F., Thiamine requirement in relation to cytokinin in "normal" and "mutant" strains of tobacco callus, *Planta,* 72, 146, 1967.

194. Dravnieks, D. E., Skoog, F., and Burris, R. H., Cytokinin activation of *de novo* thiamine biosynthesis in tobacco callus cultures, *Plant Physiol.,* 44, 866, 1969.

195. Erner, Y., Reuveni, O., and Goldschmidt, E. E., Partial purification of a growth factor from orange juice which affects citrus tissue culture and its replacement by citric acid, *Plant Physiol.,* 56, 279, 1975.

196. Kessell, R. H. J., Goodwin, C., Philp, J., and Fowler, M. W., The relationship between dissolved oxygen concentration, ATP and embryogenesis in carrot (*Daucus carota*) tissue cultures, *Plant Sci. Lett.,* 10, 265, 1977.

197. Wood, H. N. and Braun, A. C., Studies on the regulation of certain essential biosynthetic systems in normal and crown-gall tumor cells, *Proc. Natl. Acad. Sci. U.S.A.,* 47, 1907, 1961.

198. Sogeke, A. K. and Butcher, D. N., The effect of inorganic nutrients on the hormonal requirements of normal, habituated and crown-gall tissues cultures, *J. Exp. Bot.,* 27, 785, 1976.

199. Skoog, F. and Miller, C. O., Chemical regulation of growth and organ formation in plant tissues cultured in vitro, *Symp. Soc. Exp. Biol.,* 11, 118, 1957.

200. Murashige, T., Plant propagation through tissue cultures, *Annu. Rev. Plant Physiol.,* 25, 135, 1974.

201. Shabde, M. and Murashige, T., Hormonal requirements of excised *Dianthus caryophyllus* L. shoot apical meristem in vitro, *Am. J. Bot.,* 64, 443, 1977.

202. Schneider, E. A. and Wightman, F., Metabolism of auxin in higher plants, *Annu. Rev. Plant Physiol.,* 25, 487, 1974.

203. Wain, R. L. and Fawcett, C. H., Chemical plant growth regulation, in *Plant Physiology, A Treatise,* Vol. 5A, Steward, F. C., Ed., Academic Press, New York, 1969, chap. 4.

204. **Fosket, D. E. and Torrey, J. G.**, Hormonal control of cell proliferation and xylem differentiation in cultured tissues on *Glycine max* var. *Biloxi, Plant Physiol.*, 44, 871, 1969.
205. **Miller, C. O.**, Control of deoxyisoflavone synthesis in soybean tissue, *Planta*, 87, 26, 1969.
206. **Torrey, J. G. and Fosket, D. E.**, Cell division in relation to cytodifferentiation in cultured pea root segments, *Am. J. Bot.*, 57, 1072, 1970.
207. **Witham, F. H.**, Effect of 2,4-dichlorophenoxyacetic acid on the cytokinin requirement of soybean cotyledon and tobacco stem pith callus tissues, *Plant Physiol.*, 43, 1455 1968.
208. **Syōno, K. and Furuya, T.**, Effects of cytokinins on the auxin requirement and auxin content of tobacco calluses, *Plant Cell Physiol.*, 13, 843, 1972.
209. **Einset, J. W.**, Two effects of cytokinin on the auxin requirement of tobacco callus cultures, *Plant Physiol.*, 59, 45, 1977.
210. **Widholm, J. M.**, Relation between auxin autotrophy and tryptophan accumulation in cultured plant cells, *Planta*, 134, 103, 1977.
211. **Feung, C. S., Hamilton, R. H., and Witham, F. H.**, Metabolism of 2,4-dichlorophenoxyacetic acid by soybean cotyledon callus tissue cultures, *J. Agric. Food Chem.*, 19, 475, 1971.
212. **Feung, C. S., Hamilton, R. H., Witham, F. H., and Mumma, R. O.**, The relative amounts and identification of some 2,4-dichlorophenoxyacetic acid metabolites isolated from soybean cotyledon callus cultures, *Plant Physiol.*, 50, 80, 1972.
213. **Feung, C. S., Hamilton, R. H., and Mumma, R. O.**, Metabolism of 2,4-dichlorophenoxyacetic acid. V. Identification of metabolites in soybean callus tissue cultures, *J. Agric. Food Chem.*, 21, 637, 1973.
213. **Feung, C. S., Hamilton, R. H., and Mumma, R. O.**, Metabolism of 2,4-dichlorophenoxyacetic acid. V. Identification of metabolites in soybean callus tissue cultures, *J. Agric. Food Chem.*, 21, 637, 1973.
214. **Feung, C. S., Mumma, R. O., and Hamilton, R. H.**, Metabolism of 2,4-dichlorophenoxyacetic acid. VI. Biological properties of amino acid conjugates, *J. Agric. Food Chem.*, 22, 307, 1974.
215. **Leguay, J. J. and Guern, J.**, Quantitative effects of 2,4-dichlorophenoxyacetic acid on growth of suspension-cultured *Acer pseudoplatanus* cells. II. Influence of 2,4-D metabolism and intracellular pH on the control of cell division of intracellular 2,4-D concentration, *Plant Physiol.*, 60, 265, 1977.
216. **Simard, A.**, Initiation of DNA synthesis by kinetin and experimental factors in tobacco pith tissues in vitro, *Can. J. Bot.*, 49, 1541, 1971.
217. **Das, N. K., Patau, K., and Skoog, F.**, Initiation of mitosis and cell division by kinetin and indole-acetic acid in excised tobacco pith tissue, *Physiol. Plant.*, 9, 640, 1956.
218. **Nishi, A., Kato, K., Takahashi, M., and Yoshida, R.**, Partial synchronization of carrot cell culture by auxin deprivation, *Physiol. Plant.*, 39, 9, 1977.
219. **Skoog, F. and Schmitz, R. Y.**, IX. Cytokinins, in *Plant Physiology A Treatise*, Vol. 6B, Steward, F. C., Ed., Academic Press, New York, 1972, chap. 5.
220. **Fox, J. E.**, The cytokinins, in *The Physiology of Plant Growth and Development*, Wilkins, M. B., Ed., McGraw-Hill, Maidenhead, Berkshire, England, 1969, chap. 3.
221. **Hall, R. H.**, Cytokinins as a probe of developmental processes, *Annu. Rev. Plant Physiol.*, 24, 415, 1973.
222. **Szweykowska, A.**, The role of cytokinins in the control of cell growth and differentiation in culture, in *Tissue Culture and Plant Science 1974*, Street, H. E., Ed., Academic Press, London, 1974, 19.
223. **Skoog, F., Hamzi, H. Q., Szweykowska, A. M., Leonard, N. J., Carraway, K. L., Fujii, T., Helgeson, J. P., and Loeppky, R. N.**, Cytokinins: structure/activity relationships, *Phytochemistry*, 6, 1169, 1967.
224. **Mackenzie, I. A., Konar, A., and Street, H. E.**, Cytokinins and the growth of cultured sycamore cells, *New Phytol.*, 71, 633, 1972.
225. **Street, H. E., Collin, H. A., Short, K., and Simpkins, I.**, Hormonal control of cell division and expansion in suspension cultures of *Acer pseudoplatanus*, L: the action of kinetin, in *Biochemistry and Physiology of Plant Growth Substances*, Wightman, F. and Setterfield, G., Eds., Runge Press, Ottawa, 1968.
226. **Smith, R. H., Price, H. J., and Thaxton, J. B.**, Defined conditions for the initiation and growth of cotton callus in vitro. I. *Gossypium arboreum, In Vitro*, 13, 329, 1977.
227. **Price, H. J., Smith, R. H., and Grumbles, R. M.**, Callus cultures of six species of cotton (*Gossypium* L.) on defined media, *Plant. Sci. Lett.*, 10, 115, 1977.
228. **Cheng, T. Y.**, Factors effecting adventitious bud formation of cotyledon culture of Douglas fir, *Plant Sci. Lett.*, 9, 179, 1977.
229. **Miller, L. R. and Murashige, T.**, Tissue culture propagation of tropical foliage plants, *In Vitro*, 12, 797, 1976.
230. **Syōno, K. and Furuya, T.**, Effects of temperature on the cytokinin requirement of tobacco calluses, *Plant Cell Physiol.*, 12, 61, 1971.

231. **Meins, F., Jr.,** Mechanisms underlying the persistence of tumour autonomy in crown-gall disease, in *Tissue Culture and Plant Science 1974,* Street, H. E., Ed., Academic Press, London, 1974, 10.

232. **Meins, F., Jr. and Binns, A.,** Epigenetic variation of cultured somatic cells: evidence for gradual changes in the requirement for factors promoting cell division, *Proc. Natl. Acad. Sci. U.S.A.,* 74, 2928, 1977.

233. **Binns, A. and Meins, F., Jr.,** Habituation of tobacco pith cells for factors promoting cell division is heritable and potentially reversible, *Proc. Natl. Acad. Sci. U.S.A.,* 70, 2660, 1973.

234. **Meins, F., Jr.,** Cell division and the determination phase of cyto-differentiation in plants, *Results Probl. Cell Differ.,* 7, 151, 1975.

235. **Tegley, J. R., Witham, F. H., and Krasnuk, M.,** Chromatographic analysis of a cytokinin from tissue cultures of crown-gall, *Plant Physiol.,* 47, 581, 1971.

236. **Linstedt, D. and Reinert, J.,** Occurrence and properties of a cytokinin in tissues cultures of *Daucus carota, Naturwissenschaften,* 62, 238, 1975.

237. **Miller, C. O.,** Ribosyl *trans-*zeatin, a major cytokinin produced by crown gall tumor tissue, *Proc. Natl. Acad. Sci. U.S.A.,* 71, 334, 1974.

238. **Wood, H. N., Rennekamp, M. E., Bowen, D. V., Field, F. H., and Braun, A. C.,** A comparative study of cytokinesins I and II and zeatin riboside: a reply to Carlos Miller, *Proc. Natl. Acad. Sci. U.S.A.,* 71, 4140, 1974.

239. **Short, K. C. and Torrey, J. G.,** Cytokinin production in relation to the growth of pea-root callus tissue, *J. Exp. Bot.,* 23, 1099, 1972.

240. **Dyson, W. H. and Hall, R. H.,** N^6-(Δ^2-Isopentenyl)adenosine: its occurrence as a free nucleoside in an autonomous strain of tobacco tissue, *Plant. Physiol.,* 50, 616, 1972.

241. **Jouanneau, J. P. and Tandeau de Marsac, N.,** Stepwise effects of cytokinin activity and DNA synthesis upon mitotic cycle events in partially synchronized tobacco cells, *Exp. Cell Res.,* 77, 167, 1973.

242. **Jouanneau, J. P.,** Protein synthesis requirement for the cytokinin effect upon tobacco cell division, *Exp. Cell Res.,* 91, 184, 1975.

243. **Hagen, G. L. and Marcus, A.,** Cytokinin effects on growth of quiescent tobacco pith cells, *Plant Physiol.,* 55, 90, 1975.

244. **Fosket, D. E. and Short, K. C.,** The role of cytokinin in the regulation of growth, DNA synthesis and cell proliferation in cultured soybean tissues (*Glycine max* var. *Biloxi*), *Physiol. Plant.,* 28, 14, 1973.

245. **Short, K. C., Tepfer, D. A., and Fosket, D. E.,** Regulation of polyribosome formation and cell division in cultured soybean cells by cytokinin, *J. Cell Sci.,* 15, 75, 1974.

246. **Muren, R. C. and Fosket, D. E.,** Cytokinin-mediated translational control of protein synthesis in cultured cells of *Glycine max, J. Exp. Bot.,* 28, 775, 1977.

247. **Klämbt, D.,** Cytokinin effects on protein synthesis of in vitro systems of higher plants, *Plant Cell Physiol.,* 17, 73, 1976.

248. **Mass, H. and Klämbt, D.,** Cytokinin effect on protein synthesis in vivo in higher plants, *Planta,* 133, 117, 1977.

249. **Letham, D. S., Wilson, M. M., Parker, C. W., Jenkins, I. D., MacLeod, J. K., and Summons, R. E.,** Regulators of cell division in plant tissues. XXIII. The identity of an unusual metabolite of 6-benzylaminopurine, *Biochim. Biophys. Acta,* 399, 61, 1975.

250. **Deleuze, G. G., McChesney, J. D., and Fox, J. E.,** Identification of a stable cytokinin metabolite, *Biochem. Biophys. Res. Commun.,* 48, 1426, 1972.

251. **Laloue, M., Gawer, M., and Terrine, C.,** Modalités de l'utilisation des cytokinines exogènes par les cellules de Tabac cultivées en milieu liquide agité, *Physiol. Veg.,* 13, 781, 1975.

252. **Laloue, M., Terrine, C., and Guern, J.,** Cytokinins: metabolism and biological activity of N^6-(Δ^2-Isopentenyl)adenosine and N^6-(Δ^2-Isopentenyl) adenine in tobacco cells and callus, *Plant Physiol.,* 59, 478, 1977.

253. **Laloue, M.,** Cytokinins: 7-glucosylation is not a prerequisite of the expression of their biological activity, *Planta,* 134, 273, 1977.

254. **Gawer, M., Laloue, M., Terrine, C., and Guern, J.,** Metabolism and biological significance of benzyladenine-7-glucoside, *Plant Sci. Lett.,* 8, 267, 1977.

255. **Wood, H. N. and Braun, A. C.,** 8-Bromoadenosine 3′:5′-cyclic monophosphate as a promoter of cell division in excised tobacco pith parenchyma tissue, *Proc. Natl. Acad. Sci. U.S.A.,* 70, 447, 1973.

256. **Lundeen, C. V., Wood, H. N., and Braun, A. C.,** Intracellular levels of cyclic nucleotides during cell enlargement and cell division in excised tobacco pith tissues, *Differentiation,* 1, 255, 1973.

257. **Basile, D. V., Wood, H. N., and Braun, A. C.,** Programming of cells for death under defined experimental conditions: relevance to the tumor problem, *Proc. Natl. Acad. Sci. U.S.A.,* 70, 3055, 1973.

258. **Ammirato, P. V.,** The effects of abscisic acid on the development of somatic embryos from cells of caraway (*Carum carvi* L.), *Bot. Gaz. (Chicago),* 135, 328, 1974.

259. **Ammirato, P. V.**, Hormonal control of somatic embryo development from cultured cells of caraway. Interactions of abscisic acid, zeatin, and gibberellic acid, *Plant Physiol.*, 59, 579, 1977.
260. **Fujimura, T. and Komamine, A.** Effects of various growth regulators on the embryogenesis in a carrot cell suspension culture, *Plant Sci. Lett.*, 5, 359, 1975.
261. **Gregorini, G. and Lorenzi, R.**, Meristem-tip culture of potato plants as a method of improving productivity, *Potato Res.*, 17, 24, 1974.
262. **Pennazio, S. and Vecchiati, M.**, Effects of naphtalenacetic acid on potato meristem tip development, *Potato Res.*, 19, 257, 1976.
263. **Mauseth, J. D.**, Cytokinin- and gibberellic acid-induced effects on the determination and morphogenesis of leaf primordia in *Opuntia polyacantha* (Cactaceae), *Am. J. Bot.*, 64, 337, 1977.
264. **Murashige, T.**, Effects of stem-elongation retardants and gibberellin on callus growth and organ formation in tobacco tissue culture, *Physiol. Plant.*, 18, 665, 1965.
265. **Li, H. C., Rice, E. L., Rohrbaugh, L. M., and Wender, S. H.**, Effects of abscisic acid on phenolic content and lignin biosynthesis in tobacco tissue culture, *Physiol. Plant.*, 23, 928, 1970.
266. **Haddon, L. and Northcote, D. H.**, The influence of gibberellic acid and abscisic acid on cell and tissue differentiation of bean callus, *J. Cell Sci.*, 20, 47, 1976.
267. **Nésković, M., Petrović, J., Radojević, L. J., and Vujicić, R.**, Stimulation of growth and nucleic acid biosynthesis at low concentration of abcisic acid in tissue culture of *Spinacia oleracea, Physiol. Plant.*, 39, 148, 1977.
268. **Abeles, F. B.**, *Ethylene in Plant Biology*, Academic Press, New York, 1973.
269. **MacKenzie, I. A. and Street, H. E.**, Studies on the growth in culture of plant cells. VIII. The production of ethylene by suspension cultures of *Acer pseudoplatanus*, L., *J.Exp. Bot.*, 21, 824, 1970.
270. **LaRue, T. A. G. and Gamborg, O. L.**, Ethylene production by plant cell cultures. Variations in production during growing cycle and in different plant species, *Plant Physiol.*, 48, 394, 1971.
271. **Dalton, C. C. and Street, H. E.**, The role of the gas phase in the greening and growth of illuminated cell suspension cultures of spinach (*Spinacia oleracea*, L.), *In Vitro*, 12, 7, 1976.
272. **Westcott, R. J.**, Changes in the phenolic metabolism of suspension cultures of *Acer pseudoplatanus* L. caused by the addition of 2-(chloroethyl) phosphonic acid (CEPA), *Planta*, 131, 209, 1976.
273. **Kato, A., Shimizu, Y., and Nagai, S.**, Effect of initial $\kappa_L a$ on the growth of tobacco cells in batch culture, *J. Ferment. Technol.*, 53, 744, 1975.
274. **Kato, A., Kawazoe, S., Iijima, M., and Shimizu, Y.**, Continuous culture of tobacco cells, *J. Ferment. Technol.*, 54, 82, 1976.
275. **Kessell, R. H. J. and Carr, A. H.**, The effect of dissolved oxygen concentration on growth and differentiation of carrot (*Daucus carota*) tissue, *J. Exp. Bot.*, 23, 996, 1972.
276. **Lorz, H., Potrykus, I., and Thomas, E.**, Somatic embryogenesis from tobacco protoplasts, *Naturwissenschaften*, 64, 439, 1977.
277. **King, J.**, Growth characteristics of *Acer pseudoplatanus* L. cells grown in chemostat culture in the presence of urea alone as a source of nitrogen, *Plant Sci. Lett.*, 6, 409, 1976.
278. **Sakato, K. and Misawa, M.**, Effects of chemical and physical conditions on growth of *Camptotheca acuminata* cell cultures, *Agric. Biol. Chem.*, 38, 491, 1974.
279. **Reuveny, Z. and Dougall, D.** unpublished data.

Chapter 3

SECONDARY METABOLISM AND BIOTRANSFORMATION

E. John Staba

TABLE OF CONTENTS

I. INTRODUCTION

This chapter will emphasize the metabolism of organic compounds added to a growth medium by unorganized plant suspension cultures (cell cultures). It will not consider the metabolism by plant tissue cultures of nutrients or plant-growth regulators (natural and synthetic auxins, gibberellins, cytokinins, ethylene, inhibitors). However, growth regulators are very important substances in that they may repress or derepress enzyme production and affect the rate of product turnover.[17]

Plant tissue cultures that are organized contain structures such as roots and buds (organ culture), whereas those that are unorganized do not (e.g., parenchyma cells). Unorganized tissue cultures may or may not differentiate into specialized cells (e.g., meristematic centers, lacticifer cells) or differentiate intracellularly (e.g., large vacuoles, lysozymes). Some plant tissue cultures are photoautotropic.[124] Both organized (organ) or unorganized (callus) tissues are often grown in liquid medium (suspension culture) or on a medium containing agar (static culture).

Although plant tissue cultures can be grown in fermentors used for bacteria or fungi, they may have unique physical and chemical needs in order to assure that differentiated cells, tissues, or organs grow. Tissue-culture growth is affected by physical factors such as culture age[221] or light;[348] chemical factors such as type and concentration of nutrient,[43,200,201] or growth regulator added to the medium[85,303] or biosynthesized[92]; or genetic/epigenetic factors present in the plant tissue used to establish the tissue culture[362] or those selected from a tissue culture.[316]

The advantages of using tissue cultures over plants for biosynthetic studies were recently summarized. They were stated by Overton[215] to be, "(1) undifferentiated cells, simple organization: minimize problems of translocation, permeability, segregation of metabolic pools; hence good precursor incorporation; (2) can be grown under standardized conditions, often on synthetic media; (3) short growth cycles; no seasonal variation; (4) incorporation and turnover of labeled precursors can be studied over short periods; (5) sterile conditions ensure observed biosynthesis is mediated by plant tissue, not microorganisms associated with it: (6) active cell-free preparations more readily prepared — absence of enzyme-deactivating phenols and quinones (?)."

Tissue cultures may produce compounds identical to[39] or similar to[228] those present in the plant, or the compound of interest may be absent.[347] Enzymes and substrates are occasionally produced by tissue cultures that are extracellular[76] and unique.[31] Compounds are most often added to a medium to be incorporated or modified into a compound of similar or greater chemical complexity. However, such added compounds may be poorly assimilated or never reach a cellular compartment,[211] be toxic,[276] or even be degraded[17] by the tissue culture. For commercialization, a tissue-culture system must form a product faster than it is metabolized and have a low turnover rate.[283]

II. PHENYLPROPANOIDS

Phenylpropanoid units (C6-C3) are involved in the biosynthesis of (1) simple aromatic acids which are often phenolic, (2) coumarins which are lactones, and (3) various types of compounds which are often colored such as flavonoids, anthocyanins, anthraquinones, tannins, and polymeric lignins. Cinnamic acid (Figure 1) is converted into various phenylpropanoid compounds. Dehydroquinic acid and shikimic acid, which utilize phosphoenolpyruvic acid and erythrose-4-phosphate for their biosynthesis, fuse to form cinnamic acid. Phenylalanine, a product of the shikimic acid pathway, may be converted to tyrosine and, in turn, to cinnamic acid.

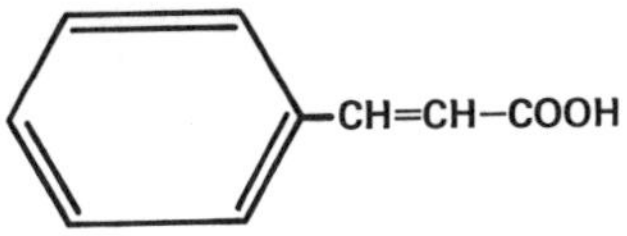

FIGURE 1.   Cinnamic acid.

A. Simple Aromatic Acids

Dehydroquinate dehydratase and shikimate dehydrogenase enzymes have been demonstrated in mung-bean tissue cultures.[89] Cinnamic acid,[39] chlorogenic acid,[232] and benzoic acid[256] have often been found in plant cell systems.

Chlorogenic acid (Figure 2) may form from quinic acid and caffeic acid directly, as in potato cell suspension,[90] or with caffeoyl coenzyme A, as in tobacco cell suspension.[289] Caffeic acid-o-methyltransferase activity is significantly greater in large cell aggregates of tobacco cells grown with kinetin.[174] Rosmarinic acid (caffeic acid ester of 3,4-dihydroxyphenyllactic acid) accumulates to levels as high as 8 to 15% of its dry weight in *Coleus* suspension cells.[232,364] Production of this acid is enhanced in the absence of plant hormones and high concentrations of sucrose (7%) and inhibited by 2-chloro-4-fluorophenoxyacetic acid.[364] Young *Coleus* suspension cells fed phenylalanine produced greater amounts of rosmarinic acid and contained increased phenylalanine ammonia-lyase (PAL) activity, but rosmarinic acid amounts did not increase with cinnamic acid, caffeic acid, p-coumaric acid, tyrosine, or DOPA.[232] Simple phenolic acids (expressed as chlorogenic acid) are at the highest concentration in the stationary growth phase of Paul's Scarlet Rose suspension cells,[8] or as caffeic, ferulic, and p-hydroxybenzoic acids in the logarithmic phase of carrot suspension cells.[305] One should not assume that increased cell growth will insure increased product production.[28]

Suspension cells of *Catharanthus, Conium* or *Apocynum* will 4-hydroxylate benzoic acid, 7-hydroxylate coumarin (exception: *Apocynum*), and N-acetylate aniline to acetanilide. Three other biotransformations were related to culture age (complete metabolism of benzoic acid, conversion of an aniline 3-hydroxyl derivative, conversion of anisole to phenol), and two biotransformations by *Conium* cells required 3 days rather than 1 day.[41]

A large number of tissue cultures can decarboxylate salicylic acid, but can not degrade its aromatic ring.[66] Cell suspensions of *Datura innoxia* will convert salicyl alcohol and salicyl aldehyde to isosalicin, convert salicylic acid to a monoglucoside or glucose ester, and efficiently convert dihydroxybenzenes (hydroquinione, resorcinol, catechol) to mono-β-glucosides.[315] Carrot cells will glycosidate vanillin to vanilloside.[93] The cell walls isolated from *Convolvulus arvensis* cell suspensions contained nine different glycosidase enzymes, one of which was a β-glucosidase.[222]

Of seven plant species established as tissue cultures and known to contain glucosinolate, two contained 2-phenylethyl glucosinolate and 2-hydroxy-2-phenylethyl glucosinolate (*Reseda luteola*), and one contained benzyl glucosinolate (*Tropaelolum majus*). All seven of the tissue cultures retained the glucosidase enzyme, myrosinase.[168]

An informative article was recently written about the degradation of organic compounds by tissue cultures, including aromatic-ring cleavage reactions.[17,24] Cinnamic acid, pheylalanine, and tyrosine were degraded by *Melilotus alba* tissue cultures. However, only phenylalanine and tyrosine were degraded by an active cinnamate strain of *Ruta graveolens*. It was suggested that tyrosine may also form the ring-fission substrate, homogentisic acid. Neither benzoic acid or salicylic acid was degraded.[67] Monohydroxybenzoic acids are decarboxylated, and benzoic acid and dihydroxy phenolic compounds may be degraded by tissue cultures.[225] In soybean cells, the peroxidase enzyme is responsible for the decarboxylation of hydroxybenzoic acid and for the deg-

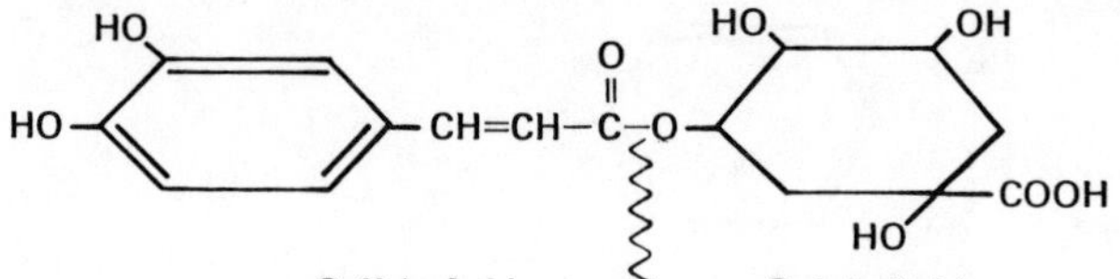

FIGURE 2.   Chlorogenic acid.

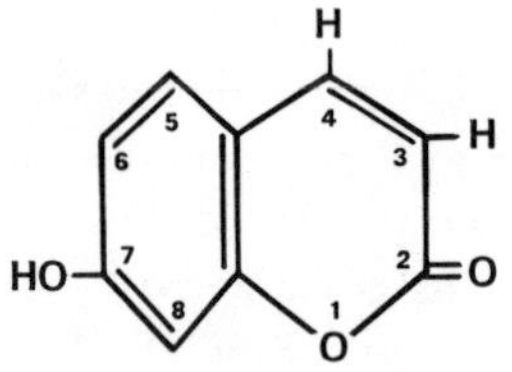

FIGURE 3.   7-Hydroxycoumarin (umbelliferone).

radation of catechol in the presence of hydrogen peroxide.[225] Four anionic isozymes isolated from peanut cells which possess peroxidase polyphenol oxidase and indole-acetic acid (IAA) oxidase activity are believed able to regulate the concentration of phenolic compounds and IAA.[273] Compounds may also be degraded by conjugation reactions with organic acids, sugars, and amino acids.

Polycyclic aromatic hydrocarbons such as benzo ($\propto$)-pyrene are degraded by *Chenopodium rubrum* tissue cultures.[102] A number of plant tissue cultures can degrade pesticides such as aldrin by epoxide and/or epoxide-glutathione complexes,[32,252] or lindane by glucosidation.[17]

The polyphenols evolving from the fermented and roasted cotyledon of the cocoa bean are considered necessary for its chocolate flavor. The meristematic tissue of the cocoa plant has a reduced capacity to synthesize polyphenols. Although callus tissue contains none of the flavonol glycosides and few of the polyphenols found in the parent tissue,[134] roasted cocoa suspension cells from the mature-death stage of the growth curve occasionally produced a chocolate aroma.[326]

B. Coumarins and Furanocoumarins

Coumaric acid (2-hydroxyl trans-cinnamic acid) will, upon isomerization by UV light and glucosylation, form coumarinic acid (2-*O*-glucoside of *cis*-cinnamic acid). Coumarins are lactones of coumarinic acid and are often isolated as 7-hydroxycoumarin (Figure 3). Furano ring fusion can occur at positions 6 and 7 with mevalonic acid to form linear furanocoumarins, and at position 7 and 8 to form angular furanocoumarins.

Isozymes (I and IV) of glucose-6-phosphate dehydrogenase were isolated from tobacco cells and decreasingly inhibited by chlorogenic acid, scopolin and esculin glucosides, and scopoletin and esculetin aglucones. The phenolic acids, caffeic and ferulic, were less inhibitory than the coumarins tested.[123] An *O*-methyltransferase enzyme was purified from tobacco cells which would both *m*- and *p*-methylate caffeic acid; 5-hydroxylate ferulic acid, quercetin, and esculetin; and *m*-methylate daphnetin.[501]

Tobacco tissue cultures incorporate phenylalanine into the coumarin scopoletin and its glycoside scopolin.[181] Both compounds are subsequently incorporated into proteins and cell wall fractions. Skimmin, the glycosylated form of umbelliferone, and the sweetner, phyllodulcin, have been isolated from amacha (*Hydrangea macrophylla*) cell

63

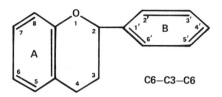

FIGURE 4. Flavonoid derivative.

cultures.[308] Crown gall tobacco cells contain large amounts of free and bound scopo-letin and esculetin, but no umbelliferone or bergapten.[36] Scopoletin is metabolically more rapidly turned over by tobacco cells, perhaps in a diphasic manner, than is sco-polin.[17] Scopoletin can be polymerized by an isoperoxidase enzyme.[234]

Coumarins, furanocoumarins, quinolines, and furanoquinolines have been isolated from cells of the garden rue (*Ruta graveolens*).[237,282] The coumarin, rutacultin, and the furanocoumarin, isopimpinellin, are not present in the garden rue plant, but are present in its cell suspensions.[35] Umbelliferone, 7-demethylsuberosin, and marmesin were very good precursors, but mevalonate was not, to four linear furanocoumarins (psoralen, xanthotoxin, bergapten, and isopimpinellin). However, in *Thamnosma montana* cell suspensions, mevalonate was a precursor to the furan ring of isopimpi-nellin, alloimperatorin methyl ether, and isoimperatorin.[175] Psoralen was a precursor to bergapten and xanthotoxin, but not dimethoxylated isopimpinellin.[11] A chloroplast localized prenyltransferase (umbelliferone:dimethylallyltransferase) was isolated from garden rue cells and is responsible for an early metabolic step in linear furanocoumarin synthesis. The enzyme catalyzes the addition of isoprenoid-derived dimethylallylpyro-phosphate to umbelliferone, which results in demethylbuberosin and psoralen.[58]

C. Flavonoids

The CoA ester of 4-hydroxy cinnamic acid (4-coumaryl CoA), or possibly 3-4 dihy-droxy cinnamic acid, will directly form the C6-C3 portion of the flavonoids. The num-bering system for a flavonoid derivative is given in Figure 4.

Flavonoids are distinguished by various increasing oxidation states of the C3 chain (catechins are least oxidized; flavanones, flavanonols, flavones, flavonols are most oxidized; leucoanthocyanidins are least oxidized, and anthocyanidins are most oxi-dized). Flavonoids are often glycosylated. Variations of the C6-C3-C6 pattern occur to form chalcones, dihydrochalcones, aurones, and isoflavones.

Phenylalanine is sequentially converted into 4-coumaryl CoA by three enzymes in soybean cells referred to as the group-I enzymes (PAL, cinnamate 4-hydroxylase, and a CoA ligase II isozyme) or by one enzyme in parsley cells.[99] It is well established that PAL is activated by UV light,[86] and that its activity will then involve the red/far red phytochrome system.[348] Also affected by light are the enzymes of group II which cat-alyze flavonoid synthesis from 4-coumaryl CoA. A flavanone-synthase enzyme has been isolated from *H. gracilis* and parsley cell suspensions. The enzyme catalyzes the formation of naringenin from 4-coumaryl-CoA and malonyl-CoA at pH 8, and eriod-ictyol from caffeyl-CoA and malonyl-CoA at pH 6.5 to 7.[250] *Glycyrrhiza echinata* cells incorporated cinnamic acid into the chalcone, isoliquiritigenin, which is then incorpo-rated into the retrochalcone, echinatin.[249]

A flavonoid-specific methyl-transferase and a UDP-glucose:flavonol 3-O-transfer-ase were isolated from soybean cells.[37,99] Cell-free extracts of citrus tissues will transfer the methyl group of S-adenosyl-L-methionine to ring-A hydroxyls of flavonoid com-pounds.[37] Twenty-four different flavonoid glycosides involving five aglycones were isolated from parsley cell-suspension cultures. The flavones (apigenin, luteolin, chry-

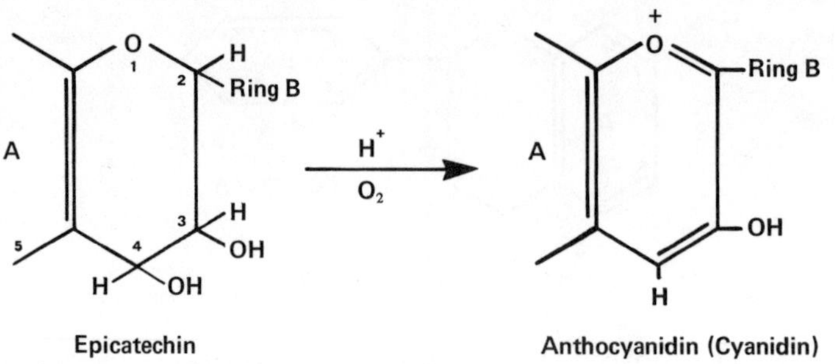

Epicatechin   Anthocyanidin (Cyanidin)

FIGURE 5.   Anthocyanidin formation.

soeriol) occurred either as 7-*O*-glucosides or as 7-*O*-apioglucosides, while the flavonols (quercetin, isorhamnetin) were 3-*O*-monoglucosides or 3,7-*O*-diglucosides.[171] *Haplopappus gracilis* cells contained a cyanidin 3-*O*-glucosyltransferase enzyme which was not specific in that it is also glucosylated other anthocyanidins and flavonols in position 3. The enzyme could not glycosylate apigenin, luteolin, naringenin, and dihydroquercetin.[251] Glucosylation of the isoflavone daidzein is favored when mungbean cell suspensions are grown anaerobically.[16]

Flavonoid degradation may not occur in some cell cultures, or the flavonoids may be degraded to chalcones and aurones and, ultimately, benzoic acid.[17] Cell suspensions, or crude cell-wall fractions from four cell strains, did not contain a specific β-glycosidase enzyme for flavanol 3-glycosides.[307]

D. Proanthocyanidins and Catechins

Proanthocyanidins are colorless compounds which form red to blue anthocyanins on heating with acid. They are classified as follows:

1. Leucoanthocyanidins. These are monomeric flavan-3,4-diols that occasionally exist as glycosides. Their immediate precursors are flavanonols.
2. Dimeric structures. These are complexes of catechin and anthocyanidin. Upon their oxidation, they may form colored polymers known as phlobaphenes or tannin reds.
3. Polymers. These may consist of only flavonoid units or a flavonoid-polysaccharide complex.

Anthocyanidins are often glycocylated at C-3 and C-5, and are formed from proanthocyanidins (e.g., epicatechin) by oxidation and dehydration reactions (Figure 5).

Catechins are highly reduced flavonoids that contain two asymmetric carbons at C-2 and C-3 that result in (+) and (−) catechins (trans) or epicatechins (cis). They may be esters of gallic acid that are mono- (e.g., afzelechin), di- (e.g., catechin) or tri- (e.g., gallocatechin) hydroxylated in ring-B.

Smaller polymerized proanthocyanidins are present in *Crateagus monogyna* cells as compared to the plant. Their production requires light and will vary with different hormones.[256] Leukoanthocyanin production is favored in the late logarithmic phase of Paul's Scarlet Rose cells grown on a low concentration of nitrogen and a high concentration of glucose.[8] *Populus* cells containing a high PAL activity produce more anthocyanins in blue light and in high levels of sucrose and/or riboflavin.[189] Blue light at 438 nm and 372 nm specifically stimulates anthocyanin production.[28] Other spectra may further promote its production.[39]

Selected carrot cell lines that produce anthocyanin (cyanidin-gluco-xyloside) will in-

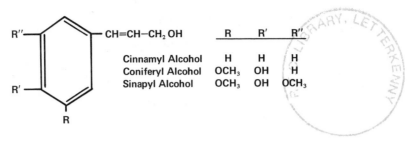

	R	R'	R''
Cinnamyl Alcohol	H	H	H
Coniferyl Alcohol	OCH₃	OH	H
Sinapyl Alcohol	OCH₃	OH	OCH₃

FIGURE 6.   Lignin units.

corporate phenylalanine rapidly in the dark. Nonanthocyanin-producing dark lines have only 15% of the PAL activity of anthocyanin-producing dark-grown lines.[261] The PAL enzyme is probably involved in those carrot lines that produce anthocyanin in the light, but not for those that produce anthocyanin in the dark.[281] Anthocyanin synthesis is inhibited by gibberellic acid, and such carrot lines will (1) contain low levels of PAL,[115] (2) poorly metabolize p-coumaric acid, and (3) efficiently incorporate phenylalanine into chlorogenic acid.[116]

Anthocyanin production in dark-grown carrot-cell lines is regulated by auxins. Non-producing anthocyanin lines grown in the dark will produce anthocyanins or chlorogenic acid when grown in the light. A growth regulator with a chlorine atom ortho to a carboxylic side chain, or one with two ring halogen atoms (e.g., 2,4-dichlorophenoxyacetic acid (2,4-D), 2-chlorophenoxyacetic acid, p-chlorophenoxyacetic acid) is required for the production of anthocyanins in the dark.[6] However, other investigators have found 2,4-D to inhibit anthocyanin synthesis.[39]

Naringerin, dihydrokaempferol, and dihydroquercetin are incorporated into cyanidin by *Haplopappus* tissue culture.[77] Microsomal fractions from illuminated cell suspensions would perform many of the reactions that convert flavonoids to cyanidin and its 3-*O*-glucoside.[138]

E. Tannins, Lignans, and Lignins

Tannins are generally considered to be either condensed (catechin tannins) or hydrolyzable tannins. Hydrolyzable tannins are yellow-brown compounds that contain phenolic acids such as gallic acid and are often esterified with sugars. Ellagic acid is formed on hydrolysis of some tannins that are esters of hexaoxydiphenic acid.

Lignans are colorless compounds formed from two phenylpropanoids through their aliphatic side chain. Their aromatic rings are oxygenated, and they may have additional ring closures and be glycosidic.

Lignins are polymers (mol wt. 2800 to 6700) of several phenypropanoids, some of which are related to coniferyl alcohol, or, in dicots, they may be related to both coniferyl alcohol and sinapyl alcohol. Glycosides of cinnamyl alcohol or its derivatives may be precursors to lignins.

An informative review of lignin biosynthesis in tissue cultures was recently written.[39] An isoenzyme (4-coumarate: CoA Ligase I) was isolated from soybean cells which converted 4-coumarate, ferulic, 5-hydroxy ferulic, and sinapic acid into lignins rather than into flavonoids.[99] Two enzymes that reduced cinnamoyl-CoA to cinnamyl alcohol (cinnamoyl-CoA: NADP oxidoreductase and cinnamyl alcohol dehydrogenase isozymes I and II)[64] were also found.

Callus tissues of *Juniperus communis* contain about 13% dry weight of condensed and hydrolyzable tannins. Precursors (cinnamic acid, ferulic acid, and sinapic acid) and dark growth conditions enhanced tannin production, but reduced cell growth.[52] Sycamore cells incorporated phenylalanine into phenolics (expressed as gallic acid equivalents) in the stationary-growth phase.[221] Their production was inhibited by the

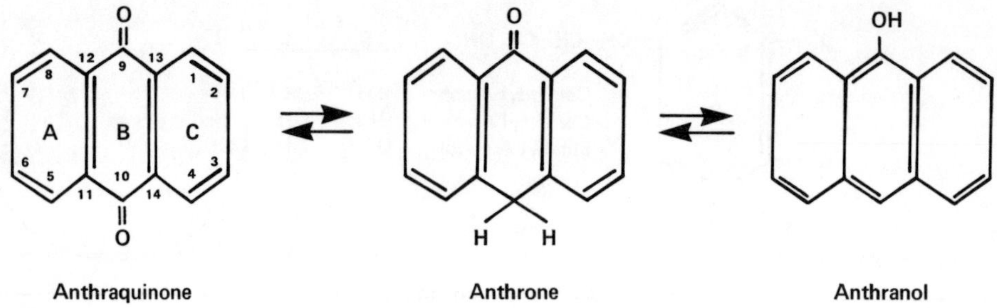

FIGURE 7.   Anthraquinone formation.

addition of a nitrogen source (urea) and/or 2,4-D. It was increased by the addition of sucrose in the stationary-growth phase. In Paul's Scarlet Rose cells, high light intensity reversed the inhibition of polyphenol synthesis by 2,4-D, and polyphenol synthesis was correlated to PAL activity. Phenylalanine and glucose stimulated the production of phyllemblin, a gallic acid compound isolated from *Emblica officinalis* cells.[208]

The lignan, sesamin, is produced by sesame cells.[152] In *Silybum marianum* cells, the flavonolignan, silybin, is formed from taxifolin and coniferyl alcohol, and the flavonolignan, hydrocarpin, is formed from luteolin and coniferyl alcohol.[257]

The cells walls from pine callus contain peroxidase which will incorporate coniferyl alcohol in the presence of hydrogen peroxide into lignin and bind it as a lignin-carbohydrate-extensin complex. The general lack of lignification in callus may be due to its low PAL activity.[349] The tannin in pine cells is associated with the smooth endoplasmic reticulum in vesicles and located within vacuoles.[20] It is suggested that the peroxidase enzyme in peanut cells is synthesized on the smooth endoplasmic reticulum.[335]

The activity of *O*-methyl transferase is considered important for lignin biosynthesis, and this enzyme is present in higher concentrations in large tobacco cell clusters than in small cell clusters.[174] An enzyme specific for the glucosylation of coniferyl alcohol was isolated from dark-grown Paul's Scarlet Rose cells and detected in six other cell cultures.[125] A large number of tissue cultures could convert protocatechuic acid and catechol to catechol β-D-glucoside and polymeric substances.[225] The lignin polymerization reactions possibly present in tissue cultures were also recently reviewed.[17]

F. Anthraquinones and Naphthoquinones

The sugar portion of anthranol C-9 glycosides may be hydrolyzed and the compound then oxidized to anthrone and anthraquinones. Anthranol glycosides at other than C-9 may be directly oxidized to anthraquinone glycosides. Some anthrones will directly bond sugars at position C-10 (e.g., barbaloin) or form dianthrones at position C-10 (e.g., sennosides). The most active laxatives are the anthranols, not the anthraquinones or its glycosides.

Acetate-mevalonate compounds can biosynthesize anthracene, anthrone, and anthraquinones that are substituted in rings A and C (e.g., emodin). It is also possible for anthraquinones that are A-ring unsubstituted to evolve from naphthoquinones originating from shikimic acid and ortho-succinylbenzoic acid (A and B rings) and then reacting with mevalonate (ring C).[349] The quinone ring of the yellow-red naphthoquinones (A and B rings) can be synthesized from either acetate of shikimic acid.

The pattern of anthraquinones produced from tissue cultures often differ[39] or are similar to that of the plant.[228] The precursors of alizarin, a substituted A-ring anthraquinone, were shikimic acid and *o*-succinylbenzoic acid in *Morinda citrifolia* cells. It was concluded that the hydroxyl groups of shikimic acid were not transferred to ring

A of morindone. Unexpectedly, a very low level of mevalonic acid was incorporated into morindone.[180] Six anthraquinones were isolated from *Digitalis lanata* cells with various substitutions on ring C and none on ring A, suggesting that the anthraquinones were biosynthesized from mevalonate.[84] Of 146 growth regulators tested, anthraquinone biosynthesis was greatest with naphthaleneacetic acid (NAA) and least with 2,4-D in *M. citrifolia* cells.[28,362] The availability of NAA was the factor controlled in order to continuously culture *Galium mollugo* cells for anthraquinones.[351] The precursor, *o*-succinylbenzoic acid, and sucrose will stimulate, and 2,4-D (22 mg/ℓ) will depress, the production of the anthraquinone lucidin-primveroside in *G. mollugo* cells. The three anthraquinone glycosides and the four anthraquinones present at the stationary-growth phase equaled that of the plant.[18] Mevalonic acid was incorporated into lucidin, but neither it nor acetate, shikimic acid, phenylalanine, leucin, or α-napthol were incorporated into 1-naphthyisopentenyl ether or 3,4-dihydro-2,2-dimethyl-naphtho (1,2-β) pyran. It was concluded that these latter two compounds were very rapidly metabolized.[19]

On media containing 2,4-D, *Cassia angustifolia* cells produced both dianthrones and five anthraquinones,[74] and *C. tora* produced more anthraquinones than that in the plant.[313]

The naphthoquinones, alkannin and its optical isomer shikionin were synthesized from *o*-hydroxybenzic acid and mevalonic acid in *Plagiobothrys arizonicus*[255] and *Lithospermum erythrorhizon*[200,201] cells, respectively. Shikonin production was stimulated by phenylalanine, but not by phenolic acids (*trans*-cinnamic, coumaric, benzoic, and *p*-hydroxybenzoic), a situation somewhat analogous to that for rosmarinic acid production.[232] Cell lines have been selected for high shikonin production from a heterogenous cell population that greatly exceed the shikonin content in whole plants.[316] Shikonin is a valued drug in the Orient for the treatment of burns, skin diseases, and hemorrhoids. Plumbagin production in *Plumbago zeylanica* cells was enhanced if 2,4-D was present.[105] Ubiquinone-40 is produced from *Parthenocissis* callus,[217] ubiquinone-10 from tobacco cells,[126] and ubiquinone-9 from safflower cells.[98] High ubiquinone-10-producing strains could be selected from a heterogenous population of tobacco cells and its production enhanced by 2,4-D.[188] Ubiquinone-10 is used in heart surgery.

III. MEVALONATES

Terpenoids and steroids are biosynthesized from isoprene or isopentane (C5) units evolving from mevalonic acid (C6). Mevalonic acid may form from the fusion of a C4-C2 unit or from L-leucine through various intermediates. Mevalonic acid is converted to isopentyl pyrophosphate via its pyrophosphate. Isomerization of isopentyl pyrophosphate results in dimethylallyl pyrophosphate and a fusion of the two form geraniol pyrophosphate (C10). A fusion of the C10 unit with a C5 unit (isopentyl pyrophosphate) results in the sesquiterpene, farnesol pyrophosphate (C15). These biochemical reactions involve microsomes and, perhaps, protein-bound substrates. Metabolic compartmentation may hinder lower (C5 to C15) terpenoid biosynthetic studies.

A. Monoterpenes (C10) and Sesquiterpenes (C15)

The term terpene refers specifically to hydrocarbon compounds. Many essential oils are monoterpenoids. Monoterpenoid compounds may be acyclic, monocyclic, bicyclic, or involved in the formation of furanochromones, iridoids, cannabinoids, or pyrethrins. Polyisoprenols (C45 to C110) such as rubber may also be formed. Examples of monocylic and dicyclic monoterpenoids are pulegone and menthofuran, respectively (Figure 8).

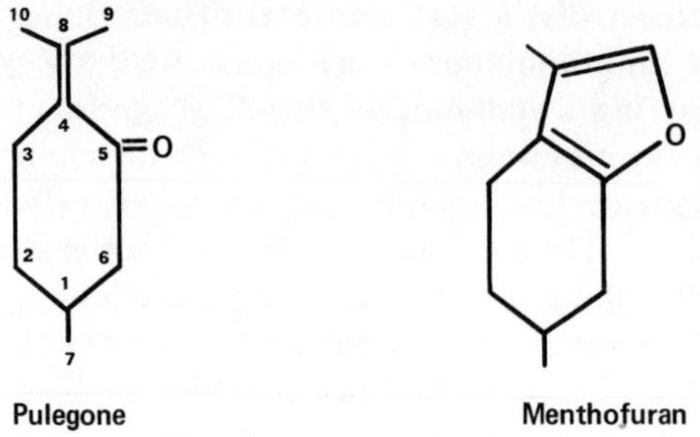

Pulegone   Menthofuran

FIGURE 8.   Monoterpenoids.

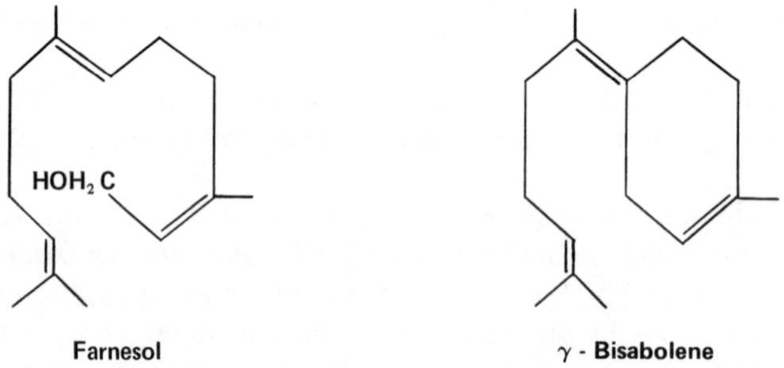

Farnesol   γ - Bisabolene

FIGURE 9.   Sesquiterpenoids.

Bonds which are perpendicular to the ring are axial (polar) or equatorial (coplanar). Groups on adjacent carbons are cis if one is axial and the other equatorial and trans if both are either axial or equatorial. The cyclohexane ring is either boat or chair shaped.

Sesquiterpenoids are often found as constituents of steam-distillable volatile oils, and may be acyclic (e.g., fanesol) and cyclic (e.g., bisabolene) (Figure 9). Some sesquiterpenoids are plant-growth regulators (e.g., caryophyllene).

1. Monoterpenes

Four umbellifere and five labiate plants established as tissue cultures did not produce volatiles similar to those in the conventionally grown plants. The volatile spectrum of *Pimpinella anisum* root- and leaf-differentiated cultures were similar to each other, and both cultures contained one volatile present in the plant.[21] Stem and leaf cultures of *Matricaria chamomilla* (chamomile) were similar to each other, but not to the volatiles from the plant.[233] Nepetalactone was not synthesized by *Nepeta cataria* cells,[63] and isothujone was not the principal monoterpene produced from *Tanacetum vulgare* cells.[15] As many as 17 different volatiles were produced from *Ocimum basicilum* cells, many of which were sugar bound.[177] Although *Rosa* cells were observed to be sweet smelling,[331] and endive plantlets to have a mild aroma, a number of rose varieties established as tissue cultures could not produce monoterpenes.[137,242] However, rose cells could convert geraniol to geranial, neral, nerol, and citronellol in both the free and β-glucosidic form. Damask rose callus synthesize terpenes such as linalool and glycoside-bound alcohols that are present in the organs of the intact plant.[167,241]

Mentha spicata and *M. piperita* tissue cultures do not produce the typical mint oil.[21,172,347] *M. piperita* cells produce high amounts of pulegone and menthofurane, low amounts of methyl acetate, menthone, and limonene, but no menthol.[220] *Mentha spicata* and *M. piperita* cells did not biotransform menthol, menthone, piperitenone, and pulegone.[276] Recent studies reported that four of six *Mentha* strains efficiently[13] and specifically[12] converted pulegone to isomenthone, and that mint callus contained more pulegone and piperitone than the intact plant.[241]

Eleven different aromatics produced by *Ruta graveolens* cells were identical to those in the plant[209] Stem-callus cultures grown in the light would green, differentiate oil passages, produce C9-C11 compounds, and produce oils found in the root (geijerene, pregeijerene, and isogeijerene production required light). Root-callus cultures would form oil cells, but not oil passages. They only produced the oils found in the root.[239]

Tobacco cells could biotransform the C-8 *trans*-methyl group of linalool and its derivatives, but not the *cis*-methyl group, to hydroxylated products.[304] Linolenic and linoleic acids were degraded by green alfalfa cells to *cis*-3-hexenal and *n*-hexanal.[262]

A number of other acetate-mevalonate-derived compounds have been studied in tissue cultures, i.e., furanochromones, iridoids, cannabinoids, pyrethrins, valepotriates, rubber, and celery flavors.

Amni visnaga cells produce the furanochromone visnagin from acetate,[48] and may[260] or may not[145] produce khellin. Gardenia cells will transform iridodial to its glucoside, 7-desoxyloganin, loganin, tarennoside, and geniposide. Iridoids normally present in *Galium mollugo* plants were absent from its cell culture.[18] Although *Cannabis sativa* cells do not produce the acetate-mevalonate-derived compound, tetrahydrocannabinol,[131,341] or the plant's essential oil,[131] they do produce phenolics and antimicrobials.[341] *C. sativa* cells contain an alcohol oxidase enzyme which is involved in the conversion of allylic alcohols to aldehydes.[131,317] Iso-pyrethrins[45] and their glycosides,[132] valepotriates,[22] and rubber[10,218] are produced, and pyrethrins not produced,[50] by plant tissue cultures. Partially differentiated celery cells produce phthalides, some of which are responsible for its characteristic flavor.[3]

2. Sesquiterpenes

The plant *Andrographis paniculata* produces sesquiterpenoids which accumulate as diterpenoids. However, *A. paniculata* cells produce three unique sesquiterpenoids (paniculide A,B,C) that do not accumulate as diterpenoids. Cell-free tissue-culture preparations would incorporate mevalonate into *cis,trans*-farnesol; *cis,cis*-farnesol; and γ-bisabolene. It was concluded that 2-*cis*,6-*trans*-farnesyl pyrophosphate was incorporarated into z-γ-bisabolene (ring carbon originated from C-2 of mevalonate and syn to the side chain) and paniculide B.[216] Chamomile cells will produce in light the ethereal oils (farnesene, α-bisabolol, bisabolol-oxide I-II, spathulenol) normally found in the plants inflorescence and root.[309,310]

Lindera strychnifolia cells produce nearly equal amounts of lindenenol, lindenenol acetate, linderane, lideralacton, and smaller amounts of lindesterene and caryophyylene.[324] Carrot (*Daucus carota*) cells did not produce daucol or carotol.[39]

B. Diterpenes (C20) and Tetraterpenes (C40)

Diterpenes are formed from four isoprene units and are normally not found in volatile oils, but in plant resins. They may be acyclic (e.g., phytol), but more often are cyclic compounds (e.g., gibberellic acid, abietic acid, gossypol, stevioside).

Tetraterpenes are formed from the fusion of two diterpene radicals and are normally trans as they are symmetrical. Carotenes are the most familiar tetraterpene. When oxygenated, they form the xanthophylls. Tetraterpenoids are acyclic, monocyclic, or bicyclic compounds which are normally yellow-red when containing a significant number of conjugated double bonds.

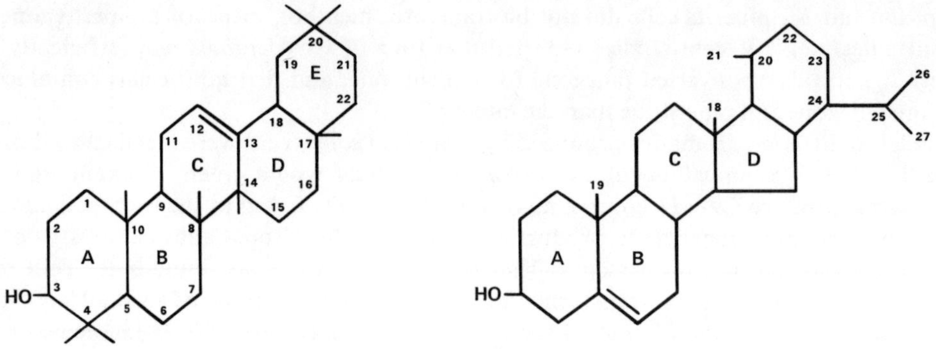

β - Amyrin   Cholesterol

FIGURE 10.   Triterpenoid and steroid.

1. Diterpenes

Tobacco and tomato cells could incorporate copalyl pyrophosphate, but not *trans*-geranylgeranyl pyrophosphate, into the diterpenoid gibberellin precursor, *ent*-kaurene. It appers that gibberellin synthesis in cell cultures is blocked at this step as germinating tomato seeds could incorporate both compounds into gibberellin. The cell cultures also incorporated mevalonate or isopentenyl pyrophosphate into *trans*-farnesol and *trans*-geranylgeraniol.[353]

Kalanchoe crenata cells grown in the light would significantly incorporate mevalonate into the acyclic diterpenoid, phytol. Light-grown cultures contain chlorophylls, the synthesis of which is dependent upon phytol and chlorophyllase. The cell cultures also contained tetraterpenoids (carotenoids and xanthophyllis).[285]

Cells from the coffee plant (*Coffea arabica*) produce two unique diterpenoid alcohols, cafestol and kahweol, in lower amounts than that in the bean.[336] A Japanese patent has been isued for the production of the sweetner, stevioside, from *Stevia rebaudiana* cells grown in light conditions.[196] *Stevia* and *Digitalis* cells will biotransform steviol to stevioside and three unknown compounds.[78]

2. Tetraterpenes

Cell cultures which have chloroplasts also contain tetraterpene-derived carotenoids. The carotenoids in Paul's Scarlet Rose cells contained four different carotenoids. *Ruta graveolens* cells contained seven different carotenoids.[39] Carrot cell lines will turn yellow on continuous light exposure.[327] The β-carotene content of cells may vary from zero in white cell cultures.[327] to 1% in orange cell lines,[205] or produce primarily lycopene.[306]. In general, the level of total carotenoids (carotenes and lycopene) in carrot cells varies from 3 to 40% of that present in yellow-orange carrot roots.[203]

C. Triterpenes (C30) and Steroids (C27) to (29)

The triterpenoids are widely distributed in plant resins and are often in association with carbohydrates (gum resins). They may be acyclic (e.g., squalene), tricyclic, or more complex (e.g., β-amyrin, cholesterol), (Figure 10). Triterpenoids may occur free or as glycosides (saponins).

Three classes of pentacyclic triterpenoids are known which are distinguished from each other by their stereochemistry and structure (ursane, oleanane, and lupane). The oleanane-type sapogenin is most common.

Steroids are similar to the triterpenoids, but with only two methyl groups attached to the ring system and are generally alcohols (e.g., β-sitosterol, see below). Sterolins

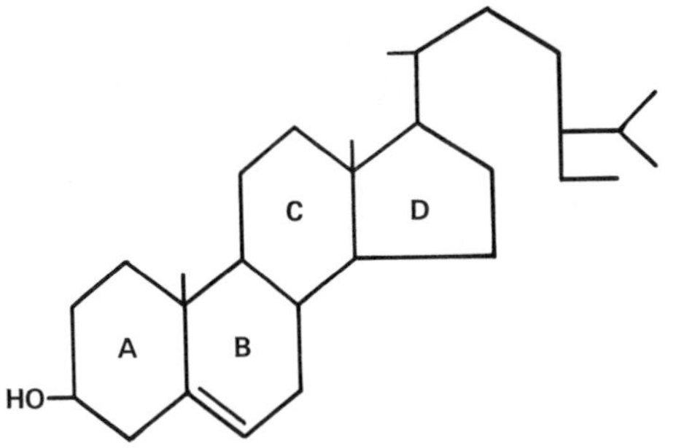

β - Sitosterol

FIGURE 11. β-Sitosterol.

(sterol glycosides) are distinguished from saponins by their insolubility in water (e.g., β-sitosterol glycoside).

Animal hormones (e.g., cholesterol, cholanic acids, estrones) and insect hormones (e.g., ecdysone) are present in plants.[92]

The organic rings may be joined to each other by trans linkages and be coplanar. If the C10 methyl group is perpendicular to the ring system, then any group trans to it is α, and any group cis to it is β. If rings A and B are trans, they may be described as 5-α as the hydrogen at C5 is below the plane.

Two farnesyl pyrophosphate units fuse to form squalene. Squalene cyclization may occur chemically to triterpenoids, or enzymatically through epoxide intermediates to steroids. Plant steroids are most often formed from cycloartenol and, occasionally, from lanosterol. The C24 ethyl group is derived from successive additions of the methyl group of methionine.

1. Triterpenes

The triterpenoid, β-amyrin, is formed from mevalonate and squalene 2,3-epoxide and is found in *Tylophora indica* and Paul's Scarlet Rose cells. Both α-amyrin and β-amyrin epoxide are found in bramble (*Rubus fruticosis*) cells.[65] Aroundoin is found in rice (*Oryza sativa*) cells.[355]

Tomita and his colleagues demonstrated that cultures of *Isodon japonicus* would incorporate labeled mevalonate into the triterpenoids maslinic acid and 3-*epi*-maslinic acid, but that the latter compound lost one sixth of the tritium label. It was suggested that the 3-*epi* compound formed from a 3-ketone intermediate, and not directly from the cyclization of (3R)-2,3-oxidosqualene. The triterpenoid, oleanolic acid, was formed via the mevalonate-β-amyrin pathway. It was theorized that the triterpenoid, ursolic acid, proceeded from mevalonate by one of two pathways. The correct pathway was established by using (1,2-^{13}C2) acetate, and that pathway used a common intermediate for both oleane and ursane triterpenoids.[216]

2. Steroids

Steroids are often present in tissue cultures as phytosterols (β-sitosterol, stigmasterol, and campesterol), with either sitosterol or stigmasterol being the dominant sterol.[299] Stigmasterol is an economically useful steroid intermediate derived from soybeans. Also detected in tissue cultures were cycloartenol and five subsequently formed metabolites in tobacco cells,[23] and trace amounts of cholesterol in digitalis cells[117] and six other cell cultures.[299] In addition, 24-methylene-cycloartanol was present in digitalis cells,[117] 24-methylene-cholesterol and 24-ethyldiene-cholesterol in *Withania somnifera* cells,[358] and 24-methylenecholesterol in *Holarrhena antidysenterica* cells.[106] The fol-

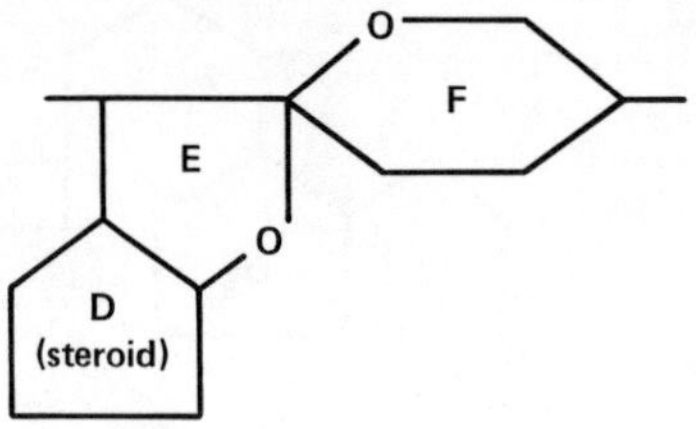

FIGURE 12.   Spiroketal side chain.

lowing sterols and as many as 50 others[159,299] are also present in cell cultures: (1) *iso*-fucosterol (in *Helianthus*[39] and digitalis[117]), (2) spinasterol (in pumpkin[354]), (3) phy-toecdysone (in *Trianthema portulacastrum*[265]), (4) various oxidized sterols (in *Stephania cepharantha*[130] and *Momordica charantia*[159]), and (5) lanosterol in three different cultures.[299]

Tobacco cells will incorporate acetate and cycloartenol into sterols,[23] as will Jerusalem artichoke (*Helianthus tuberosus*) cells exposed to far-red light.[103] Presqualene pyrophosphate and presqualene alcohol were identified as steroid intermediates in bramble cell cultures.[114] Tobacco cells[69] grown anaerobically, and their microsomes, converted squalene-2,3-epoxide(oxidosqualene) to cycloartenol.[112] Parkeol incubated with tobacco cells was converted to 24,25-epoxy-lanost-9(11)-en-3β-ol, but not into either cycloartenol or lanosterol.[253] The C-24 side chain of phytosterols is formed from two successive trans-methylations from adenosyl methionine. Bramble (*Rubus fruticosus*) cell microsome preparations completed a second C-methylation reaction upon the substrate 24-methylene lophenol.[73] Olefins are intermediate compounds to sigmasterol in tobacco, dioscorea cells,[321] and to poriferasterol in *Ochromonas malhamensis* cells.[100] Tobacco and dioscorea tissue cells do not incorporate cycloartenol into stigmasterol. It was concluded that stigmasterol biosynthesis involves a $\Delta24$-25 compound.[321] Bramble-cell microsome preparations, but not rabbit-liver microsomes, converted cycloeucalenol (9β,19β-cyclopropane sterol) to obtusifoliol.[113]

It is possible that lanosterol is particle-bound, or has a high turn-over rate, as it is converted differently to sterols than is cycloartenol.[118] Sterols (cholesterol, ergosterol, sitosterol) were not biotransformed by tobacco, digitalis, and *Sophora* cells,[120] but cholesterol was biotransformed by dioscorea[292] and *Holarrhena* cells.[107] The cholesterol-derived compound, cholest-4-en-3-one.[293] is converted by four different cell cultures into 5α-cholestan-3-one, but not 5β-cholestan-3-one.[293] Cells of *Vinca rosea* will biotransform progesterone to 14α-progesterone.[88] The growth regulators kinetin and IAA stimulated β-sitosterol and stigmasterol production in *Trigonella foenum-graecum* cells.[150] In *Solanum xanthocarpum*, kinetin and 2,4-D stimulated β-sitosterol production. The addition of cyclic AMP to a medium containing 2,4-D increased sitosterol and decreased compesterol yields in *Corchorus olitorius* cells.[303] In cells of *T. foenumgraecum*, kinetin increased growth, but not the free-sterol concentration, whereas 2,4-D increased both growth and free-sterol concentration. The concentration of the bound (glycosidic) sterol was always low.[33]

D. Saponins

Saponins may be either triterpenoid glycosides, or glycosides of steroids with a spiroketal side chain (Figure 12).

The aglycones (sapogenins) are occasionally cis-A/B-ring junctured. Glycosylation normally occurs at C3 and with a wide variety of different sugars. The nonacylated, water-soluble form of cholesterol glycoside may be an important precursor to some plant steroids and to the cardenolides (cardenolide saponins, cardiac glycosides).

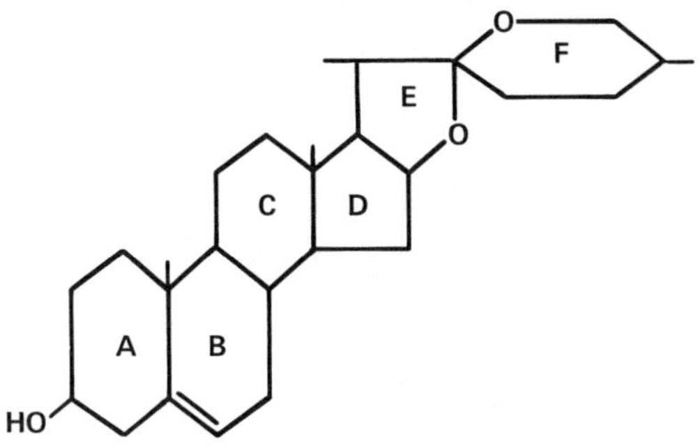

FIGURE 13. Diosgenin.

The structure of cardenolides resemble sterols, but are distinguished from them by a five-membered, unsaturated lactone ring at C17, cis-A/B-ring juncture, a 14β hydroxyl group, and by the sugars attached (e.g., digitoxose, cymarose). Cardenolides from squill and helleborus have a six-membered, unsaturated lactone ring.

1. Triterpenoid Saponins

Triterpenoid glycosides of panaxadiol, panaxatriol, and oleanolic acid have been identified as present in unorganized cells of *Panax ginseng*[86] and *Panax quinquefolium*[135] in concentrations similar to that in the root. A Japanese[82] and a German patent[195] were issued for the production of crude saponins and sapogenins from *Panax* plant tissue cultures, and a Japanese patent was issued for the use of 3-indole-caproic acid or caprylic acid for increasing saponin production.[214] Habituated *P. ginseng* callus produce considerably lower amounts of saponins as compared to that produced on a medium containing 2,4-D.[212] *Panax* cells will biotransform panaxatriol to 3β- and 6β-glucosides and an unknown compound.[78]

Oleanolic acid has been isolated from *Isodon japonicus* callus cultures.[320] Induced roots, but not unorganized s, of *Bupleurum falcatum* produced saikosaponins a, b, c, and d.[311] A U.S. patent has been granted to produce a licorice-like material containing glycyrrhizin from *Glycyrrhiza* cells which is to be used as tobacco flavoring.[318]

2. Steroid Saponins

The steroid saponin, diosgenin (Figure 13) is found in many plants,[275] but it is obtained principally from *Dioscorea* roots (4 to 6% dry weight) for conversion to commercially useful drugs. Tissue cultures of *D. floribunda* may be used to develop somatic embryoids[7] or to asexually propagate the plant.[271]

Diosgenin can exist as the glycoside dioscin and be dehydrated during acid hydrolysis to form the artifact, 25-D-spirosta-3,5-diene.[187] Diosgenin is produced from various species of dioscorea cells in yields less than 1.0%[146,194,275] and from 1 to 2.5% dry weight if grown on media containing cholesterol and 2,4-D.[147,275,298] Chemical mutagens have been used on *D. deltoidea* somatic-cell cultures.[140] A U.S. patent has been issued for the production of diosgenin by plant tissue cultures.[278] Diosgenin is also produced by cells of *Dioscorea tokoro*,[325] *Momordica charantia* (1.4% dry weight),[159] *Daucus carota* (0.6% dry weight),[156] *Trigonella foenum-graecum* (reported as 2.5% dry weight in kinetin medium[150] or absent[33]), *T. occulta* (0.37% dry weight), and *Solanum* sp. (0.2% dry weight).[70] Gitogenin and tigogenin have been detected in *Trigonella* cells.[133,153] Prototokoronin,[323] tokorogenin, and yonogenin have been detected in *D. tokoro* cells,[325] and gitogenin and manogenin have been found in *Yucca* cells.[303]

Dioscorea deltoidea cells will incorporate (4[14]-C) and (26[14]-C)-cholesterol[298] and sitosterol[301] into diosgenin. Studies with *D. tokoro* cells suggest the following biosyn-

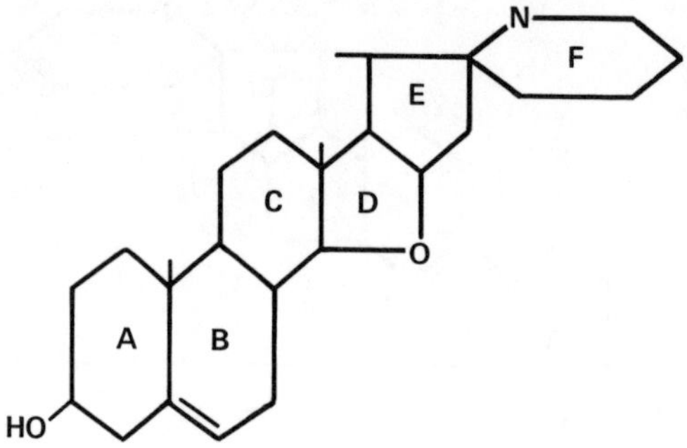

FIGURE 14.   Solasodine.

thetic sequence: mevalonate, cycloartenol, cholesterol, cholest-5-ene-3β, 16,26-triol, cholest-5-ene-3β,16,22,26-tetrol, diosgenin, yonogenin, tokorogenin,[322] and prototo-koronin.[323] Cells of *D. deltoidea* wil biotransform progesterone to 5α-pregnan-3-β-ol-20-one and 5α-pregnan-3β,20β-diol,[295] and 4-androsten-3,17-dione to 5α-androstan-3β-ol,17-one and 5α-androstan-3β,17β-diol.[294]

Daucus carota (0.6% dry weight),[156] *Trigonella foenum-graecum* (reported as 2.5% dry weight in kinetin medium[150] or absent[33]), *T. occulta* (0.37% dry weight), and *Solanum* sp. (0.2% dry weight).[70] Gitogenin and tigogenin have been detected in *Trigonella* cells.[133,153] Prototokoronin,[323] tokorogenin, and yonogenin have been detected in *D. tokoro* cells,[325] and gitogenin and manogenin have been found in *Yucca* cells.[303]

   Dioscorea deltoidea cells will incorporate (4[14]-C) and (26[14]-C)-cholesterol[298] and sitosterol[301] into diosgenin. Studies with *D. tokoro* cells suggest the following biosynthetic sequence: mevalonate, cycloartenol, cholesterol, cholest-5-ene-3β, 16,26-triol, cholest-5-ene-3β,16,22,26-tetrol, diosgenin, yonogenin, tokorogenin,[322] and prototo-koronin.[323] Cells of *D. deltoidea* wil biotransform progesterone to 5α-pregnan-3-β-ol-20-one and 5α-pregnan-3β,20β-diol,[295] and 4-androsten-3,17-dione to 5α-androstan-3β-ol,17-one and 5α-androstan-3β,17β-diol.[294]

3. Nitrogen-Containing Steroid Saponins

   Tissue cultures produce the following N-containing sapogenins (steroidal glycoalkaloids): solasodine (Figure 14), *S. xanthocarpum,* [104] *S. acculeatissimum,*[139] *S. aviculare,* *S. elaegnifolium, S. khasianum, and S. nigrum.*[165] Solasonine, *Solanum xanthocarpum*[104] solanine, chaconine, and dehydrocommersonine, *S. chacoense;*[359] their glycosides solamargine, *S. acculeatissimum,*[139] and tomatine, *Lycopersicon esculentum.*[244] Upon acid extraction, solasodine can form the artifact, solasodiene.[259] Diosgenin may be present in some *Solanum* cultures (*S. xanthocarpum* and *S. aviculare*),[65] and solasodine may be absent in others (*S. laciniatum*).[338] Plant leaves of *S. aurantiacobaccatum* contain 2.6% diosgenin on a dry-weight basis.[44] Root organ differentiation significantly increased yields of the steroidal glycoalkaloids in *S. khasianum,*[169] *S. tuberosum* (potato),[360] and *S. chacoense* cultures.[359,360] Studies with potatoes established that solanidine biosynthesis is dependent upon chlorophyll synthesis,[227] and that *S. dulcamara* plants will incorporate cholestenol compounds into solasodine and coladulcidine.[330] The production of solasodine was significantly increased by a cholesterol supplement to *S. xanthocarpum* cells.[157] Solasonine production yields of 2.5% dry weight and greater occurred in approximately four of 143 cell strains.[361]

4. Cardenolide Saponins

   Tissue cultures established from more than eight different cardenolide plants did

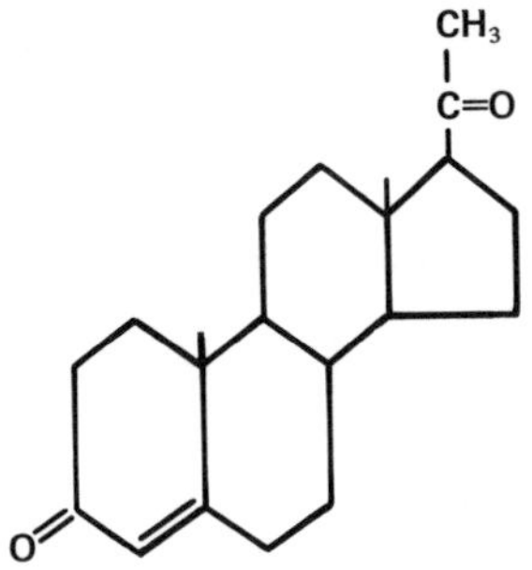

FIGURE 15.   Progesterone.

not produce,[4,117,269] or contained trace amounts of cardenolides.[182,193,247,275,299] Of cardenolides detected in *Digitalis purpurea* plants, nine occurred in suspension cultures,[141] and 15 in newly established cultures.[142] However, these cultures lost their ability to produce cardenolides after 18 passages. Very low concentrations of cardenolides are reported to persist in *D. lanata* tissue cultures.[182] Biological tests indicate that tissue cultures of cardenolides plants do have some cardiac activity.[148,192] Cells of *D. purpurea* produce steroids, such as cholesterol and progesterone[96] (Figure 15), and sapogenins, such as tigogenin and gitogenin.[96,224] Many of the established cell cultures produce unusual sugars and/or glycosides.[101,235] Kedde-positive substances reported present in digitalis cells[276] have been stated to be anthraquinone pigments.[83]

Cardenolides are believed to be biosynthesized from cholesterol via 3-keto reduction, hydroxylation, C5 reduction, and pyran-ring-closure reactions. The side chain would then be cleaved at C21-C22 to form pregnenolone, and an acetate addition to progesterone would form the ring D lactone.[243,292] Mevalonic acid is incorporated into both cycloartenol and cholesterol by excised shoots of digitalis seedlings.[62] Although cholesterol is metabolized in plants to cardenolides,[109] Δ7-, Δ8-, Δ8(14)-, and 14α-hydroxy progesterone precursors are not involved.[1] Digitalis plants can also convert sitosterol to progesterone and progesterone to deoxycorticosterone.[109]

Cardenolide production is strongly correlated with the presence of leaf-like structures. Leaf organs from *D. purpurea* can produce cardenolides,[122,247] but newly formed roots and callus produce low amounts of cardenolides or none at all.[247] Sucrose (5%) inhibited root formation,[247] and sucrose (0.25 to 3%) with cultures in various light conditions was without effect on cardenolide production.[122]

Cells of *D. mertonensis* formed positive Baljet, but not positive Kedde, compounds when grown on a medium containing solubilized lanolin fraction or cholesterol.[193] The compounds were tentatively identified as *Digitalinum verum* and verodoxin.[192] *Digitalis, Cheiranthus,* and *Strophanthus* leaf homogenates[297] and cell cultures will reduce cholesterol to cholest-4-en-3-one, and digitalis and *Cheiranthus* leaf homogenates will metabolize pregnenolone to progesterone and 5α-pregnan-3,20-dione.[296] *Digitalis* and other cell cultures will often reduce the C4 double bond and the C3 keto group of pregnenolone and progesterone,[94,121] and are able to form 5α-compounds from pregnenolone and progesterone.[79,235] Although *D. purpurea* seeds contain a cholesterol side-chain-cleavage ability, this activity could not be demonstrated in cell cultures.[223]

Digitalis lanata and *D. purpurea* cells biotransform digitoxigenin[302] to 3-dehydrodigitoxigenin.[299] After 26 days, *D. purpurea* cells biotransform digitoxin to gitoxin and smaller amounts of purpurea glycoside A and B.[80] Cells of *D. lanata* transform digitoxin to the therapeutically important drug digoxin (12β-hydroxylation). See Figure 15. Also formed from digitoxin are the compounds purpurea glycoside A (glucosilation), and desacetyllanatoside C (12β-hydroxylation).[5,235] Glucosilation reactions occur

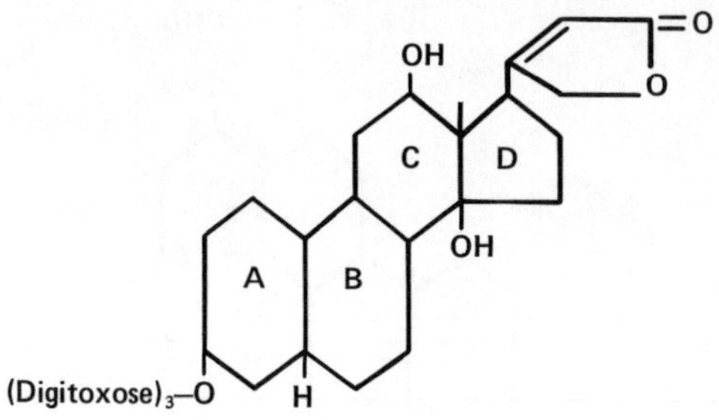

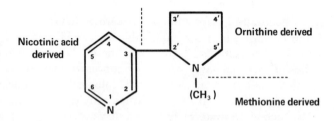

FIGURE 16.   Digoxin.

FIGURE 17.   Nicotine.

within the first day of fermentation. Acetylation and desacetylation occur within the first to sixth day, and 12β-hydroxylation occurs after the sixth day.[236]

There is no correlation between the digoxin content of *D. lanata* leaves and the hydroxylation rate of the corresponding cell culture. However, there is a correlation between the *hydroxylation* rate of *D. lanata* leaves and the hydroxylation rate of the cell cultures.[110] By using selected cell strains (No. 291) large amounts (4 gm) of β-methyldigoxin was made from β-methyldigitoxin after 12 days in a 20 ℓ airlift fermentor.[111] Under specified fermentation conditions, 1 g (dry weight) of *D. lanata* cells would yield 8 mg of β-methyldigoxin within 24 hr.[238,276] Glycosylation and C19 reduction reactions of cardenolides is performed by both *D. lanata* and *Thevetia neriifolia* cells.[61] Cells of *Cannabis, Ipomoea,* and *Daucus* would oxidize, hydroxylate, and reduce cardenolides (digitoxigenin, gitoxigenin, etc.). *Daucus* cells biotransformed gitoxigenin to a new cardenolide, 5β-hydroxygitoxigenin.[343]

IV. ALKALOIDS

Alkaloids are plant nitrogenous compounds that are often physiologically active in man. They are most often organic bases which form more water-soluble salts with mineral or organic acids.

In general, alkaloids are not produced in cell cultures in as high a concentration as that in the plant, and may not be structurally identical to those in the plant. Alkaloids may[213,262] or may not[2] be produced upon reorganization of cell cultures to organs.

A. Betaines, Acyclics, and Pyridines

The pyridine, nicotinic acid, is biosynthesized from glycerol and aspartic acid. Nicotinic acid reacts with an ornithine equivalent to form nicotine (Figure 17) or with lysine to form anabasine. Nicotine and anabasine are primarily products of root metabolism, with demethylation reactions occurring in the leaves. The compound, nornicotine, can function as a direct precursor to nicotine.

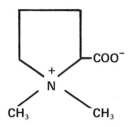

FIGURE 18.   Stachydrine.

Plants and their tissue cultures[263] contain some of the nitrogenous substances that are common in animals (e.g., acetylcholine, serotonin, norepinephrine). The concentration of the acyclic compound, choline, is eight times higher in *Cannabis* cells than in its leaves.[341] The nonaromatic ring betaine compound, stachydrine (Figure 18), is produced from chlorophyllous cells of *Medicago sativa* (alfalfa), but not the betaines homostachydrine and trigonelline.[263] Trigonelline (*N*-methylnicotinicacid) is biosynthesized from nicotinic acid and is produced by *Trigonella foenum-graecum* cells.[151] The compound, psuedo-ephedrine is produced from *Ephedra foliata* cells.[166]

A patent in the U.K. was issued to produce nicotine from tobacco-root organ cultures,[51] and Japanese patents were issued to regulate and grow tobacco sheets and cells without nicotine.[196] Considerable effort has been devoted to improving the efficiency of growing tobacco cells on an industrial scale.

Studies with a number of tissue-culture systems indicate that nicotinic acid is probably assimilated into the cell as the *N*-α-L-arabinopyranoside[17] and then metabolized to form NAD and nicotinic acid.[178,179] The compounds nicotinic acid and nicotinamide form *N*-methyl nicotinic acid (trigonelline) which functions as a methyl donor.[108] Degradation of nicotinic acid does not involve the intermediate 6-hydroxy nicotinic acid.[179]

Nicotiana tabacum var. *Bright Yellow* callus produced nicotine, anatabine, and anabasine when grown on a medium with IAA, but not with 2,4-D.[85] In another study, cells from the same variety of tobacco were inhibited by high concentrations of either IAA, NAA, or 2,4-D. Tobacco callus tissue grown on a medium with 0.1 ppm NAA produced 0.5% nicotine or more, which is similar to that produced by the root of the plant.[266] Tobacco cells that do not produce nicotine produce the ornithine-derived compounds *p*-coumaroylputrescine, caffeoylputrescine, and feruloylputrescine, principally because high concentrations of growth regulators inhibit putrescine-*N*-methyl transferase.[202] Tobacco cell lines have been selected from cells subcultured for more than 10 years on a 2,4-D-containing medium that were able to produce significant amounts of nicotine.[312]

A cell-squash technique has been developed to screen tobacco cells efficiently for alkaloid content, and a cell line was found that produced as high as 3.4% dry weight of alkaloids. High and low alkaloid-producing strains were reorganized into plants, and the plants retained the same general level of alkaloid production. Tissue cultures reestablished from these plants retained their general propensity for producing alkaloids.[316]

The ornithine-derived pyrrolizidine alkaloid, junceine, is produced by *Crotalaria juncea* cells.[158]

B. Tropanes

The tropane alkaloids scopolamine (hyoscine) and 1-hyoscyamine (*dl*-atropine) are biosynthesized from the base moiety, tropine, and the acid moiety, tropic acid, (Figure

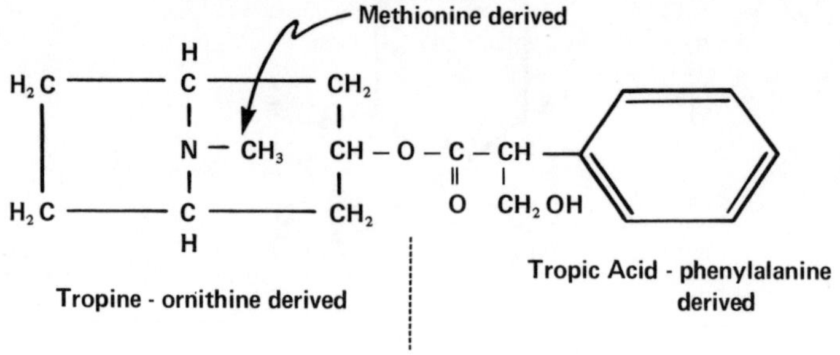

FIGURE 19.   1-Hyoscyamine.

19). The precursors to tropine are ornithine, acetoacetate, and methionine, and the precursor to tropic acid is pheylalanine.

Normally, plants contain total tropane alkaloids from 100 to 1000 mg% dry weight, cell cultures from 1 to 35% dry weight, and root organ cultures from 500 to 1000 mg% dry weight.[274,275] The following tropane-alkaloid-containing plants have been studied as tissue cultures: *Atropa belladonna*,[163,319] *Datura ferox*,[68] *D. innoxia*,[46,254] *D. metel*,[49] *D. quercifolia*,[46] *D. stramonium*,[46] *Dubosia myoporoides*,[346] *Hyoscyamus niger*,[54] *Scopolia japonica*, and *S. parviflora*.[119,314]

The fusion of tropine and tropic acid may be accomplished by either tobacco or datura cells,[291] and scopolamine and hyoscyamine appear interconvertable[274] with the epoxide scopolamine favored.[46] Epoxidase/epoxide hydrase activity is present in *Phaseolus vulgaris* cells,[246] and arginase, transaminase, and esterase activity is in *Datura* cells.[136]

In *Datura* tissue cultures, the minor alkaloids cuscohygrine, choline, and psuedotropine are present.[277] Cells of *D. ferox* lack the ability to convert ornithine and acetoacetate to hygrine α-carboxylate.[68] It is known that *D. innoxia* plants will incorporate both D(+)- and L(−)-hygrine into cuscohygrine, but only D(+)-hygrine into the tropane alkaloids.[190]

In *Datura* and *Scopolia* cells, tropic acid increased tropane-alkaloid production significantly, but tropine yielded only acetyl tropine.[119,170] Efficient incorporation of phenylalanine into tropic acid and the tropane alkaloids probably requires root structures.[68,119,270,314] Nevertheless, acetate,[345] phenylalanine,[46,345] and tyrosine[161,207] are reported to increase the total tropane-alkaloid content of tissue cultures. A tyrosine ammonialyase enzyme is present in *Arachis* cells,[230] and melanin is present in *D. metal* cells.[160]. The major alkaloids identified in *Dubosia myoporoides* cells were valtropine, scopolamine, and atropine.[170]

C. Isoquinoline

Opium (*Papaver somniferum*) plants will join two tyrosine units to form papaverine, narcoteine, or morphine (Figure 20) via the following intermediates: norlaudansoline, reticuline, salutaridine, salutaridinol-1, thebaine, codeinone, and codeine.

Methylation reactions are required for the formation of the phenanthrene, salutaridine, and demethylation reactions for the formation of morphine from thebaine. *Papaver bracteatum* plants apparently lack demethylation enzymes and accumulate thebaine. The alkaloid, berberine (Figure 21) and jatrorrhizine are also formed from two tyrosine molecules in *Coptis* or *Hydrastis* plants, and sanguinarine is formed from reticuline in *Macleaya* plants.

Tissue cultures of *P. somniferum* are reported not to produce the major opium alkaloids[81,204,274] and to produce the major alkaloids papaverine, thebaine, codeine, and

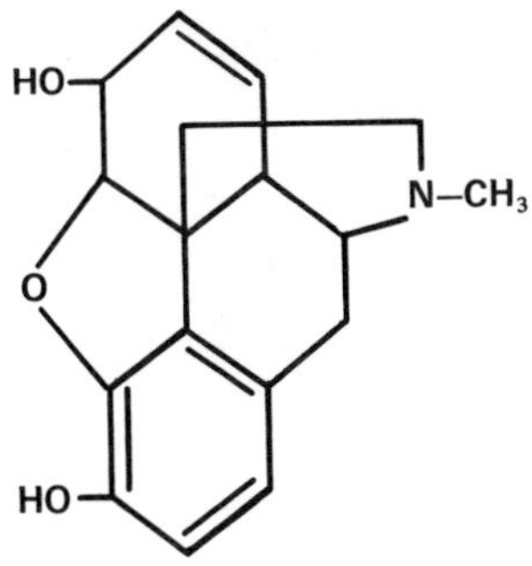

FIGURE 20. Morphine.

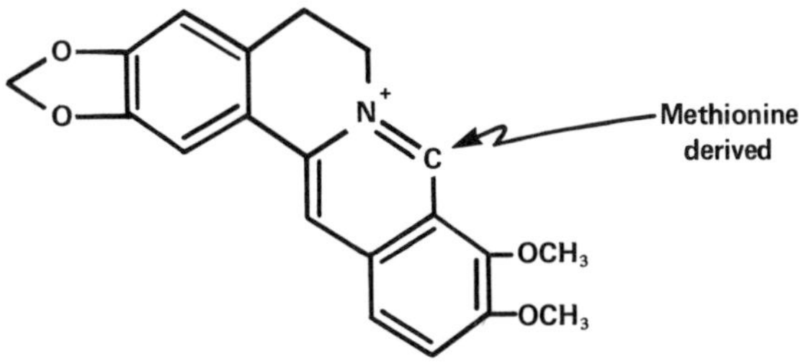

Methionine
derived

FIGURE 21. Berberine.

morphine.[70,154] Tyrosine would stimulate *P. somniferum* cells to produce more alkaloids, but would also inhibit growth.[155] *Papaver* cell cultures that produce the major alkaloids contained tracheid-like cells.[70] A new alkaloid, norsanguinarine, and others (benzophenanthridine, protopine, and aporphine) accumulate in cell cultures that do not produce the major opium alkaloids.[81] The alkaloid, norsanguinarine was absent in *Papaver* plantlets.[127]

Cells of *Papaver bracteatum* are reported to produce[267] and not to produce, thebaine.[127] In the order given, the following precursors stimulate thebaine production, but reduce *P. bracteatum* cell growth: L-tyrosine, L-DOPA, L-phenylalanine, L-dopamine, DL-tropic acid. The ability for these cells to produce thebaine was lost upon repeated subculturing, but was regained upon cell organization.[72] Opium alkaloid vesicles appear derived from the endoplasmic reticulum of lactifer cells.[210]

Cells of *Coptis japonica* produce berberine and jatrorrhizine in smaller amounts than that in the rhizome.[128] However, processes have been patented in Japan for berberine productions.[340] Cells of *Macleaya microcarpa* produce sanguinarine and are accumulated preferentially in some suspension cells.[29]

Cells of *Papaver* may lack phenol oxidation enzymes which can catalyze the reaction from (−)-(R)-reticuline to salutaridine. However, *Papaver* and *Macleaya* both can convert (+)-(S)-reticuline to scoulerine, and *Papaver* cells can stereospecifically reduce (−)-codeinone to (−)-codeine.[87]

Enzymes controlling specific methylations and methylenedioxy formation are absent in *Stephania cepharantha* cells as the biscoclavrine alkaloids berbamine and aromorine are present in the cells, but absent in the plant.[2]

Betalaines are nitrogenous pigments that are probably related to tyrosine metabolism. Cells of *Beta vulgaris* (sugar beet) produce betalaines.[53] The red pigment, betanin, is produced by *Phytolacca americana* cells, and additional red pigments are produced from *B. vulgaris* var. *rubra, Chenopodium album* L. var. *centro-rubrum,* and *Spinacia oleraceae.*[340]

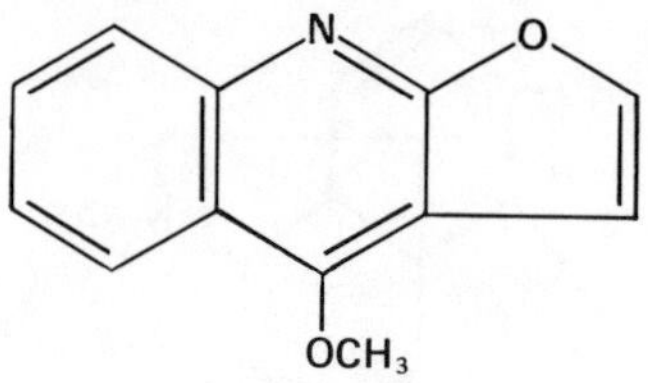

Dictamnine

FIGURE 22.   Quinoline alkaloid

D. Quinoline

Tryptophan is the major precursor to quinoline alkaloids. Chorismic acid can be converted to either phenylalanine and tyrosine or to anthranilic acid and tryptophan. The amide nitrogen of anthranilic acid is derived from glutamine, and the amine nitrogen of tryptophan is derived from serine. Quinolines evolve from monoterpenoids interacting with tryptophan to form the *Corynanthe*-type of indole alkaloids.

Rue (*Ruta graveolens*) cells will form significant amounts (up to 0.6% dry weight) of the furoquinoline alkaloids dictamnine (Figure 22) and 8-methoxydictamnine from 4-hydroxy-2-quinoline.[284] Eduline was specifically made from *N*-methyl-4-hydroxy-2-quinoline.[30] Dictamnine was catabolized to γ-fagarine.[284] Four acridone alkaloids and an alkaloid glycoside were produced from rue cultures. A yellow tissue culture of hypocotyl origin contained up to 1.5% dry weight of rutacridone.[176]

E. Indoles

The indole alkaloids are formed from tryptophan-derived tryptamine fusing with monoterpenoid precursors. There are three general classes of monoterpenoid precursors: *Aspidosperma, Corynanthe,* and *Iboga*. Ajmalicine (Figure 23) is biosynthesized from tryptamine and a *Corynanthe*-type monoterpenoid, the iridoid glycoside, secologanin.

Cell suspensions of *Phaseolus vulgaris* produce β-carboline (nor-harman) and 1-methyl-β-arboline (harman),[339] the production of which is significantly increased by the addition of tryptophan to the medium.[342] Callus cultures of *Peganum harmala* produced harmine and 8-hydroxy-glucosyl harmaline when grown on a medium without growth regulators, but not if grown on a medium with 2,4-D. Another callus strain produced 5-hydroxytryptamine rather than harmine. Various phenolic substrates (5- and 6-hydroxytryptophan) were not metabolized by the *P. harmala* cultures.[211] Some tissue cultures will take up tryptophan less efficiently than either phenylalanine or tyrosine and degrade it to carbon dioxide.[67]

Trace amounts of lysergic-acid-type alkaloids are present in *Ipomoea* tissue cultures,[59] and ergot alkaloid production is increased when the *Claviceps* fungus is grown on rye callus.[274] *Ipomoea* cell suspensions biotransformed tryptophan to tryptophol more effectively at a pH of 6.3 than a pH of 4.8.[340]

The indole alkaloid, reserpine, is produced by tissue cultures of *Alstonia constricta*[40] and *Rauwolfia serpentina*.[274] A Japanese patent has been issued for the production of *Rauwolfia* alkaloids.[357]

The monomeric alkaloid, ajmalicine, occurs in *Rauwolfia, Catharanthus,* and a number of other plant genus and species.[362] Ajmalicine is used extensively to improve blood circulation and to reduce blood pressure when combined with *Rauwolfia* alkaloids. Ajmalicine is biologically oxidized to serpentine, and serpentine may be chemically reduced to form ajmalicine.

A radioimmunoassay (RIA) technique was used to screen *Catharanthus roseus* cell

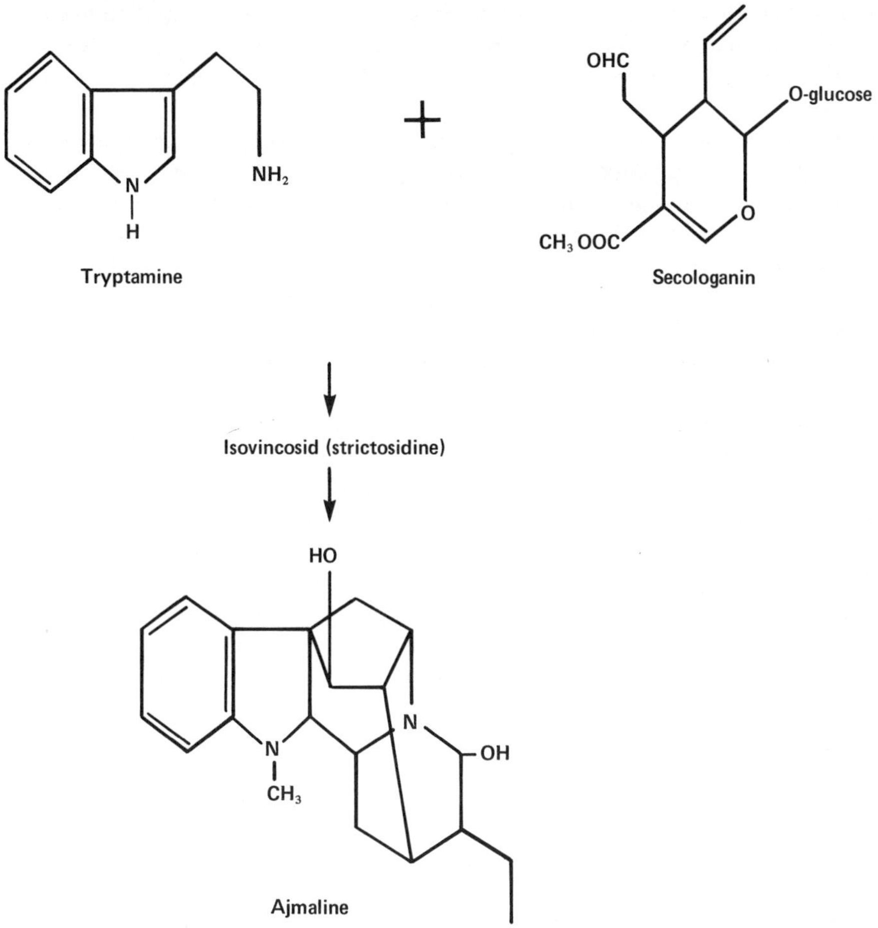

FIGURE 23. Ajmaline biosynthesis.

cultures established from high serpentine-yielding plants (0.93% alkaloid) and low ser-pentine-yielding plants (0.17% alkaloid).[328,362] The precursors, L-tryptophan (0.05%) and loganin (0.025%), significantly increased alkaloid production in selected *Cathar-anthus* strains. Strains were established that produced ajmalicine (264 mg/ℓ) and low amounts of serpentine (77 mg/ℓ), or serpentine (162 mg/ℓ) and no ajmalicine.[362] In other studies, serpentine production in the plant could not be correlated with serpen-tine formation in the corresponding tissue culture,[245] and tryptophan was not an effec-tive precursor in one cell line of *C. roseus*.[60] With time, selected *C. roseus* cell strains will vary in their alkaloid production, possibly because of the degradation of produced alkaloids.[57] *Vinca minor* cells produce the lignan, lirioresnol-B, and not vincamine.[91]

A soluble-enzyme system that required tryptamine, secologanin, and NADH or NADPH was prepared from *C. roseus* tissue cultures that could synthesize ajmalicine and geissoschizine[248,258] or ajmalicine, 19-epiajmalicine, and tetrahydroalsonine.[288] Such cell-free systems can be 1000 times more efficient than differentiated seedlings or plants.[362] It is now established that strictosidine [isovincoside, 3α(S)], and not vin-coside [3β(R)], is a major precursor to the indole alkaloids,[34,290] that cathenamine(20,21-didehydroajmalicine) accumulates in cell-free systems of *C. roseus* without NADPH or NADH,[286,287,290] and that a β-glucosidase enzyme is involved in the formation of cathenamine from strictosidine.[328] The "isovincoside synthetase" and "ajmalicine synthetase" enzymes are distinct in their pH optima and stability.[287] Efforts are being made to select cell strains of *C. roseus*,[25,26] *Solanum tuberosum*, *N. tabacum*, and *D. carota*[350] that are resistant to 5-methyltryptophan and accumulate tryptophan.

The plant, *Catharanthus roseus*, is the major source of the antineoplastic dimeric alkaloids, vincaleukoblastine and leurocristine. Efforts to produce the dimeric alkaloids from *C. roseus* tissue cultures have been unsuccessful, although many monomeric alkaloids are produced.[219] Tryptamine had greater effect than L-tryptophan in stimulating alkaloidal formation, and secologanin was without effect. When both tryptamine and secologanin were fed, two new metabolites formed, one of which was tentatively identified as sitsirikine.[173] Cells of *C. roseus* could biotransform vindoline hydrochloride into desacetylvindoline and three other unidentified products,[27] and into desacetylvindoline and dihydrovindoline.[42] The alkaloid catharanthine was not metabolized, and the alkaloid vincaleukoblastine was converted to two other dimeric alkaloids and a third unidentified compound.[42]

The antineoplastic alkaloids, camptothecin and 10-methoxycamptothecin, are produced by *Camptotheca acuminta* cells. The cells contained $2.5 \times 10^{-4}\%$ camptothecin. The plant contained $5 \times 10^{-3}\%$ camptothecin on a dry-weight basis. Tissue cultures of the Japanese plumyew, *Cephalotaxus harringtonia* produced four 1-leucine-biosynthesized antineoplastic alkaloids and the new alkaloid homodeoxyharringtonine.[55,56] Antineoplastic activity was detected in the extracts of callus derived from two of three plants (*Tripterygium wilfordii, Maytenus buchananii*, and *Putterlickia verrucosa*).[47]

F. Purines

Caffeine is produced by tea tissue cultures (0.1% dry weight) and released extracellularly by coffee tissue cultures (1.0 to 1.6% dry weight).[76,149] If the medium contains more than 1.0% caffeine, both cell growth and caffeine production will be inhibited. There is a free exchange between cells and medium for both theobromine and caffeine.[75] Considerably less caffeine (0.039%) was produced by El Salvador *Coffee arabica* suspension cells, but large amounts of chlorogenic acid (1.3% dry weight) was present when cell multiplication stopped.[38]

Sycamore callus can be used as a source of polyphenol-oxidase enzymes to produce brown-tea-containing theaflavins from green tea.[71]

Soybean cells produce the purine compound zeatin riboside.[337]

V. MISCELLANEOUS

A. Carbohydrates

Small amounts of β-glucosidase enzymes are present in the medium of peanut cells,[334] and these enzymes are principally localized in the walls of *Convolvulus arvensis* cells. In addition, β-1,3-glucanase,[144,183] invertase,[333] and low levels of amylase[344] are produced by plant tissue cultures.

Extracellular polysaccharides resembling the plant gums leiocarpan A and ghatti are secreted into the medium by tobacco cells.[143] A Japanese patent has been issued for the production of agar by callus tissues of algae.[206]

B. Lipids

The lipids of plant tissue cultures have recently been reviewed.[226] Heterotrophic cell cultures are characterized by relatively large amounts of sterols and complex lipids containing sterols and low levels of glycerol-derived lipids.[184] The predominant fatty acids in tissue cultures were linolinic, linoleic, and palmitic acid.[268]

Erucic acid, a major fatty acid in rape and turnip seeds, was more significantly produced in callus with embryo-like structures[137] than in callus.[280] The subcellular site of straight-chain fatty acids is located in proplastids.[272]

Cyclopentenyl fatty acids[272] and Jojoba wax[231] are produced from tissue cultures. *Pharbitis nil* excised apices[95] also convert arachidonic acid to various prostaglandins. It has been suggested that plant cell cultures be used to prepare unusual labeled lipid compounds.[185]

C. Amino Acids and Nucleotides

The tyrosine related product, L-DOPA, is reported largely produced extracellularly by *Mucuna* tissue cultures in amounts exceeding 1%.[31,229] Tobacco cells will isomerize D-tryptophan to L-tryptophan,[199] and *Ipomoea* cells will significantly convert tryptophan to tryptophol.[342] The peptide inhibitor, glutathionine, has been isolated from a conditioned soybean culture medium.[240]

Cells of *Vinca rosea* and *Phytolacca americana* are used to produce 5′-phosphodiesterase enzymes for 5′-ribonucleotide formation from RNA. A number of other plant tissue cultures can be used to degrade RNA and DNA directly to food-seasoning 5′-nucleotides.[340]

D. Proteins

The presence of antimicrobials in plant tissue cultures is well established.[164] Nitrogen-containing compounds from *P. americana* cells were antibiotic against *B. subtilis, S. faecalis,* and tobacco mosaic virus.[197] Also, cells of *Vinca rosea* inhibited coccidium protozoan infections in chickens.[196] The nonnitrogen phytoalexins, mediacarpin[97] and rishitin,[360] were produced by *Conavalis ensiformis* cells challenged with *Pithomyces chartarum* spores and by *Solanum tuberosum* cells challenged with *Phytophthora infestans.*

Scopolia japonica cells produce a protein plasmin inhibitor and a proteinase inhibitor more effective than a bovine trypsin-kallikrein inhibitor.[198] *Isodon japonicus* cells produce an anti-peptic-ulcer substance.[196] Papaya callus can be redifferentiated to plants[356] and produce proteolytic enzymes.[191]

Protein allergens are produced by ragweed cell cultures.[264,279,352] *Momordica charantia* fruits and tissue cultures produce a v-insulin (vegetable)[14,162] that has been tested in humans.[14] Although many of the necessary flavor enzymes are present, redifferentiation is necessary before *Allium cepa* (onion) cells will produce S-propenyl cysteine sulphoxide.[332]

A number of plant callus cultures, particularly if supplemented with 2% natural mulberry-leaf powder, can be used to feed silkworms and result in an increased cocoon shell weight and a decrease in diseased silkworms.[196]

ACKNOWLEDGMENT

The author wishes to gratefully acknowledge the assistance of Joseph H. C. Lui in the acquisition of many of the articles cited.

REFERENCES

1. **Aberhart, D. J., Lloyd-Jones, J. G., and Caspi, E.,** Biosynthesis of cardenolides in *Digitalis lanata, Phytochemistry,* 12, 1065, 1973.

2. **Akusu, M., Itokawa, H., and Fujita, M.,** Bioscoclaurine alkaloids in callus tissues of *Stephania cepharantha, Phytochemistry,* 15, 471, 1976.

3. **Al-Abta, S., Galpin, I., and Collin, H. A.,** Secondary product fornation during embryogenesis in celery tissue cultures, in *Abstr. — 4th Int. Congr. Plant Tissue and Cell Culture,* Thorpe, T. A., Ed., University of Calgary, Canada, 1978.

4. **Alfermann, A. W.,** Biotransformation of cardiac glycosides by digitalis cell cultures, in *Abstr. — 4th Int. Congr. Plant Tissue and Cell Culture,* Thorpe, T. A., Ed., University of Calgary, Canada, 1978, 79.

5. **Alfermann, A. W., Boy, H. M., Döller, P. C., Hagedorn, W., Heins, M., Wahl, J., and Reinhard, E.,** Biotransformation of cardiac glycosides by plant cell cultures, in *Plant Tissue Culture and Its Bio-technological Application,* Barz, W., Reinhard, E., and Zenk, M. H., Springer-Verlag, New York, 1977, 125.

6. **Alfermann, A. W. and Reinhard, E.,** Influence of phytohormones on secondary product formation in plant cell cultures, in *Secondary Metabolism and Coevolution,* Luckner, M., Mothes, K., and Nover, L., Eds., Deutsche Akademie der Naturforscher Leopoldina, Halle, 1976, 345.

7. **Ammirato, P. V.,** Somatic cell embryogenesis in suspension cultures of the medicinal yam, *Dioscorea floribunda,* in *Abstr. — 4th Int. Congr. Plant Tissue and Cell Culture,* Thorpe, T. A., Ed., University of Calgary, Canada, 1978, 134.

8. **Amorim, H. V., Dougall, D. K., and Sharp, W. R.,** The effect of carbohydrate and nitrogen concentration on phenol synthesis in Paul's Scarlet Rose cells grown in tissue culture, *Physiol. Plant.,* 39, 91, 1977.

9. **Applewhite, P. B.,** Serotonin and norepinephrine in plant tissues, *Phytochemistry,* 12, 191, 1973.

10. **Arreguin, B. and Bonner, J.,** The biochemistry of rubber formation in guayule. II. Rubber formation on aseptic tissue culture, *Arch. Biochem.,* 26, 178, 1950.

11. **Austin, D. J. and Brown, S. A.,** Furanocoumarin biosynthesis in *Ruta graveolens* cell cultures, *Phytochemistry,* 12, 1657, 1973.

12. **Aviv, D. and Galun, E.,** Conversion of pulegone to isomenthone by cell suspension lines of *Mentha* chemotypes, in *Production of Natural Compounds by Cell Culture Methods,* Alfermann, A. W. and Reinhard, E., Eds., Gesellschaft fur Strahlen und Umweltforschung MBH, Munich, 1978, 60.

13. **Aviv, D. and Galun, E.,** Biotransformation of monoterpenes by *Mentha* cell lines: conversion of pulegone to isomenthone, *Planta Medica,* 33, 70, 1978.

14. **Baldwa, V. S., Bhandari, C. M., Pangaria, A., and Goyal, R. K.,** Clinical trial in patients with diabetes mellitus of an insulin-like compound obtained from plant source, *Upsala J. Med. Sci.,* 82, 39, 1977.

15. **Banthorpe, D. V. and Wirz-Justice, A.,** Terpene biosynthesis. VI. Monoterpenes and carotenoids from tissue cultures of *Tanacetum vulgare* L., *J. Chem. Soc. Perkin Trans. 1,* 1769, 1972.

16. **Barz, W.,** Abbau von aromatischen und heterocyclischen pflanzeninhaltsstoffen durch zellsuspensionskulturen, *Planta Medica,* Suppl., 117, 1975.

17. **Barz, W.,** Catabolism of endogenous and exogenous compounds by plant cell cultures, in *Plant Tissue Culture and Its Bio-technological Application,* Barz, W., Reinhard, E., and Zenk, M. H., Eds., Springer-Verlag, New York, 1977, 153.

18. **Bauch, H. J. and Leistner, E.,** Aromatic metabolites in cell suspension cultures of *Galium mollugo* L., *Planta Medica,* 33(2), 105, 1978.

19. **Bauch, J. J. and Leistner, E.,** Attempts to demonstrate incorporation of labelled precursors into aromatic metabolites in cell suspension cultures of *Galium mollugo* L., *Planta Medica,* 33, 124, 1978.

20. **Baur, P. S. and Walkinshaw, C. H.,** Fine structure of tannin accumulations in callus cultures of *Pinus elliotti* (slash pine), *Can. J. Bot.,* 52, 615, 1974.

21. **Becker, H.,** Untersuchungen zur frage der bildung flüchtiger stoffwechselprodukte in calluskulturen, *Biochem. Physiol. Pflanz.,* 161, 425, 1970.

22. **Becker, H., Schrall, R., and Hartmann, W.,** Cultivation of tissue cultures of *Valeriana wallichii* DC and first analytical determination, *Arch. Pharm. (Weinheim),* 310, 481, 1977.

23. **Benveniste, P., Hirth, L., and Ourisson, G.,** La biosynthese des sterols dans les tissus de tabac cultives in vitro. I. *Phytochemistry,* 5, 31, 1966.

24. **Berlin, J. and Barz, W.,** Degradation of phenolic compounds in plant cell cultures, *FEBS Lett.,* 16, 141, 1971.

25. **Berlin, J., Schallenberg, J., Mutert, U., and Matuszak, U.,** Characterization of 5-methyltryptophan resistant cell lines, of *Catharanthus roseus,* in *Abstr. — 4th Int. Congr. Plant Tissue and Cell Culture,* Thorpe, T. A., Ed., University of Calgary, Canada, 1978, 127.

26. **Berlin, J. and Widholm, J. M.,** Amino acid analog resistant cell lines. A tool for studying secondary metabolism in plant cell cultures ?, in *Production of Natural Compounds in Cell Culture Methods,* Alfermann, A. W. and Reinhard, E., Eds., Gesellschaft fur Strahlen und Umweltforschung MBH, Munich, 1978, 171.

85

27. Boder, G. B., Gorman, M., Johnson, I. S., and Simpson, P. J., Tissue culture studies of *Catharanthus roseus* crown gall, *Lloydia*, 27, 328, 1964.
28. Böhm, H., II. Secondary metabolism in cell cultures of higher plants and problems of differentiation, in *Secondary Metabolism and Cell Differentiation*, Luckner, M., Nover, L., Böhm, H., Eds., Springer-Verlag, New York, 1977, 103.
29. Böhm, H., Regulation of alkaloid production in cell cultures, in *Abstr. — 4th Int. Congr. Plant Tissue and Cell Culture*, Thorpe, T. A., Ed., University of Calgary, Canada, 1978, 11.
30. Boulanger, D., Bailey, B. K., and Steck, W., Formation of edulinine and furoquinoline alkaloids from quinoline derivatives by cell suspension cultures of *Ruta graveolens*, *Phytochemistry*, 12, 2399, 1973.
31. Brain, K. R., Accumulation of L-DOPA in cultures from *Mucuna pruriens*, *Plant Sci. Lett.*, 7, 157, 1976.
32. Brain, K. R. and Lines, D. S., Uptake and metabolism of aldrin in plant tissue cultures, in *Plant Tissue Culture and Its Bio-Technological Application*, Barz, W., Reinhard, E., and Zenk, M. H., Eds., Springer-Verlag, New York, 1977, 197.
33. Brain, K. R. and Lockwood, G. B., Hormonal control of steroid levels in tissue cultures from *Trigonella foenumgraecum*, *Phytochemistry*, 15, 1651, 1976.
34. Brown, R. T., Leonard, J., and Sleigh, S. K., The role of strictosidine in monoterpenoid indole alkaloid biosynthesis, *Phytochemistry*, 17, 899, 1978.
35. Brown, S. A. and Sampathkumar, S., The biosynthesis of isopimpinellin, *Can. J. Biochem.*, 55, 686, 1977.
36. Brown, S. A. and Tenniswood, M., Aberrant coumarin metabolism in crown gall tumor tissue of tobacco, *Can. J. Bot.*, 52, 1091, 1974.
37. Brunet, G. and Ibrahim, R. K., O-Methylation of ring-A of flavonoids by cell-free extracts of citrus tissues, in *Plant Tissue Culture and Its Bio-technological Application*, Barz, W., Reinhard, E., and Zenk, M. H., Eds., Springer-Verlag, New York, 1977, 121.
38. Buckland, E. and Townsley, P. M., Coffee cell suspension cultures caffeine and chlorogenic content, *Can. Inst. Food Sci. Technol. J.*, 8(3), 164, 1975.
39. Butcher, D. N., Secondary products in tissue cultures, in *Plant Cell, Tissue, and Organ Culture*, Reinert, J. and Bajaj, Y. P. S., Eds., Springer-Verlag, New York, 1977, 668.
40. Carew, D. P., Reserpine in a tissue culture of *Alstonia constricta* F. Muell., *Nature (London)*, 207, 89, 1965.
41. Carew, D. P. and Bainbridge, T., Biotransformation with plant tissue cultures, *Lloydia*, 39, 204, 1976.
42. Carew, D. P. and Krueger, R. J., Metabolism of vindoline, catharanthine HCl, and vincaleukoblastine sulfate by suspension cultures of *Catharanthus roseus*, *Phytochemistry*, 16, 1462, 1977.
43. Carew, D. P. and Kreuger, R. J., *Catharanthus roseus* tissue culture: the effects of medium modifications on growth and alkaloid production, *Lloydia*, 40, 326, 1977.
44. Carle, R., Alfermann, A. W., and Reinhard, E., Diosgenin from *Solanum aurantiacobaccatum* de Wild, *Planta Med.*, 32, 195, 1977.
45. Cashyap, M. M., Kueh, J. S. H., Mackenzie, I. A., and Pattenden, G., In vitro synthesis of pyrethrins from tissue cultures of *Tanacetum cinerarifolium*, *Phytochemistry*, 17(3), 544, 1978.
46. Chan, W. N. and Staba, E. J., Alkaloid production by *Datura* callus and suspension tissue cultures, *Lloydia*, 28, 55, 1965.
47. Chen, P. K., Davis, P., Lin, P., Dujack, L., Chorghade, M., and Hammer, C. F., Plant tissue cultures of some neoplastic agents producing plants, in *Abstr. — 4th Int. Congr. Plant Tissue and Cell Culture*, Thorpe, T. A., Ed., University of Calgary, Canada, 1978, 130.
48. Chen, S., Stohs, S. J., and Staba, E. J., The biosynthesis of visnagin from 2-14C-acetate by *Ammi visnaga* suspension cultures and the metabolism of 14C-visnagin and 14C-khellin by *A. visnaga* and *A. majus*, *Lloydia*, 32, 339, 1969.
49. Chokashi, S. J. and Mehta, A. R., Growth and alkaloid production in suspension cultures of *Datura metel* L. anther, *Indian J. Pharm.*, 38(1), 13, 1976.
50. Chumsri, P. and Staba, E. J., Pyrethrins content and larvicidal activity of *Chrysanthemum* plants and tissue cultures, *Acad. Pharm. Sci. Abstr.*, 5, 169, 1975.
51. Comber, R., Georgina, D., and Newell, E., Improvements Relating to Smoking Materials, British Patent 1,466,912, 1977.
52. Constabel, F., Phenolics in tissue cultures derived from *Juniperus communis* L. studies on tannin synthesis, in *Proceedings — Int. Conf. Plant Tissue Culture*, White, P. R., Ed., McCuthan Publishing, Berkeley, Calif., 1965, 183.
53. Constabel, F. and Nassif-Makki, H., Betalainbildung in Beta-calluskulturen, *Ber. Dtsch. Bot. Ges.*, 84, 629, 1971.

54. **Corduan, G. and Spix, C.**, Another culture of a hybrid of the genus *Hyoscyamus*, a rapid method to obtain homozygous recombinants, in *Production of Natural Compounds by Cell Culture Methods*, Alfermann, A. W. and Reinhard, E., Eds., Gessellschaft fur Strahlen und Umweltforschung MBH, Munich, 1978, 295.

55. **Delfel, N. E.**, Alkaloid metabolism and growth of *Cephalotaxus harringtonia* cultures, in *Abstr. — 4th Int. Congr. Plant Tissue and Cell Culture*, Thorpe, T. A., Ed., University of Calgary, Canada, 1978, 124.

56. **Delfel, N. E. and Rothfus, J. A.**, Antitumor alkaloids in callus cultures of *Cephalotaxus harringtonia*, *Phytochemistry*, 16, 1595, 1977.

57. **Deus, B.**, Cellkulturen von *Catharanthus roseus*, in *Production of Natural Compounds by Cell Culture Methods*, Alfermann, A. W. and Reinhard, E., Eds., Gesellschaft for Strahlen und Umweltforschung MBH, Munich, 1978, 118.

58. **Dhillon, D. S. and Brown, S. A.**, Localization, purification, and characterization of dimethylallylpyrophosphate: umbelliferone dimethylallytransferase from *Ruta graveolens*, *Arch. Biochem. Biophys.*, 177, 74, 1976.

59. **Dobberstein, R. H. and Staba, E. J.**, *Ipomoea, Rivea* and *Argyreia* tissue cultures: influence of various chemical factors on indole alkaloid production and growth, *Lloydia*, 32, 141, 1969.

60. **Döller, G.**, Influence of the medium on the production of serpentine by suspension cultures of *Catharanthus roseus* (L.) G. Don, in *Production of Natural Compounds by Cell Culture Methods* Alfermann, A. W. and Reinhard, E., Eds., Gesellschaft fur Strahlen und Umweltforschung MBH, Munich, 1978, 109.

61. **Döller, P. C., Alfermann, A. W., and Reinhard, E.**, Biotransformation von cardenoliden durch zellsuspensionskulturen von *Digitalis lanata* und *Thevetia nerhfolia, Planta Med.*, 31, 1, 1977.

62. **Douglas, T. J. and Paleg, L. G.**, Amo 1618 effects on incorporation of ^{14}C-MVA and ^{14}C-acetate into sterols in *Nicotiana* and *Digitalis* seedlings and cell-free preparations from *Nicotiana*, *Phytochemistry*, 17, 713, 1978.

63. **Downing, M. R. and Mitchell, E. D.**, Mevalonate-activating enzymes in callus culture cells from *Nepeta cataria*, *Phytochemistry*, 14, 369, 1975.

64. **Ebel, J. and Grisebach, H.**, Enzymology and regulation of lignin formation in cultured cells, in *Abstr. — 4th Int. Congr. Plant Tissue and Cell Culture*, Thorpe, T. A., Ed., University of Calgary, Canada, 1978, 122.

65. **Elder, J., Benveniste, P., and Fonteneau, P.**, *In vitro* cyclization of squalene 2,3-epoxide to *a*-amyrin by microsomes from bramble cell suspension cultures, *Phytochemistry*, 16, 490, 1977.

66. **Ellis, B. E.**, A survey of catechol ring cleavage by sterile plant tissue cultures, *FEBS Lett.*, 18(2), 228, 1971.

67. **Ellis, B. E. and Towers, G. H. N.**, Degradation of aromatic compounds by sterile plant tissues, *Phytochemistry*, 9, 1457, 1970.

68. **Elze, H. and Teuscher, E.**, in *Biochem. Physiol. Alkaloide, 4th Int. Symp.*, Mothes, K., Ed., Akademie Verlag, Berlin, 1972, 239.

69. **Eppenberger, U., Hirth, L., and Ourisson, G.**, Anaerobische cyclisierung von squalen-2,3-epoxyd zu cycloartenol in gewebekulturen von *Nicotiana tabacum* L., *Eur. J. Biochem.*, 8, 180, 1969.

70. **Erdelsky, K.**, Secondary compounds of callus from *Papaver somniferum*, in *Abstr. — 4th Int. Congr. Plant Tissue and Cell Culture*, Thorpe, T. A., Ed., University of Calgary, Canada, 1978.

71. **Fairley, C. J. and Swaine, D.**, Green Tea Fermentation by Callus Tissue Enzyme Preparations, British Patent 1,318,035, 1973.

72. **Famimura, S., Akutsu, M., and Nishikawa, M.**, Formation of thebaine in the suspension culture of *Papaver bracteatum*, *Agric. Biol. Chem.*, 40, 913, 1976.

73. **Fonteneau, P., Hartmann-Bouillon, M. A., and Benveniste, P.**, A 24-methylene lophenol C-28 methyltransferase from suspension cultures of bramble cells, *Plant Sci. Lett.*, 10, 147, 1977.

74. **Friedrich, H. and Baier, S.**, Anthracen-derivate in kalluskulturen aus *Cassia angustifolia*, *Phytochemistry*, 12, 1459, 1973.

75. **Frischknecht, P. M., Baumann, T. W., and Wanner, H.**, Purine alkaloid metabolism in suspension cultures of *Coffea arabica*, in *Abstr. — 4th Int. Congr. Plant Tissue and Cell Culture*, Thorpe, T. A., University of Calgary, Canada, 1978, 124.

76. **Frischknecht, P. M., Baumann, T. W., and Wanner, H.**, Tissue culture of *Coffea arabica* growth and caffeine formation, *Planta Med.*, 31, 346, 1977.

77. **Fritsch, H. and Griesbach, H.**, Biosynthesis of cyanidin in cell cultures of *Haplopappus gracilis*, *Phytochemistry*, 14, 2437, 1975.

78. **Furuya, T.**, Biotransformation by plant cell cultures, in *Abstr. — 4th Int. Congr. Plant Tissue and Cell Culture*, Thorpe, T. A., Ed., University of Calgary, Canada, 1978, 11.

79. **Furuya, T., Hirotani, M., and Kawaguchi, K.**, Biotransformation of progesterone and pregnenolone by plant suspension cultures, *Phytochemistry*, 10, 1013, 1971.

80. **Furuya, T., Hirotani, M., and Shinohara, T.,** Biotransformation of digoxin by suspension callus culture of *Digitalis purpurea, Chem. Pharm. Bull.,* 18(5), 1080, 1970.

81. **Furuya, T., Ikuta, A., and Syōno, K.,** Alkaloids from callus tissue of *Papaver somniferum, Phytochemistry,* 11, 3041, 1972.

82. **Furuya, T. and Ishii, T.,** Production of ginseng radix, Japan Patent (Kokai), 73-31917, 1973.

83. **Furuya, T. and Kojima, H.,** 4-Hydroxydigitolutein, A new anthraquinone from callus tissue of *Digitalis lanata, Phytochemistry,* 10, 1607, 1971.

84. **Furuya, T., Kojima, H., and Katsuta, T.,** 3-Methylpurpurin and other anthraquinones from callus tissue of *Digitalis lanata, Phytochemistry,* 11, 1073, 1972.

85. **Furuya, T., Kojima, H., and Syōno, K.,** Regulation of nicotine biosynthesis by auxins in tobacco callus tissues, *Phytochemistry,* 10, 1529, 1971.

86. **Furuya, T., Kojima, H., Syōno, K., and Ishii, T.,** Isolation of panatriol from *Panax ginseng* callus, *Chem. Pharm. Bull.,* 18, 2371, 1970.

87. **Furuya, T., Nakano, M., and Yoshikawa, T.,** Biotransformation of (RS)-reticuline and morphinan alkaloids by cell cultures of *Papaver somniferum, Phytochemistry,* 17, 891, 1978.

88. **Gallili, G. E., Yagen, B., and Metales, R. I.,** Hydroxylation of progesterone by plant cell suspension cultures of *Vinca rosea, Phytochemistry,* 17, 578, 1978.

89. **Gamborg, O. L.,** Aromatic metabolism in plants. IV. The interconversion of shikimic acid and quinic acid by enzymes from plant cell cultures, *Phytochemistry,* 6, 1067, 1967.

90. **Gamborg, O.,** Aromatic metabolism in plants. V. The biosynthesis of chlorogenic acid and lignin in potato cell cultures, *Can. J. Biochem.,* 45, 1451, 1967.

91. **Garnier, J., Kunesch, N., Siou, E., Poisson, J., Kunesch, G., and Koch, M.,** Study of cultures of tissues of *Vinca minor.* Isolation of a lignan lirioresorcinol B, *Phytochemistry,* 14, 1385, 1975.

92. **Geuns, J. M. C.,** Steroid hormones and plant growth and development, *Phytochemistry,* 17, 1, 1978.

93. **Goris, A.,** Toxicite comparee de las vanilline et du vanilloside sur les cultures *in vitro* de tissue de carotte, *Ann. Pharm. Fr.,* 23(4), 275, 1965.

94. **Graves, J. M. H. and Smith, W. K.,** Transformation of pregnenolone and progesterone by cultured plant cells, *Nature (London),* 214, 1248, 1967.

95. **Groenewald, E. G. and Visser, J. H.,** Possible conversion of arachidonic acid to prostaglandins F2a, E2, A2 and B2 by aseptic excised apices of *Pharbitis nil,* in *Abstr. — 4th Int. Congr. Plant Tissue and Cell Culture,* Thorpe, T. A., Ed., University of Calgary, Canada, 1978, 155.

96. **Gurny, L. and Kapetanidis, I.,** Steran-derivate in gewebekulturen von *Digitalis purpurea* L., Abstr. Int. Meet., *Planta Med.,* 286, 1978.

97. **Gustine D. L., Sherwood, R. T., and Vance, C. P.,** Regulation of phytoalexin synthesis in jackbean callus cultures, *Plant Physiol.,* 61, 226, 1978.

98. **Hagimori, M., Matsumoto, T., and Noguchi, M.,** Isolation and identification of ubiquinone 9, from cultured cells of safflower (*Carthamus tinctorius* L.), *Agric. Biol. Chem.,* 42, 499, 1978.

99. **Hahlbrock, K.,** Regulatory aspects of phenylpropanoid biosynthesis in cell cultures, in *Plant Tissue Culture and Its Bio-technological Application,* Barz W., Reinhard, E., and Zenk, M. H., Eds., Springer-Verlag, New York, 1977, 95.

100. **Hall, J., Smith, A. R. H., Goad, L. J., and Goodwin, T. W.,** The conversion of lanosterol, cycloartenol and 24-methylenecycloartanol into poriferasterol by *Ochromonas malhamensis, Biochem. J.,* 112, 129, 1969.

101. **Harris, A. L., Nylund, H. B., and Carew, D. P.,** Tissue culture studies of certain members of the Apocynaceae, *Lloydia,* 27, 322, 1964.

102. **Harms, H., Dehnen, W., and Monch, W.,** Benzo(a)pyrene metabolites formed by plant cells, *Z. Naturforsch.,* 32, 321, 1977.

103. **Hartmann, M. A., Benveniste, P., and Durst, F.,** Biosynthesis of sterols in Jerusalem artichoke tuber tissue, *Phytochemistry,* 11, 3003, 1972.

104. **Heble, M. R., Narayanaswamy, S., and Chadha, M. S.,** Solasonine in tissue cultures of *Solanum xanthocarpum, Naturwissenschaften,* 7, 350, 1968.

105. **Heble, M. R., Narayanaswamy, S., and Chadha, M. S.,** Tissue differentiation and plumbagin synthesis in variant cell strains of *Plumbago zeylanica* L. in vitro, *Plant Sci. Lett.,* 2, 405, 1974.

106. **Heble, M. R., Narayanaswamy, S., and Chadha, M. S.,** Studies on growth and steroid formation in tissue cultures of *Holarrhena antidysenterica, Phytochemistry,* 15, 681, 1976.

107. **Heble, M. R., Narayanaswamy, S., and Chadha, M. S.,** Metabolism of cholesterol by callus culture of *Holarrhena antidysenteric, Phytochemistry,* 15, 911, 1976.

108. **Heeger, V., Leienbach, K., and Barz, W.,** Metabolism of nicotinic acid in plant cell suspension cultures. III. Formation and metabolism of trigonelline, *Z. Physiol. Chem.,* 357, 1081, 1976.

109. **Heftmann, E.,** Steroid hormones in plants, *Lloydia,* 38, 195, 1975.

110. **Heins, M.,** Screening of *Digitalis lanata* plants and cell cultures for hydroxylation capacity, in *Production of Natural Compounds by Cell Culture Methods,* Alfermann, A. W. and Reinhard, E., Eds., Gesellschaft fur Strahlen und Umwelttforschung MBH, Munich, 1978, 39.

111. **Heins, M., Wahl, J., Lerch, H., Kaiser, F., and Reinhard, E.,** Preparation of β-methyldigoxin by hydroxylation of β-methyldigitoxin in fermentor cultures of *Digitalis lanata, Planta Medica,* 33, 57, 1978.

112. **Heintz, R. and Benveniste, P.,** Cyclisation de l'epoxyde-2,3 de squalene par des microsomes extraits de tissus de tabac cultives *in vitro, Phytochemistry,* 9, 1499, 1970.

113. **Heintz, R. and Benveniste, P.,** Plant sterol metabolism; enzymatic cleavage of the 9β,19β-cyclopropane ring of cyclopropyl sterols in bramble tissue cultures, *J. Biol. Chem.,* 249(13), 4267, 1974.

114. **Heintz, R., Benveniste, P., Robinson, W. H., and Coates, R. M.,** Demonstration and identification of a biosynthetic intermediate between farnesyl PP and squalene in a higher plant, *Biochem. Biophys. Res. Commun.,* 49(6), 1547, 1972.

115. **Heinzmann, U. and Seitz, U.,** Synthesis of phenylalanine ammonia-lyase in anthocyanin-containing and anthocyanin-free callus cells of *Daucus carota* L., *Planta,* 135, 63, 1977.

116. **Heinzmann, U., Seitz, U., and Seitz, U.,** Purification and substrate specificities of hydroxycinnamate: CoA ligase from anthocyanin-containing and anthocyanin-free carrot cells, *Planta,* 135, 313, 1977.

117. **Helmbold, H., Voelter, W., and Reinhard, E.,** Sterols in cell cultures of *Digitalis lanata, Planta Medica,* 33, 185, 1978.

118. **Hewlins, M. J. E., Ehrhardt, J. D., Hirth, L., and Ourisson, G.,** The conversion of (14C) cycloartenol and (14C) lanosterol into phytosterols by cultures of *Nicotiana tabacum, Eur. J. Biochem.,* 8, 184, 1969.

119. **Hiraoka, N., Tabata, M., and Konoshima, M.,** Formation of acetyltropine in *Datura* cellus cultures, *Phytochemistry,* 12, 795, 1973.

120. **Hirotani, M. and Furuya, T.,** Biotransformation of testosterone and other androgens by suspension cultures of *Nicotiana tabacum* "Bright Yellow", *Phytochemistry,* 13, 2135, 1974.

121. **Hirotani, M. and Furuya, T.,** Metabolism of 5 β-pregnane-3,20-dione and 3 β-hydroxy-5 β-pregnan-20-one by *Digitalis* suspension cultures, *Phytochemistry,* 14, 2601, 1975.

122. **Hirotani, M. and Furuya, T.,** Restoration of cardenolide-synthesis in redifferentiated shoots from callus cultures of *Digitalis purpurea, Phytochemistry,* 16, 610, 1977.

123. **Hoover, J. D., Wender, S. H., and Smith, E. C.,** Effect of phenolic compounds on glucose-6-phosphate dehydrogenase isoenzymes, *Phytochemistry,* 16, 199, 1977.

124. **Husemann, W. and Barz, W.,** Photoautotrophic growth and photosynthesis in cell suspension cultures of *Chenopodium rubrum, Physiol. Plant.,* 40, 77, 1977.

125. **Ibrahim, R. K. and Grisebach, H.,** Purification and properties of UDP-glucose: coniferyl alcohol glucosyltransferase from suspension cultures of Paul's Scarlet Rose, *Arch. Biochem. Biophys.,* 176, 700, 1976.

126. **Ikeda, T., Matsumoto, T., and Noguchi, M.,** Formation of ubiquinone by tobacco plant cells in suspension culture, *Phytochemistry,* 15, 568, 1971.

127. **Ikuta, A., Syōno, K., and Furuya, T.,** Alkaloids of callus tissues and redifferentiated plantlets in the Papaveraceae, *Phytochemistry,* 13, 2175, 1974.

128. **Ikuta, A., Syōno, K., and Furuya, T.,** Plant tissue cultures. XXIV. Alkaloids in plants regenerated from *Coptis* callus cultures. *Phytochemistry,* 14, 1209, 1975.

129. **Inouye, H.,** Neuere ergebnisse über die biosynthese der glucoside der irioidreihe, *Planta Medica* 33, 193, 1978.

130. **Itokawa, H., Akasu, M., and Fujita, M.,** Several oxidized sterols isolated from callus tissue of *Stephania cepharantha, Chem. Pharm. Bull.,* 21(6), 1386, 1973.

131. **Itokawa, H., Takeya, K., and Mihashi, S.,** Biotransformation of cannabinoid precursors and related alcohols by suspension cultures of callus induced from *Cannabis sativa* L., *Chem. Pharm. Bull.,* 25 (8), 1941, 1977.

132. **Jain, S. C.,** Chemical investigation of *Tagetes* tissue cultures, *Planta Medica,* 31, 68, 1977.

133. **Jain, S. C., Rosenberg, H., and Stohs, S. J.,** Steroidal constituents of *Trigonella occulta* tissue cultures, *Planta Medica,* 31, 109, 1977.

134. **Jalal, M. A. F. and Collin, H. A.,** Polyphenols of mature plant, seedling and tissue cultures of *Theobroma cacao, Phytochemistry,* 16, 1377, 1977.

135. **Jhang, J. J., Staba, E. J., and Kim, J. Y.,** American and Korean ginseng tissue cultures: growth, chemical analysis, and plantlet production, *In Vitro,* 9, 253, 1974.

136. **Jindra, A. and Staba, E. J.,** *Datura* tissue cultures: arginase, transaminase and esterase activities, *Phytochemistry,* 7, 79, 1968.

137. **Jones, L. H.,** Plant cell culture and biochemistry: studies for improved vegetable oil production, in *Industrial Aspects of Biochemistry,* Spencer, B., Ed., Federation European Biochemical Societies, Elsevier North-Holland, Amsterdam, 1974, 813.

138. **Jurd, L.,** The acid catalyzed conversion of 3-hydroxyflavanones to anthocyanidins, *Phytochemistry,* 8, 2421, 1969.

139. **Kadkade, P. G. and Madrid, T. .**, Glycoalkaloids in tissue cultures of *Solanum acculeatissimum, Naturwissenschaften*, 64, 147, 1977.

140. **Karanova, S. L. and Samina, Z. B.**, Chemical mutagenesis in *Dioscorea deltoidea* Wall. somatic cell culture, in *Use of Tissue Cultures in Plant Breeding*, Novak, F. J., Ed., Ceskoslovenska Academie Ved Ustav Experimentalni Botaniky, Prague, 1977, 325.

141. **Kartnig, T. and Kobosil, P.**, Observations on the occurrence and the formation of cardenolides in tissue cultures of *Digitalis purpurea* and *Digitalis lanata, Planta Medica*, 31, 221, 1977.

142. **Kartnig, T., Russheim, U., and Maunz, B.**, Cardenolide in oberflachenkulturen aus keim- und laubblattern von *Digitalis purpurea, Planta Medica*, 29, 275, 1976.

143. **Kato, K., Watanabe, F., and Eda, S.**, Interior chains of glucuronomannan from extracellular polysaccharides of suspension-cultured tobacco cells, *Agric. Biol. Chem.*, 41(3), 539, 1977.

144. **Kato, K., Yamada, A., and Noguchi, M.**, Purification and some properties of β-1,3-glucanase of suspension-cultured tobacco cells, *Agric. Biol. Chem.*, 37(6), 1269, 1973.

145. **Kaul, B. and Staba, E. J.**, Visnagin: biosynthesis and isolation from *Ammi visnaga* suspension cultures, *Science*, 150, 1731, 1965.

146. **Kaul, B. and Staba, E. J.**, Dioscorea tissue cultures. I. Biosynthesis and isolation of diosgenin from *Dioscorea deltoidea* callus and suspension cells, *Lloydia*, 31(2), 171, 1968.

147. **Kaul, B., Stohs, S. J., and Staba, E. J.**, Dioscorea tissue cultures. III. Influence of various factors on diosgenin production by *Dioscorea deltoidea* callus and suspension cultures, *Lloydia*, 32(3), 347, 1969.

148. **Kaul, B., Wells, P., and Staba, E. J.**, Production of cardioactive substances by plant tissue cultures and their screening for cardiovascular activity, *J. Pharm. Pharmacol.*, 19, 760, 1967.

149. **Keller, H., Wanner, H., and Baumann, T. W.**, Caffeine synthesis in fruits and tissue cultures of *Coffea arabica, Planta*, 108, 339, 1972.

150. **Khanna, P., Bansal, R., and Jain, S. C.**, Effect of various hormones on production of sapogenins and sterols in *Trigonella foenum-graecum* L. suspension cultures, *Indian J. Exp. Biol.*, 13(6), 582, 1975.

151. **Khanna, P. and Jain, S. C.**, Effect of nicotinic acid on growth and production of trigonelline by *Trigonella foenum-graecum* L. tissue cultures, *Indian J. Exp. Biol.*, 10(3), 248, 1972.

152. **Khanna, P. and Jain, S. C.**, Isolation and identification of sesamin from *Sesamum indicum* tissue cultures, *Curr. Sci.*, 42(7), 252, 1973.

153. **Khanna, P. and Jain, S. C.**, Diosgenin, gitogenin, and tigogenin from *Trigonella foenum-graecum* tissue cultures, *Lloydia*, 36(1), 96, 1973.

154. **Khanna, P. and Khanna, R.**, Production of major alkaloids from *in vitro* tissue cultures of *Papaver somniferum* Linn, *Indian J. Exp. Biol.*, 14(5), 628, 1976.

155. **Khanna, P., Khanna, R., and Sharma, M.**, Production of free ascorbic acid and effect of exogenous ascorbic acid and tyrosine on production of major opium alkaloids from *in vitro* tissue culture of *Papaver somniferum* Linn., *Indian J. Exp. Biol.*, 16(1), 110, 1978.

156. **Khanna, P., Khanna, R., Sogani, M., and Manot, S. K.**, *Daucus carota* L. seedling callus a new source of diosgenin, *Indian J. Exp. Biol.*, 15(7), 586, 1977.

157. **Khanna, P. and Manot, S. K.**, Effect of cholesterol on suspension culture of *Solanum xanthocarpum* Schrad and Wendl, *Indian J. Exp. Biol.*, 14, 631, 1976.

158. **Khanna, P. and Manot, S. K.**, Production of pyrrolizidine alkaloid from *in vitro* tissue culture of *Crotalaria juncea* Linn., *Indian J. Exp. Biol.*, 15(9), 807, 1977.

159. **Khanna, P. and Mohan, S.**, Isolation and identification of diosgenin and sterols from fruits and *in vitro* cultures of *Momordica charantia* L., *Indiana J. Exp. Biol.*, 11, 58, 1973.

160. **Khanna, P. and Nag, T. N.**, Melanogenesis in *Datura* tissue cultures, *Curr. Sci.*, 41(3), 115, 1972.

161. **Khanna, P. and Nag, T. N.**, Incorporation of dl-tyrosine-1-14C in the biosynthesis of tropane alkaloids in tissue cultures of *Datura metel* L., *Indian J. Exp. Biol.*, 12(1), 109, 1974.

162. **Khanna, P., Nag, T. N., Jain, S. C., and Mohan, S.**, Extraction of insulin from plant cultures *in vitro, 3rd Int. Congr. Plant Tissue and Cell Culture, Abstr.*, University of Leicester, 1974, 257.

163. **Khanna, P., Sharma, G. L., and Uddin, A.**, Atropine from *Atropa belladonna* Linn. tissue culture, *Indian J. Exp. Biol.*, 15(4), 323, 1977.

164. **Khanna, P. and Staba, E. J.**, Antimicrobials from plant tissue cultures, *Lloydia*, 31, 180, 1968.

165. **Khanna, P., Uddin, A., Sharma, G. L., Manot, S. K., and Rathore, A. K.**, Isolation and characterization of sapogenin and solasodine from *in vitro* tissue cultures of some solanaceous plants, *Indian J. Exp. Biol.*, 14, 694, 1976.

166. **Khanna, P., Uddin, A., and Sogani, M.**, Pseudoephedrine from *in vivo* and *in vitro* tissue cultures of *Ephedra foliate* Boiss., *Indian J. Pharm.*, 38(6), 140, 1976.

167. **Kireeva, S. A., Bugorskii, P. S., and Reznikova, S. A.**, Cultivation of Damask rose tissue and accumulation of terpenoids in them, *Sov. Plant Physiol.*, 24(4), 824, 1977.

168. **Kirkland, D. R., Matsuo, M., and Underhill, E. W.**, Detection of glucosinolates and myrosinase in plant tissue cultures, *Lloydia*, 34, 195, 1971.

169. **Kokate, C. K. and Radwan, S. S.**, Steroidal glycoalkaloids in tissue cultures of *Solanum khasianum* during organogenesis, Abstr. of the Int. Meet., *Planta Med.,* 301, 1978.

170. **Konoshima, M., Tabata, M., Yamamoto, H., and Hiraoka, N.**, Growth and alkaloid production of *Datura* tissue cultures, *Yakugaku Zasshi,* 90(3), 370, 1970.

171. **Kreuzaler, F. and Hahlbrock, K.**, Flavonoid glycosides from illuminated cell suspension cultures of *Petroselinum hortense, Phytochemistry,* 12, 1149, 1973.

172. **Krikorian, A. D. and Steward, F. C.**, Biochemical differentiation: the biosynthetic potentialities of growing and quiescent tissue, in *Plant Physiology,* Vol. 5 B, Steward, F. C., Ed., Academic Press, New York, 1969, 225.

173. **Krueger, R. J. and Carew, D. P.**, *Catharanthus roseus* tissue culture: the effects of precursors on growth and alkaloid production, *Lloydia,* 41(4), 327, 1978.

174. **Kuboi, T. and Yamada, Y.**, Caffeic acid-*O*-methyltransferase in a suspension of cell aggregates of tobacco, *Phytochemistry,* 15, 397, 1976.

175. **Kutney, J. P., Salisbury, P. J., and Verma, A. K.**, Biosynthetic studies in the coumarin series. III. Studies in tissue cultures of *Thamnosma montana* Torr. and Frem. the role of mevalonate, *Tetrahedron,* 29, 2673, 1973.

176. **Kuzavkina, I. N., Smirnov, A. M., Szendrei, K., Rozsa, Z., and Reisch, J.**, Acridone alkaloids in callus tissues of *Ruta graveolens* L., in *Abstr. — 4th Int. Congr. Plant Tissue and Cell Culture,* Thorpe, T. A., Ed., University of Calgary, Canada, 1978, 125.

177. **Lang, E. and Horster, H.**, Sugar bound regular monoterpenes. II. Production and accumulation of essential oils in *Ocimum basilicum* callus and suspension cultures, *Planta Medica,* 31, 112, 1977.

178. **Leienbach, K. and Barz, W.**, Metabolism of nicotinic acid in plant cell suspension cultures. III. Isolation characterization and enzymology of nicotinic acid *N*-α-arabinoside, *Z. Physiol. Chem.,* 357, 1069, 1976.

179. **Leienbach, K., Heeger, V., and Barz, W.**, Metabolism of nicotinic acid in plant cell suspension cultures, IV. Occurrence and metabolism of nicotinic acid *N*-α-arabinoside, *Z. Physiol. Chem.,* 357, 1089, 1976.

180. **Leistner, E.**, Biosynthesis of morindone and alizarin in intact plants and cell suspension cultures of *Morinda citrifolia, Phytochemistry,* 12, 1669, 1973.

181. **Loewenberg, J. R.**, Observations of scopoletin and scopolin metabolism, *Phytochemistry,* 9, 361, 1970.

182. **Lui, J. H. C. and Staba, E. J.**, Presence of cardenolides in *Digitalis lanata* tissue cultures, in *Abstr. — 4th Int. Congr. Plant Tissue and Cell Culture,* Thorpe, T. A., Ed., University of Calgary, Canada, 1978, 80.

183. **Mandels, M., Parrish, F. W., and Reese, E. T.**, β (1→3) Glucanases from plant callus cultures, *Phytochemistry,* 6, 1097, 1967.

184. **Mangold, H. K.**, The common and unusual lipids of plant cell cultures, in *Plant Tissue Culture and Its Bio-technological Application,* Barz, W., Reinhard, E., and Zenk, M. H., Eds., Springer-Verlag, New York, 1977, 55.

185. **Mangold, H. K. and Radwan, S. S.**, Use of cell cultures for the preparation of labelled compounds, in *Abstr. — 4th Int. Congr. Plant Tissue and Cell Culture,* Thorpe, T. A., Ed., University of Calgary, Canada, 1978, 81.

186. **Margna, U.**, Control at the level of substrate supply — an alternative in the regulation of phenylpropanoid accumulation in plant cells, *Phytochemistry,* 16, 419, 1977.

187. **Marshall, J. G. and Staba, E. J.**, Steroids and an artifact from *Dioscorea deltoidea* tissue cultures, *Lloydia,* 39, 84, 1976.

188. **Matsumoto, T., Ikeda, T., and Noguchi, M.**, Formation of ubiquinone-10 by tobacco plant cells in suspension culture, in *Abstr. — 4th Int. Congr. Plant Tissue and Cell Culture,* Thorpe, T. A., Ed., University of Calgary, Canada, 1978, 130.

189. **Matsumoto, T., Koh, N., Noguchi, M., and Tamaki, E.**, Some factors affecting the anthocyanin formation by *Populus* cells in suspension culture, *Agric. Biol. Chem.,* 37(3), 561, 1973.

190. **McGaw, B. A. and Woolley, J. G.**, Stereochemistry of tropane alkaloid formtion in *Datura, Phytochemistry,* 17, 257, 1978.

191. **Medora, R. S., Campbell, J. M., and Mell, G. P.**, Proteolytic enzymes in papaya tissue cultures, *Lloydia,* 36, 214, 1973.

192. **Medora, R., Kosegarten, D., Tsao, D. P. N., and de Feo, J. J.**, Cardiotonic activity in callus tissue of *Digitalis mertonensis, J. Pharm. Sci.,* 56, 540, 1967.

193. **Medora, R. S., Tsao, D. P. N., and Albert, L. S.**, Tissue culture of *Digitalis mertonensis* I. Effect of certain steroids on the callus growth and formation of Baljet positive substances in *D. Mertonensis, J. Pharm. Sci.,* 56, 67, 1967.

194. **Mehta, A. R. and Staba, E. J.**, Presence of diosgenin in tissue cultures of *Dioscorea composita* Hemsl. and related species, *J. Pharm. Sci.,* 59(6), 864, 1970.

195. Metz, H. and Lang, H., Verfahren zur Zuchtung von Differenziertem Wurzelgewebe, German Patent 1,216,009, 1966.
196. Misawa, M., Production of natural substances by plant cell cultures described in Japanese patents, in *Plant Tissue Culture and Its Bio-technological Application*, Barz, W., Reinhard, E., and Zenk, M. H., Eds., Springer-Verlag, New York, 1977, 17.
197. Misawa, M., Hayashi, M., Tanaka, H., Ko, K., and Misato, T., Production of plant virus inhibitor by *Phytolacca americana* suspension culture, *Biotechnol. Bioeng.*, 17, 1335, 1975.
198. Misawa, M., Tanaka, H., Chiyo, O., and Mukai, N., Production of a plasmin inhibitory substance by *Scopolia japonica* suspension cultures, *Biotechnol. Bioeng.*, 17, 305, 1975.
199. Miura, G. A. and Mills, S. E., The conversion of D-tryptophan to L-tryptophan in cell cultures of tobacco, *Plant Physiol.*, 47, 483, 1971.
200. Mizukami, H., Konoshima, M., and Tabata, M., Effect on nutritional factors on shikonin derivative formation in *Lithospermum* callus cultures, *Phytochemistry*, 16, 1183, 1977.
201. Mizukami, H., Konoshima, M., and Tabata, M., Variation in pigment production in *Lithospermum erythrorhizon* callus cultures, *Phytochemistry*, 17, 95, 1978.
202. Mizusaki, S., Tanabe, Y., Noguchi, M., and Tamaki, E., *p*-Coumaroylputrescine, caffeoylputrescine and feruloylputrescine from callus tissue culture of *Nicotiana tabacum*, *Phytochemistry*, 10, 1347, 1971.
203. Mok, M. C., Gabelman, W. H., and Skoog, F., Carotenoid synthesis in tissue cultures of *Daucus carota* L., *J. Am. Soc. Hortic. Sci.*, 101(4), 442, 1976.
204. Mothes, K., Die alkaloide im stoffwechsel der pflanze, *Experientia*, 25, 225, 1969.
205. Naef, J. and Turian, G., Sur les carotenoides du tissu cambial de racine de carotte cultive in vitro, *Phytochemistry*, 2, 173, 1963.
206. Nakamura, T., Production of Agar, Japan Patent (Kokai) 74-101561, 1974.
207. Nag, T. N., Role of tyrosine in *Datura* tissue culture, in *Abstr. — 4th Int. Congr. Plant Tissue and Cell Culture*, Thorpe, T. A., Ed., University of Calgary, Canada, 1978, 126.
208. Nag, T. N. and Khanna, P., Effect of phenylalanine and glucose on growth and phyllemblin production in *Emblica officinalis* Gaertn tissue cultures, *Indian J. Pharm.*, 35(5), 154, 1973.
209. Nagel, M. and Reinhard, E., The volatile oil of tissue cultures of *Ruta graveolens*. II. Physiology of production of the volatile oil, *Planta Medica*, 27, 264, 1975.
210. Nessler, C. L. and Mahlberg, P. G., Ontogeny and cytochemistry of alkaloidal vesicles in laticifers of *Papaver somniferum* L., *Am. J. Bot.*, 64(5), 541, 1977.
211. Nettleship, L. and Slaytor, M., Limitations of feeding experiments in studying alkaloid biosynthesis in *Peganum harmala* callus cultures, *Phytochemistry*, 13, 735, 1974.
212. Nishio, M., Zushi, S., Ishii, T., Furuya, T., and Syōno, K., Mass fragmentographic determination of indole-3-acetic acid in callus tissues of *Panax ginseng* and *Nicotiana tabacum*, *Chem. Pharm. Bull.*, 24(9), 2038, 1976.
213. Noguchi, M., Matsumoto, T., Hirata, Y., Yamamoto, K., Katsuyama, A., Kato, A., Azechi, S., and Kato, K., Improvement of growth rates of plant cell cultures, in *Plant Tissue Culture and Its Bio-technological Application*, Barz, W., Reinhard, E., and Zenk, M. H., Eds., Springer-Verlag, New York, 1977, 85.
214. Okamoto, A., Kawasaki, Y., and Teramoto, T., Production of *Panax ginseng* cells. Japan. Patent (Kokai), 75-135276, 1975.
215. Overton, K. H., Biosynthesis of mevalonoid-derived compounds in cell cultures, in *Plant Tissue Culture and Its Bio-technological Application*, Barz, W., Reinhard, E., and Zenk, M. H., Eds., Springer-Verlag, New York, 1977, 66.
216. Overton, K. H. and Picken, D. J., Studies in secondary metabolism with plant tissue cultures, in *Progress in the Chemistry of Organic Natural Products — 34*, Herz, W., Grisebach, H., and Kirby, G. W., Eds., Springer-Verlag, New York, 1977, 249.
217. Pandya, K. P., Mascarenhas, A. F., and Sayagaver, B. M., Ubiquinone (coenzyme Q) of normal and crown gall tissue cultures of *Parthenocissus* sp., *Indian J. Biochem.*, 3(2), 127, 1966.
218. Paranjothy, K. and Othman, R., Embryoid and plantlet development from cell cultures of *Hevea*, in *Abstr. — 4th Int. Congr. Plant Tissue and Cell Culture*, Thorpe, T. A., Ed., University of Calgary, Canada, 1978, 42.
219. Patterson, B. D. and Carew, D. P., Growth and alkaloid formation in *Catharanthus roseus* tissue cultures, *Lloydia*, 32(2), 131, 1969.
220. Paupardin, C., Sur la differenciation d'un tissu secreteur et la formation d'huile essentielle par des tissus vegetaux cultives *in vitro*, *Congr. Natl. Soc. Savantes Lille Sci.*, 1, 619, 1976.
221. Phillips, R. and Henshaw, G. G., The regulation of synthesis of phenolics in stationary phase cell cultures of *Acer pseudoplatanus* L., *J. Exp. Bot.*, 28(105), 785, 1977.
222. Pierrot, H. and van Wielink, J. E., Localization of glycosidases in the wall of living cells from cultures *Convolvulus arvensis* tissue, *Planta*, 137, 235, 1977.

223. **Pilgrim, H.,** "Cholesterol side-chain cleaving enzyme." Aktivität in keimlingen und *in vitro* kultivierten geweben von *Digitalis purpurea, Phytochemistry,* 11, 1725, 1972.

224. **Pilgrim, H.,** Sapogeninbildung in suspensionkulturen von *Digitalis purpurea, Phytochemistry,* 16, 1311, 1977.

225. **Prasad, S. and Ellis, B. E.,** *In vivo* characterization of catechol ring-cleavage in cell cultures of *Glycine max, Phytochemistry,* 17, 187, 1978.

226. **Radwan, S. S. and Mangold, H. K.,** The lipids of plant tissue cultures, *Adv. Lipid Res.,* 14, 171, 1976.

227. **Ramaswamy, N., Behere, A. G., and Nair, P. M.,** A novel pathway for the synthesis of solanidine in the isolated chloroplast from greening potatoes, *Eur. J. Biochem.,* 67, 275, 1976.

228. **Rai, P. P.,** The production of anthraquinones in callus cultures of *Rheum palmatum, Lloydia,* 41, 114, 1978.

229. **Rai, P. P.,** Production of L-DOPA from callus cultures of *Mucuna sloanei,* in *Abstr. — 4th Int. Congr. Plant Tissue and Cell Culture,* Thorpe, T. B., Ed., University of Calgary, Canada, 1978, 129.

230. **Rao, S. and Mehta, A. R.,** Tyrosine ammonia-lyase in tissue cultures of *Arachis hypogaea* L., in *Abstracts All India Symp. 3rd Confr. Plant Tissue Culture,* Mehta, A. R., Ed., The Maharaja Sayajirao University, Baroda, India, 1978, 21.

231. **Rast, T. L., Lambert, C., Wrightson, M., and Paterson, K.,** Production of wax from jojoba (*Simmondsia chinensis*) cotyledon derived callus: morphogenesis and physiology of explants during first 30 days, in *Abstr. — 4th Int. Congr. Plant Tissue and Cell Culture,* Thorpe, T. A., Ed., University of Calgary, Canada, 1978, 86.

232. **Razzaque, A. and Ellis, B. E.,** Rosmarinic acid production in *Coleus* cell cultures, *Planta,* 137, 287, 1977.

233. **Reichling, J. and Becker, H.,** Tissue culture of *Matricaria chamomilla* L., I. Communication: isolation and maintenance of the tissue culture. Preliminary phytochemical investigations, *Planta Med.,* 30, 258, 1976.

234. **Reigh, D. L., Wender, S. H., and Smith, E. C.,** Scopoletin: a substrate for an isoperoxidase from *Nicotiana tabacum* tissue culture W-38, *Phytochemistry,* 12, 1265, 1973.

235. **Reinhard, E.,** Biotransformations by plant tissue cultures, in *Tissue Culture and Plant Science,* Street, H. E., Ed., Academic Press, New York, 1974, 443.

236. **Reinhard, E., Boy, M., and Kaiser, F.,** Umwandlung von digitalis-glycosiden durch zellsuspensionskulturen, *Planta Med.,* Suppl., 163, 1975.

237. **Reinhard, E., Corduan, G., and Brocke, W. V.,** Untersuchungen über das atherische ol und die cumarine in gewebekulturen von *Ruta graveolens, Herba Hung.,* 10(2—3), 9, 1971.

238. **Reinhard, E., Heins, M., Helmbold, U., and Wahl, J.,** Production of β-methyl-digoxin by cell cultures of *Digitalis lanata,* in *Abstr. — 4th Int. Congr. Plant Tissue and Cell Culture,* Thorpe, T. A., Ed., University of Calgary, Canada, 1978, 79.

239. **Reinhard, E. and Nagel, M.,** The composition of the volatile oil of *Ruta*-callus tissue in relation to culture conditions and differentiation, in *Secondary Metabolism and Coevolution,* Luckner, M., Mothes, K., and Nover, L., Eds., Deutsche Akademie der Naturforscher Leopoldina, Halle, 1976, 335.

240. **Rennenberg, H.,** Gluthathione in conditioned media of tobacco suspension cultures, *Phytochemistry,* 15, 1433, 1976.

241. **Reznickova, S. A., Kireeva, S. A., Bugorsky, P. S., and Melnikov, V. N.,** Terpene accumulation in tissue cultures of rose and mint, in *Abstr. — 4th Int. Congr. Plant Tissue and Cell Culture,* Thorpe, T. A., Ed., University of Calgary, Canada, 1978, 81.

242. **Robinson, N. E.,** The use of protoplastics and cell suspension cultures for the isolation of mutants with altered terpenoid metabolism, in *Abstr. — 4th Int. Congr. Plant Tissue and Cell Culture,* Thorpe, T. A., Ed., University of Calgary, Canada, 1978, 150.

243. **Robinson, T.,** *The Organic Constituents of Higher Plants,* Cordus Press, North Amherst, Mass., 1975.

244. **Roddick, J. G. and Butcher, D. N.,** Isolation of tomatine from cultured excised roots and callus tissues of tomato, *Phytochemistry,* 11, 2019, 1972.

245. **Roller, U.,** Selection of plants and plant tissue cultures of *Catharanthus roseus* with high content of serpentine and ajmalicine, in *Production of Natural Compounds by Cell Culture Methods,* Alfermann, A. W. and Reinhard, E., Eds., Gesellschaft fur Strahlen und Umweltforschung MBH, Munich, 1978, 95.

246. **Ross, S. F., Lines, D. S., Stevens, R. G., and Brain, K. R.,** Epoxidase/epoxide hydrase activity in cell cultures of *Phaseolus vulgaris, Phytochemistry,* 17, 45, 1978.

247. **Rücker, W., Jentzsch, K., and Wichtl, M.,** Root differentiation and glycoside formation in tissues of *Digitalis purpurea* L. cultured *in vitro, Z. Pflanzenphysiol.,* 80, 323, 1976.

248. Ryan, R. C. and Dahl, L. F., Biosynthesis of the indole alkaloids. A cell-free system from *Catharanthus roseus, J. Am. Chem. Soc.*, 97(23), 6906, 1975.

249. Saitoh, T. and Shibata, S., New type chalcones from licorice root, *Tetrahedron Lett.*, 50, 4461, 1975.

250. Saleh, N. A. M., Fritsch, H., Kreuzaler, F., and Grisebach, H,. Flavanone synthase from cell suspension cultures of *Haplopappus gracilis* and comparison with the synthase from parsley, *Phytochemistry*, 17, 183, 1978.

251. Saleh, N. A. M., Fritsch, H., Witkop, P., and Grisebach, H., UDP-glucose: cyanidin 3-*O*-glucosyltransferase from cell cultures of *Haplopappus gracilis, Planta*, 133, 41, 1976.

252. Sandermann, H., Jr., Diesperger, H., and Scheel, D., Metabolism of xenobiotics by plant cell cultures, in *Plant Tissue Culture and Its Bio-technological Application*, Barz, W., Reinhard, E., and Zenk, M. H., Eds., Springer-Verlag, New York, 1977, 178.

253. Schaefer, P. C., de Reinach, F., and Ourisson, G., The conversion of parkeol into its 24-epoxide by tissue cultures of *Nicotiana tabacum, Eur. J. Biochem.*, 14, 284, 1970.

254. Schieder, O., Haploids from *Datura innoxia* as a tool for the production of homozygous lines with high content of scopolamine and for the induction of mutants, in *Production of Natural Compounds by Cell Culture Methods,* Alfermann, A. W. and Reinhard, E., Eds., Gesellschaft fur Strahlen und Umwelforschung MBH, Munich, 1978, 330.

255. Schmid, H. V. and Zenk, M. H., *p*-Hydroxybenzoic acid and mevalonic acid as precursors of the plant naphthoquinone alkannin, *Tetrahedron Lett.*, 44, 4151, 1971.

256. Schrall, R. and Becker, H., Production of catechins and oligomeric proanthocyanidins in tissue and suspension cultures of *Crataegus monogyna, C. oxyacantha* and *Ginkgo biloba, Planta Medica*, 32, 297, 1977.

257. Schrall, R. and Becker, H., Tissue and suspension cultures of *Silybum marianum*. II. Communication: the formation of flavonolignans by feeding suspension cultures with flavonoids and coniferyl alcohol, *Planta Medica*, 32, 27, 1977.

258. Scott, A. I. and Lee, S. L., Biosynthesis of the indole alkaloids. A cell-free system from *Catharanthus roseus, J. Am. Chem. Soc.*, 97(23), 6906, 1975.

259. Segal, R., Breuer, A., and Milo-Goldzweig, I., Solasodine stability under conditions of saponin hydrolysis, *J. Pharm. Sci.*, 67(8), 1169, 1978.

260. Seitz, K., Quantitative Bestimmungsmethoden der Inhaltsstoffe von *Ammi visnaga* durch Direktauswertung von DC-Chromatogrannen und der Nachweis Ihrer Bildung in Gwebekulturen, *Doktarate Dissertation*, Universität Tübingen, 1973.

261. Seitz, U., Accumulation of anthocyanin in *Daucus carota* cell cultures, in *Secondary Metabolism and Coevolution*, Luckner, M., Mothes, K., and Nover, L., Eds., Deutsche Akademie der Naturforscher Leopoldina, Halle, 1976, 89.

262. Sekiya, J. and Hatanaka, A., *Cis*-3-hexenal and *n*-hexanal formation from linolenic and linoleic acids in alfalfa cells cultured *in vitro, Plant Sci. Lett.*, 10, 165, 1977.

263. Sethi, J. K. and Carew, D. P., Growth and betaine formation in *Medicago sativa* tissue cultures, *Phytochemistry*, 13, 321, 1974.

264. Shafiee, A. and Staba, E. J., Allergens from short ragweed leaf tissue cultures, *In Vitro*, 9, 19, 1973.

265. Shankar, G. A. R. and Mehta, A. R., Phytoecdysone production by tissue culture of Trianthema, in *Abstr. Papers, All India Symp. 3rd Confr. Plant Tissue Culture*, Mehta, A. R., Ed., The Maharaja Sayajirao University, Baroda, India, 1978, 26.

266. Shio, I. and Ohta, S., Nicotine production by tobacco callus tissues and effect of plant growth regulators, *Agric. Biol. Chem.*, 37, 1857, 1973.

267. Shafiee, A., Lalezari, I., and Yassa, N., Thebaine in tissue culture of *Papaver bracteatum* Lindl. population Arya. II, *Lloydia*, 39, 380, 1976.

268. Shin, B. S., Mangold, H. K., and Staba, E. J., Lipids of selected plant tissue cultures, in *Colloq. Int. C.N.R.S.*, 193, 51, 1973.

269. Shyr, S. E. and Staba, E. J., Examination of squill tissue cultures for bufadienolides and anthocyanins, *Planta Medica*, 30, 86, 1976.

270. Simola, L. K., Changes in the activity of several enzymes during root differentiation in cultured cells of *Atropa belladonna., Z. Pflanzenphysiol.*, 68, 373, 1973.

271. Sita, G., Bammi, R. K., and Randhawa, G. S., Clonal propagation of *Dioscorea floribunda* by tissue culture *J. Hortic. Sci.*, 51, 551, 1976.

272. Spener, F., Nothelfer, H. G., and Buchhalz, S,. Biosynthesis of straight-chain fatty acids and cyclopentenyl fatty acids in cell suspension cultures, in *Abstr. — 4th Int. Congr. Plant Tissue and Cell Culture*, Thorpe, T. A., Ed., University of Calgary, Canada, 1978, 85.

273. Srivastava, O. M. P. and van Huystee, R. B., IAA oxidase and polyphenol oxidase activities of peanut peroxidase isozymes, *Phytochemistry*, 16, 1527, 1977.

274. **Staba, E. J.,** Plant tissue culture as a technique for the phytochemist, in *Recent Advances in Phytochemistry,* Vol. 2, Seikel, M. K. and Runeckles, V. C., Eds., Appleton-Century-Crofts, New York, 1969, 75.

275. **Staba, E. J.,** Tissue culture and pharmacy, in *Plant Cell, Tissue, and Organ Culture,* Reinert, J. and Bajaj, Y. P. S., Eds., Springer-Verlag, New York, 1977, 694.

276. **Staba, E. J., Laursen, P., and Büchner, S. A.,** Medicinal plant tissue cultures, in *Proceedings of an Inter. Confr. on Plant Tissue Culture,* White, P. R., Ed., McCuthan Publishing, Berkeley, Calif., 1965, 191.

277. **Staba, E. J. and Jindra, A.,** *Datura* tissue cultures: production of minor alkaloids from chlorophyllous and nonchlorophyllous strains, *J. Pharm. Sci.,* 57(4), 701, 1968.

278. **Staba, E. J. and Kaul, B.,** Production of Diosgenin by Plant Tissue Culture Technique, U.S. Patent 3628,287, 1971.

279. **Staba, E. J. and Shafiee, A.,** Production of Allergens by Plant Tissue Culture Technique, U.S. Patent 3,846,937, 1974.

280. **Staba, E. J., Shin, B. S., and Mangold, H. K.,** Lipids in plant tissue cultures. I. The fatty acid composition of triglycerides in rape and turnip rape cultures, *Chem. Phys. Lipids,* 6, 291, 1971.

281. **Stark, V. D., Alfermann, A. W., and Reinhard, E.,** Phenylalanine-ammonia-lyase activity and biosynthesis of anthocyanins and chlorogenic acid in tissue cultures of *Daucus carota, Planta Med.,* 30, 104, 1976.

282. **Steck, W., Bailey, B. K., Shyluk, J. P., and Gamborg, O. L.,** Coumarins and alkaloids from cell cultures of *Ruta graveolens, Phytochemistry,* 10, 191, 1971.

283. **Steck, W. and Constabel, F.,** Biotransformations in plant cell cultures, *Lloydia,* 37, 2, 1974.

284. **Steck, W., Gamborg, O. L., and Bailey, B. K.,** Increased yields of alkaloids through precursor biotransformations in cell suspension cultures of *Ruta graveolens, Lloydia,* 36, 1, 1973.

285. **Stöbart, A. K., Weir, N. R., and Thomas, D. R.,** Phytol in tissue cultures of *Kalanchoe crenata, Phytochemistry,* 8, 1089, 1969.

286. **Stöckigt, J., Husson, H. P., Kan-Fan, C., and Zenk, M. H.,** Cathenamine, a central intermediate in the cell free biosynthesis of ajmalicine and related indole alkaloids, *J. Chem. Soc. Chem. Commun.,* 164, 1977.

287. **Stöckigt, J., Rueffler, M., Zenk, M. H., and Hoyer, G. A.,** Indirect identification of 4,21-dehydrocorynantheine aldehyde as an intermediate in the biosynthesis of ajmalicine and related alkaloids, *Planta Medica,* 33, 188, 1978.

288. **Stöckigt, J., Treimer, J., and Zenk, M. H.,** Synthesis of ajmalicine and related indole alkaloids by cell free extracts of *Catharanthus roseus* cell suspension cultures, *FEBS Lett.,* 70, 1, 1976.

289. **Stöckigt, J. and Zenk, M. H.,** Enzymatic synthesis of chlorogenic acid from caffeoyl co-enzyme A and quinic acid, *FEBS Lett.,* 42(2), 131, 1974.

290. **Stöckigt, J. and Zenk, M. H.,** Isovincoside (strictosidine), the key intermediate in the enzymatic formation of indole alkaloids, *FEBS Lett.,* 79, 2, 1977.

291. **Stohs, S. J.,** Production of scopolamine and hyoscyamine by *Datura stramonium* L. suspension cultures, *J. Pharm. Sci.,* 58(6), 703, 1969.

292. **Stohs, S. J.,** Metabolism of steroids in plant tissue cultures, in *Plant Tissue Culture and Its Biotechnological Application,* Barz, W., Reinhard, E., and Zenk, M. H., Eds., Springer-Verlag, New York, 1977, 142.

293. **Stohs, S. J. and el-Olemy, M. M.,** Cholesterol metabolism by *Cheiranthus cheiri* leaf and tissue culture homogenates, *J. Steroid Biochem.,* 2, 293, 1971.

294. **Stohs, S. J. and el-Olemy, M. M.,** 4-Androsten-3,17-dione metabolism by *Dioscorea deltoidea* suspension cultures, *Lloydia,* 35 (1), 81, 1972.

295. **Stohs, S. J. and el-Olemy, M. M.,** Metabolism of progesterone by *Dioscorea deltoidea* suspension cultures, *Phytochemistry,* 11, 1397, 1972.

296. **Stohs, S. J. and el-Olemy, M. M.,** Pregnenolone and progesterone metabolism by cardenolide producing leafs, *Phytochemistry,* 11, 2409, 1972.

297. **Stohs, S. J. and Haggerty, J. A.,** Metabolism of 4-cholesten-3-one to 5α-cholestan-3-one by leaf homogenates, *Phytochemistry,* 12, 2869, 1973.

298. **Stohs, S. J., Kaul, B., and Staba, E. J.,** The metabolism of ^{14}C-cholesterol by *Dioscorea deltoidea* suspension cultures, *Phytochemistry,* 8, 1679, 1969.

299. **Stohs, S. J. and Rosenberg, H.,** Steroids and steroid metabolism in plant tissue cultures, *Lloydia,* 38(3), 181, 1975.

300. **Stohs, S. J., Rosenberg, H., and Billetts, S.,** Sterols of *Yucca glauca* tissue cultures and seeds, *Planta Med.,* 28, 257, 1975.

301. **Stohs, S. J., Sabatka, J. J., and Rosenberg, H.,** Incorporation of 4-^{14}C-22,23-^{3}H-sitosterol into diosgenin by *Dioscorea deltoidea* tissue suspension cultures, *Phytochemistry,* 13, 2145, 1974.

302. **Stohs, S. J. and Staba, E. J.,** Production of cardiac glycosides by plant tissue cultures, IV. Biotransformation of digitoxigenin and related substances, *J. Pharm. Sci.,* 54, 56, 1964.

303. **Stohs, S. J., Tarng, C. S., and Rosenberg, H.,** Influence of cyclic AMP on growth and steroid formation in *Corchorus olitorius* L. suspension cultures, *Lloydia,* 40, 4, 1977.

304. **Suga, T., Hirata, T., Hirano, Y., and Ito, T.,** Biotransformation of monoterpenes by tobacco tissue cultures. Selective hydroxylation of trans-methyl group in isopropyridene group, *Chem. Lett.,* 1245, 1976.

305. **Sugano, N., Iwata, R., and Nishi, A.,** Formation of phenolic acid in carrot cells in suspension culture, *Phytochemistry,* 14, 1205, 1975.

306. **Sugano, N., Miya, S., and Nishi, A.,** Carotenoid synthesis in a suspension culture of carrot cells, *Plant Cell Physiol.,* 12, 525, 1971.

307. **Surholt, E. and Hoesel, W.,** Screening for flavonol 3-glycoside specific β-glycosidases in plants using a spectrophotometric enzymatic assay, *Phytochemistry,* 17, 873, 1978.

308. **Suzuki, H., Ikeda, T., Matsumoto T., and Noguchi, M.,** Isolation and identification of phyllodulcin and skimmin from the cultured cells of *Amacha, Agric. Biol. Chem.,* 41(4), 719, 1977.

309. **Szoke, E., Kuzovkina, I. N., Verzar-Petri, G., and Smirnov, A. M.,** Cultivation of wild chamomile tissue, *Sov. Plant Physiol.,* 24(4), 832, 1977.

310. **Szoke, E., Verzar-Petri, G., and Shavarda, A. L.,** Biosynthesis of volatile oils in tissue cultures of *Matricaria chamomilla* L., in *Abstr. — 4th Int. Congr. Plant Tissue and Cell Culture,* Thorpe, T. A., Ed., University of Calgary, Canada, 1978, 82.

311. **Tabata, M.,** Recent advances in the production of medicinal substances by plant cell cultures, in *Plant Tissue Culture and Its Bio-technological Applicaion,* aearz, W., Reinhard, E., and Zenk, M. H., Eds., Springer-Verlag, New York, 1977, 3.

312. **Tabata, M. and Hiraoka, N.,** Variation of alkaloid production in *Nicotiana rustica* callus cultures, *Physiol. Plant.,* 38, 19, 1976.

313. **Tabata, M., Hiraoka, N., Ikenoue, M., Sano, Y., and Konoshima, M.,** The production of anthraquinones in callus cultures of *Cassia tora, Lloydia,* 38, 2, 1975.

314. **Tabata, M., Yamamoto, H., Hiraoka, N., and Konoshima, M.,** Organization and alkaloid production in tissue cultures of *Scopolia parviflora, Phytochemistry,* 11, 949, 1972.

315. **Tabata, M., Ikeda, F., Hiroaka, N., and Konoshima, M.,** Glucosylation of phenolic compounds by *Datura innoxia* suspension cultures, *Phytochemistry,* 15, 1225, 1976.

316. **Tabata, M., Ogino, T., Yoshioka, K., Yoshikawa, N., and Hiraoka, N.,** Selection of cell lines with higher yield of secondary products, in *Abstr. — 4th Int. Congr. Plant Tissue and Cell Culture,* Thorpe, T. A., Ed., University of Calgary, Canada, 1978, 12.

317. **Takeya, K. and Itokawa, H.,** Stereochemistry in oxidation of allylic alcohols by cell-free system of callus induced from *Cannabis sativa* L., *Chem. Pharm. Bull.,* 25(8), 1947, 1977.

318. **Tamaki, E., Morishita, I., Nishida, K., Kato, K., and Matsumoto, T.,** Process for Preparing Licorice Extract-Like Material for Tobacco Flavoring, U.S. Patent 3,710,512, 1973.

319. **Thomas, E. and Street, H. E.,** Organogenesis in cell suspension cultures of *Atropa belladonna* L. and *Atropa belladonna* cultivar *lutea* Döll., *Ann. Bot. (London),* 34(136), 657, 1970.

320. **Tomita, Y. and Seo, S.,** Biosynthesis of terpenes maslinic acid and 3-epimaslinic acid in tissue cultures of *Isodon japonicus* Hara, *J. Chem. Soc. Chem. Commun.,* 707, 1973.

321. **Tomita, Y. and Uomori, A.,** Mechanism of biosynthesis of the ethyl side-chain at C-24 of stigmasterol in tissue cultures of *Nicotiana tabacum* and *Dioscorea* tokoro, *J. Chem. Soc. Chem. Commun.,* 1416, 1970.

322. **Tomita, Y. and Uomori, A.,** Biosynthesis of sapogenins in tissue cultures of *Dioscorea tokoro* Makino, *J. Chem. Soc. Chem. Commun.,* 284, 1971.

323. **Tomita, H. and Uomori, A.,** Structure and biosynthesis of protookoronin in tissue cultures of *Dioscorea tokoro, Phytochemistry,* 13, 729, 1974.

324. **Tomita, Y., Uomori, A., and Minato, H.,** Sesquiterpenes and phytosterols in the tissue cultures of *Lindera strychnifolia, Phytochemistry,* 8, 2249, 1969.

325. **Tomita, Y., Uomori, A., and Minato, H.,** Steroidal sapogenins and sterols in tissue culture of *Dioscorea tokoro, Phytochemistry,* 9, 111, 1970.

326. **Townsley, P. M.,** Chocolate aroma from plant cells, *J. Inst. Can. Sci. Technol. Aliment.,* 7 (1), 76, 1974.

327. **Townsley, P. M.,** The development of secondary by-products from plant cell cultures, *Dev. Ind. Microbiol.,* 18, 619, 1977.

328. **Treimer, J. F. and Zenk, M. H.,** Enzymic synthesis of Corynanthe-type alkaloids in cell cultures of *Catharanthus roseus*: quantitation of radioimmunoassay, *Phytochemistry,* 17, 227, 1978.

329. **Tsang, Y. F. and Ibrahim, R. K.,** O-Methyltransferase (OMT) of tobacco cell suspension cultures, in *Abstr. — 4th Int. Congr. Plant Tissue and Cell Culture,* Thorpe, T. A., Ed., University of Calgary, Canada, 1978, 122.

330. **Tschesche, R. and Spindler, M.,** Zur biogenese des aza-oxa-spiran-systems der steroidalkaloide vom spirosolan-typ in solanaceen, *Phytochemistry,* 17, 251, 1978.

331. **Tulecke, W.,** Growth of tissues of higher plants in continuous liquid culture and their use in a nutritional experiment, Rep. No. AMRL-TR-65-101, Aerospace Medical Division, Wright-Patterson Air Force Base, Ohio, 1965.

332. **Turnbull, A. and Collin, H. A.,** Flavour production in onion tissue cultures, in *Abstr. — Int. Congr. Plant Tissue and Cell Culture,* Thorpe, T. A., Ed., University of Calgary, Canada, 1978, 83.

333. **Ueda, Y., Ishiyama, H., Fukui, M., and Nishi, A.,** Invertase in cultured *Daucus carota* cells, *Phytochemistry,* 13, 383, 1974.

334. **van Huystee, R. B.,** Immunological studies on proteins released by a peanut (*Arachis hypogaea* L.) suspension culture, *Bot. Gaz. (Chicago),* 137(4), 325, 1976.

335. **van Huystee, R. B.,** Peroxidase synthesis in and membranes from cultured peanut cells, *Phytochemistry,* 17, 191, 1978.

336. **van de Voort, F. and Townsley, P. M.,** A comparison of the unsaponifiable lipids isolated from coffee cell cultures and from green coffee beans, *J. Inst. Can. Sci. Technol. Aliment,* 8, 4, 1975.

337. **van Staden, J. and Davey, J. E.,** The metabolism of zeatin and zeatin riboside by soya bean callus, *Ann. Bot. (London),* 41, 1031, 1977.

338. **Vagujfalvi, D., Maroti, M., and Tetenyi, P.,** Presence of diosgenin and absence of solasodine in tissue cultures of *Solanum laciniatum, Phytochemistry,* 10, 1389, 1971.

339. **Veliky, I. A.,** Synthesis of carboline alkaloids by plant cell cultures, *Phytochemistry,* 11, 1405, 1972.

340. **Veliky, I. A.,** Effect of pH on tryptophol formation by cultured *Ipomoea* sp. plant cells, *Lloydia,* 40, 5, 1977.

341. **Veliky, I. A. and Genest, K.,** Growth and metabolites of *Cannabis sativa* cell suspension cultures, *Lloydia,* 35(4), 450, 1972.

342. **Veliky, I. A. and Barber, K. M.,** Biotransformation of tryptophan by *Phaseolus vulgaris* suspension culture, *Lloydia,* 38(2), 125, 1975.

343. **Veliky, I. A. and Jones, A.,** Biotransformation of cardiotonic aglycones by plant cell suspension cultures of non-digitalis species, in *Abstr. — 4th Int. Congr. Plant Tissue and Cell Culture,* Thorpe, T. A., Ed., University of Calgary, Canada, 1978, 78.

344. **Veliky, I., Sandkvist, A., and Martin, S. M.,** Physiology of, and enzyme production by, plant cell cultures, *Biotechnol. Bioeng.,* 11(6), 1247, 1969.

345. **Verzar-Petri, G. and Szoke, E.,** Alkaloid production and biosynthesis in different tissue cultures from *Datura innoxia* Mill., in *Abstr. — 4th Int. Congr. Plant Tissue and Cell Culture,* Thorpe, T. A., Ed., University of Calgary, Canada, 1978, 126.

346. **von Sipply, K. J. and Friedrich, H.,** Alkaloide im kallus von *Dubosia myoporoides, Planta Medica,* Suppl., 186, 1978.

347. **Wang, C. and Staba, E. J.,** Peppermint and spearmint tissue culture. II. Dual carboy culture of spearmint tissues, *J. Pharm. Sci.,* 52, 1058, 1963.

348. **Wellmann, E. and Schopfer, P.,** Phytochrome-mediated *de novo* synthesis of phenylalanine ammonia-lyase in cell suspension cultures of parsley, *Plant Physiol.,* 55, 822, 1975.

349. **Whitmore, F. W.,** Lignin-carbohydrate complex formed in isolated cell walls of callus, *Phytochemistry,* 17, 421, 1978.

350. **Widholm, J. M.,** Relation between auxin autotrophy and tryptophan accumulation in cultured plant cells, *Planta,* 134, 103, 1977.

351. **Wilson, G.,** The application of the chemostat technique to the study of growth and anthraquinone synthesis by *Galium mollugo* cells, in *Production of Natural Compounds by Cell Culture Methods,* Alfermann, A. W. and Reinhard, E., Eds., Gesellschaft fur Strahlen und Umwelforschung MBH, Munich, 1978, 147.

352. **Wu, W. L., Staba, E. J., and Blumenthal, M.,** Multi-liter production and immunochemical cross-reactivity of plant tissue culture antigens, *J. Pharm. Sci.,* 65, 102, 1976.

353. **Yafin, Y. and Shechter, I.,** Comparison between biosynthesis of *ent*-kaurene in germinating tomato seeds and cell suspension cultures of tomato and tobacco, *Plant. Physiol.,* 56, 671, 1975.

354. **Yanagawa, H., Kato, T., and Kitahara, Y.,** Chemical components of callus tissues of pumpkins, *Phytochemistry,* 10, 2775, 1971.

355. **Yanagawa, H., Kato, T., and Kitahara, Y.,** Chemical components of callus tissues of rice, *Phytochemistry,* 11, 1893, 1972.

356. **Yie, S. T. and Liaw, S. I.,** Plant regeneration from shoot tips and callus of papaya, *In Vitro,* 13(9), 564, 1977.

357. **Yoshikawa, K., Suzuki, M., and Maruoka, M.,** Production of *Rauwolfia* Alkaloids, Japan Patent (Kokai) 73-80789, 1973.

358. **Yu, P. L. C., el-Olemy, M. M., and Stohs, S. J.,** A phytochemical investigation of *Withania somnifera* tissue cultures, *Lloydia,* 37(4), 593, 1974.

359. **Zacharius, R. M. and Osman, S. F.,** Glycoalkaloids in tissue culture of *Solanum* species. Dehydrocommersonine from cultured roots of *Solanum chacoense, Plant Sci. Lett.,* 10, 283, 1977.

360. **Zacharius, R. M., Osman, S. F., and Varns, J. L.,** Behavior of potato callus in secondary metabolite development, in *Abstr. — 4th Int. Congr. Plant Tissue and Cell Culture,* Thorpe, T. A., Ed., University of Calgary, Canada, 1978, 129.

361. **Zenk, M. H.,** The impact of plant tissue culture on industry, in *Abstr. — 4th Int. Congr. Plant Tissue and Cell Culture,* Thorpe, T. A., Ed., University of Calgary, Canada, 1978, 1.

362. **Zenk, M. H., el-Shagi, H., Arens, H., Stöckigt, J., Weiler, E. W., and Deus, B.,** Formation of the indole alkaloids serpentine and ajmalicine in cell suspension cultures of *Catharanthus roseus,* in *Plant Tissue Culture and Its Bio-technological Application,* Barz, W., Reinhard, E., and Zenk, M. H., Eds., Springer-Verlag, New York, 1977, 27.

363. **Zenk, M. H., el-Shagi, H., and Schulte, U.,** Anthraquinone production by cell suspension cultures of *Morinda citrifolia, Planta Medica,* Suppl., 79, 1975.

364. **Zenk, M. H., el-Shagi, H., and Ulbrich, B.,** Production of rosmarinic acid by cell-suspension cultures of *Coleus blumei, Naturwissenschaften,* 64, 585, 1977.

Chapter 4

SELECTION OF PLANT CELL LINES WHICH ACCUMULATE CERTAIN COMPOUNDS

J. M. Widholm

TABLE OF CONTENTS

I. SCOPE

This chapter will propose a fundamentally different approach to the problem of compound production by tissue cultures. This approach involves the exploitation of the natural or induced variability among cells by selecting variant cell lines which produce the desired compounds. These lines may be selected at a low frequency from large populations. This is in contrast to the usual approach where attempts are made to induce the entire wild type culture to produce the compound. Once a variant line is selected, the assumption is made that the production ability will be carried to each progeny cell. Various methods of selecting this infrequent variant will be discussed along with a review of the past selection work with plant cell cultures. General tissue culture methodology and the types of culture systems which are available will also be discussed.

Throughout this chapter, the term "line" will be used to describe a cell culture which has certain defined characteristics. These would include such designations as wild type, resistant, autotrophic, slow growing, etc., even though every cell in the line may not be identical.

II. DESIRED GOALS

Since the proposed selection schemes are relatively specific as to which compounds are likely to be produced, a consideration of the compounds which are desired must be made before beginning to design the selection method and before choosing the cell lines to use.

If the compounds desired are primary compounds (i.e., are present in all species at all times), like amino acids or nucleotides, then the choice of the cell line to use may not be limited to any particular species. In this case, the main consideration would be how desirable the culture growth and handling characteristics are. If the desired compounds are secondary compounds (i.e., are not present in all species at all times), like pigments, polyphenolics, or alkaloids, then the culture used should most probably be initiated from a species known to normally produce the desired compound. Whether cultures should be initiated from high-yielding plants for best results or not has not been thoroughly studied. However, Zenk et al.[1] did show that cultures from seedlings of plants yielding high serpentine and ajmalicine levels did contain higher levels of these compounds than cultures from low alkaloid-containing plants.

The design of the selection system must take into account all available knowledge of the biosynthetic pathway of the desired compound. For example, the biosynthesis of most amino acids in plants has been shown to be under end-product feedback control. This feedback control maintains the desired level of that amino acid in the cell. Several systems have been used, however, to screen large numbers of cells for individuals which have an altered feedback-control enzyme which allows a buildup of the end-product amino acid.[2] Toxic amino acid analogs are used to inhibit cell growth. It is known that the corresponding natural free amino acid will reverse the growth inhibition if the analog is truly an analog. Thus, cells that accumulate higher than normal levels of the corresponding amino acid will be resistant to growth inhibition by the analog. These resistant cells will grow under normally inhibitory conditions so will be selected from the wild type population.

This method of selection for the accumulation of some compound requires that the analog inhibition be reversible by the corresponding natural compound no matter what the mechanism of growth inhibition of the analog is. The natural compound must also be required for cell survival, or the analog should not be toxic in the first place.

The requirement that the desired compound be necessary for survival might imply that this selection method cannot be used to select for secondary compounds, since they may not always be needed by the cell. Several studies have shown, however, that overproduction of certain precursors (amino acids) may lead to the synthesis of certain secondary compounds (polyphenolics, indoleacetic acid) which are derived from the precursor molecules. These examples will be discussed later. Thus, these methods may be applicable to most compounds found in plants.

Selection for pigment production can be done by visually picking out colonies which show the highest pigment production. In similar fashion, production of other compounds which can be measured analytically can be selected after analysis of many colonies for the compound.

The general methodology proposed, then, must be tailored to the compound desired and the known characteristics of it and its' biosynthetic and degradative pathways.

III. CULTURE SYSTEMS

In order to design a selection system, one must consider not only the biochemical aspects of the desired compound and the plant species to be cultured, but one also must consider the culturing systems which are available.

Most tissue culture media contain minerals, an energy source (usually sucrose), one or a few vitamins, and hormones. The hormones almost invariably include an auxin such as 2,4-dichlorophenoxyacetic acid (2,4-D) or indoleacetic acid (IAA) and, sometimes, a cytokinin is found to be necessary. Other simple components, like amino acids or inositol, or undefined mixtures, like casamino acids, yeast extract, malt extract, potato extract, or coconut milk, may also be included. These may be necessary for or may stimulate growth, but when present they complicate the culture system biochemically. This may or may not matter, depending upon the goals of the work.

The use of the callus cultures in many studies is hampered by the lack of direct cell contact with the medium since the cells are piled upon each other. It is also difficult to make uniform transfers, both in terms of mass of tissue and uniformity of cell type, when transferring tissue pieces with a spatula. The callus system has, however, been used successfully in screening for streptomycin, 5-bromodeoxyuridine, and corn-blight-toxin resistance.[3,4,5]

Suspension culture systems have certain advantages including: (1) faster growth rate, (2) relatively uniform transfers can be made with widebore pipettes, (3) almost any cell can be easily viewed in the microscope, (4) the liquid medium is in direct contact with almost every cell, (5) the medium can be altered easily by additions or can be rinsed away and fresh medium added, and (6) the cells can be plated directly. Suspension-culture systems have been used to select cell lines resistant to many amino acid analogs[6,7,8,9,10] and to NaCl.[11]

Plating cells in agar-solidified medium has many uses and can be accomplished with callus, suspension cultures, or protoplasts. Callus can be shaken apart in liquid medium or pushed through a screen before suspending in liquid medium for plating. Suspension-cultured cells can be used directly if the suspended cell clumps are not too large. Freshly prepared protoplasts can also be plated after preparation from tissue cultures, leaves, or about any other plant part using enzymes which remove the cell wall. Once the protoplasts are plated, the cell wall is reformed and the cells divide and form colonies. Plated protoplasts and cells have been used to select NaCl,[12] amino-pterin-,[13] methionine sulfoximine-,[14] and 5-bromodeoxyuridine-resistant lines.[15]

Cloning is a useful technique whereby a cell line is initiated from a single cell so that all the cells in the resulting line should be genetically equivalent. This can be very important to insure purity and stability of desirable lines. If protoplasts or single cells can be induced to divide, the colonies that form from each would be a clone. Cell division may not occur, however, when cells are plated at a low population density unless special techniques are used to eliminate this obstacle. Complex components such as conditioned medium can be added to the medium. A feeder layer of cells[16] or a callus with a filter paper to separate a single isolated cell (nurse culture[17]) have been used successfully to obtain clones. In general, cloning techniques are far from being efficient or routine.

A potentially useful technique which has not been generally successful with plant cells is replica plating. With bacteria, colonies growing on plates can be blotted with a velvet cloth and stamped onto other plates to give the same colony pattern on each. The effect of different media can then be ascertained easily by noting the growth on each medium. This is usually done one colony at a time with plant tissue cultures, although Schulte and Zenk[18] have reported a method for transferring the colony pattern to one plate from another with 80% efficiency using a nylon net.

Recently, isolated microspores of *Nicotiana tabacum, N. sylvestris* and *Datura innoxia* have been induced to form embryos and, in turn, plants.[19] This system can provide single, separated haploid cells which might be very useful for screening. The feasibility of this method depends upon the numbers of embryos which can be obtained. Nitsch[19] finds that an average of about 5% of *N. tabacum* microspores develop into plantlets. Since there are five anthers in each flower, and each anther contains about 30,000 microspores, an average of about 7500 plantlets can be produced from each flower. Thus, a reasonably large number of developing embryos can be obtained using this system. No selection work has been accomplished to date with any microspore system, however.

Despite several direct comparisons of plant cell cultures to microbes, the fact remains that the plant cell is not as easy to work with as the microbe. The plant cells generally grow more slowly, form clumps of cells, do not grow if plated at low density, lack stable haploidy, and show chromosome and ploidy instability. These problems do not exclude the successful manipulations of plant cells, but do make progress slower and more difficult.

IV. VISUAL SELECTION

Many cell lines which accumulate high levels of various colored compounds have been selected over the years by visual selection. Cells which show the desired coloration are picked out and subcultured until a pure line is established.

Eichenberger, in 1951,[20] reported the isolation of a *Daucus carota* callus line high in β-carotene. This high level was maintained in the line for more than 10 years.[21] Differences in anthocyanin content in *Zea mays* endosperm callus led to the isolation of stable lines with different pigment levels.[22] *Haplopappus gracilis* cultures with high levels of anthocyanin were likewise isolated.[23] Stable strains which accumulated high levels of red betalain pigments were selected from the normally white callus of *Beta vulgaris* by visual selection.[24] Strains of *Macleaya microcarpa* with both high and low levels of protopine alkaloids were selected using pigmentation as a marker.[25] Cell clones of *Atropa belladonna* were also shown to give different pigmentation patterns.[26]

Recently, variant *D. carota* strains have been selected in several different laboratories. Four clones with varying β-carotene and lycopene levels were isolated from mutagenized, plated cells.[27] The alterations persisted for at least 1 year, and variants were observed only after mutagen treatment. The lines were isolated from two lines which had different and stable carotenoid compositions. Alfermann et al.[28] isolated lines with different anthocyanin levels which correlated positively with the phenylalanine-ammonia-lyase activity of the cells. These traits were stable for over six years. Mok et al.[29] initiated cultures from several carrot-root-pigment phenotypes (red, dark orange, orange, light orange, yellow, and white). Variations in coloration were noted in lines derived from different sources and also in lines from the same source. However, some relationship to the source of the culture was noted as carotenes predominated in cultures from red and orange roots, while xanthophylls predominated in cultures from yellow and white roots. The levels of the carotenes varied, but the main component was the same as that of the root. Lycopene was the main component in red-root-derived cultures, and β-carotene was the component in orange ones. Kinetin and 2,4-D treatments were found to affect the pigment levels. While cultures initiated from a single root were often of widely different colors and carotenoid contents, plants regenerated from these variant lines all had the same phenotype as the original root. Thus, the variation seen in the pigmentation of these cultured *D. carota* cells would either not appear to be due to a mutation, or the regenerated plants did not originate from the altered, pigmented-cell types.

While the pigments which have been selected for in culture are not especially valuable economically, a method might be devised to select for more desirable uncolored compounds if a correlation can be established with the valuable compound and that of a pigment which can be selected visually. Such a scheme might even utilize UV light or fluorescence for detection, depending upon the compound in question.

V. CHEMICAL ANALYSIS SELECTION

Another method of selection similar to visual selection is one in which compounds are measured chemically in cell colonies in order to identify high-producing lines. This method was used by Zenk et al.[1] to select *Catharanthus roseus* strains which produce much higher than normal levels of the indole alkaloids, serpentine and ajmalicine.

Zenk et al.[1] developed a highly sensitive and specific radioimmunoassay (RIA) for both serpentine and ajmalicine. Besides specificity and sensitivity, the successful application of chemical analysis methods to selection also requires rapidity so that large numbers of samples can be analyzed. Zenk's method was applied to crude extracts where more than 200 samples per day could be processed. This RIA was capable of detecting down to 0.1 ng in 0.1 mℓ samples. Serpentine and ajmalicine were not cross reactive, and no other compounds were found to be cross reactive except the diastereomers of the haptans (about 10%). These compounds are known to be present in only trace amounts, if at all, in *C. roseus*, however.

With this analytical method in hand, Zenk et al.[1] used the following strategy to select high serpentine- and ajmalicine-producing strains of *C. roseus* : (1) use callus derived from high-producing plants, (2) select variant strains capable of high production, and (3) develop the optimal production medium.

The content of the two alkaloids were first determined in root extracts from 184 *C. roseus* plants with different geographic origins which were grown under controlled conditions. Large differences in alkaloid levels were found. Callus was initiated from seedlings from self-fertilized plants of both high and low alkaloid potential. These calli were placed in a culture medium which was known to cause the production of alkaloids in a previously established line. The seven calli from individual seedlings from the high-producing plant did, on the average, produce more serpentine than did calli from seedlings from a low-producing plant. The high-producing plant root contained 0.93% dry weight serpentine, and cultures from its seedlings had an average of 70 mg/ℓ. The low-producing plant contained 0.17% serpentine, and the cultures had 16 mg/ℓ. There was considerable variation between calli, however, indicating that additional selection might pick out higher-producing strains.

Selection of high-producing strains was accomplished by filtering suspension cultures to obtain single cells and small aggregates which were then plated in agar-solidified medium. The colonies which formed were analyzed for alkaloid content, and as expected, wide variations were noted (from 0 to 1.4% serpentine and 0 to 0.8% ajmalicine on a dry-weight basis). Stable high-producing strains were isolated after high-producing colonies were cultured in liquid medium, replated, and retested.

Production was optimized by varying the medium composition and by adding various precursors. Optimal production was obtained with Linsmaier and Skoog[30] basic medium with 10^{-6} M indoleacetic acid, 5×10^{-6} M benzyladenine, 5% sucrose, and 0.05% L-tryptophan. Production rates of 162 mg/l serpentine by one strain, and 77 mg/l serpentine and 264 mg/l ajmalicine by another, were attained. This production occurred during a growth period of, apparently, about 30 days. The production of the strains was found to fluctuate, but high production could always be reestablished.

An example of an ideal analysis system is the nuclear magnetic resonance (NMR) corn-seed-oil analysis system of Alexander et al.[31] The system has been improved to the point that seed samples down to 30 mg in weight are automatically and nondestructively analyzed for oil content in 2 sec. The single seed can then be grown for further testing. This system may not be applicable, in a nondestructive manner, to tissue-culture testing since the water content of the samples must be below 4.5% during the analysis.

Selection for overproduction can be done visually if a system can be devised whereby the desired compound diffuses from the cell and reacts with some reagent in the agar medium to form a colored compound. High-producing colonies could then be identified and recovered.

Crossfeeding of an indicator organism like bacteria which requires a certain compound for growth might also be effective in identifying oversynthesis. We found that wild type carrot and tobacco cells feed amino acid auxotrophic *Escherichia coli* about the same as lines which overproduce several amino acids, however (unpublished).

It would seem that the general methods discussed in this section have shown promise for developing desired high-producing lines. They should be continued and expanded.

VI. RESISTANCE SELECTION

Lines which accumulate certain compounds can be isolated from large cell populations by selecting for resistance to certain growth-inhibitory substances. The inhibitor should be a toxic analog of a required cell metabolite whose toxicity can be reversed by the corresponding natural compound. In some cases, the accumulation of one compound is shown to affect the level of other compounds which are derived from the first.

The use of amino acid analogs which inhibit cell-culture growth serve to illustrate this technique. Several analogs have been used which may act by incorporation into protein, by false feedback inhibition of a biosynthetic enzyme, or by some other mechanism. The reason for the toxicity is not important to the selection procedure as long as the inhibitory effect can be reversed by the addition of the corresponding natural amino acid. If this happens, then mutants which accumulate the natural amino acid will be resistant to growth inhibition. Resistant lines can be selected by growing large numbers of cells in the presence of the inhibitory analog. The biosynthesis of most amino acids is controlled by feedback inhibition, and only part of the control-enzyme molecules need to be less resistant to feedback inhibition to allow oversynthesis of the endproduct. Thus, the resistance to analog growth inhibition caused by the oversynthesis of a compound should be a dominant trait and, therefore, should be selectable from diploid or higher ploidy cells.

The best-studied system in plants is 5-methyltryptophan (5MT) resistance which has been selected from several suspension-cultured lines.[2] Most cell lines resistant to 5MT

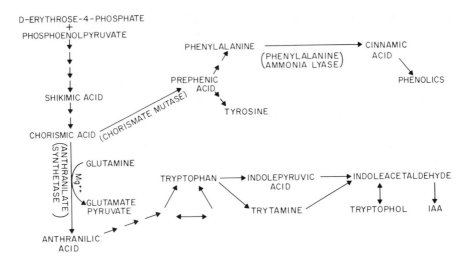

FIGURE 1. Shikimate pathway for phenylalanine and tryptophan synthesis with additional reactions leading to phenolics and indoleacetic acid.

have much higher than normal levels of free tryptophan. Tryptophan is synthesized in plants by the shikimate pathway. This pathway utilizes erythrose-4-phosphate and phosphoenolpyruvate to make chorismate through several enzymatic steps with shikimate as an intermediate (Figure 1). Chorismate is the branchpoint compound which can be converted by chorismate mutase to prephenate. Prephenate leads to phenylalanine and tyrosine. Chorismate can also be utilized by anthranilate synthetase to make anthranilate, which can be converted to tryptophan by the action of four enzymes (Figure 1). Chorismate mutase is feedback inhibited by phenylalanine and tyrosine, while anthranilate synthetase is inhibited by tryptophan. Repression of enzyme synthesis does not appear to operate with the enzymes in this pathway in higher plants.[32,33]

Anthranilate synthetase from *E. coli,* like the enzyme from higher plants, is feedback inhibited by tryptophan as well as by 5MT. Moyed[34] and Somerville and Yanofsky[35] selected *E. coli* mutants resistant to growth inhibition by 5MT. Some of the resistant lines accumulated higher than normal levels of tryptophan and also had altered anthranilate synthetase activity which was less sensitive to feedback inhibition by tryptophan and 5MT. The altered control enzyme presumably led to the accumulation of free tryptophan.

Cell lines of *D. carota, N. tabacum,* and *Solanum tuberosum* have also been selected which are resistant to growth inhibition by 5MT[8,9] (unpublished). 5MT false feedback inhibits anthranilate synthetase from these species,[36] and the addition of tryptophan, anthranilate, or indole (the immediate tryptophan precursor) relieves the growth inhibition. Resistant lines were selected by incubating suspension-cultured cells for up to 60 days in the presence of 5MT concentrations which are known to be completely inhibitory in 10- to 14-day growth studies. After the long incubation, some cells grew, and these would usually grow rapidly when reinoculated into the normally inhibitory medium. The resistant cells were selected with a frequency of about 3×10^{-7} for *D. carota*[9] and 1.5×10^{-6} for *N. tabacum.*[8] The resistance is usually stable, and two cloned *D. carota* lines have maintained the resistance for over 250 generations away from 5MT.[2] Thus far in all but one case,[10] the resistance to 5MT is also correlated with an altered anthranilate synthetase activity which is less sensitive to feedback inhibition by tryptophan and 5MT. Apparently as a result of the altered enzymes, the cell lines contain about 30 times the normal level of free tryptophan. Thus, many lines have been selected as resistant to 5MT which accumulate high levels of free tryptophan.

Recent work[37] indicates that the accumulation of high levels of free tryptophan in some of the *D. carota* cell lines results in the synthesis of indoleacetic acid. This is surmised from the fact that many of these 5MT-resistant lines are also auxin-autotrophic while the wild type and lines resistant to other analogs require auxin for growth. Added tryptophan can partially fulfill the auxin requirement with most cell lines. Preliminary measurements show that a 5MT-resistant auxin-autotrophic line does contain significant amounts of indoleacetic acid (unpublished).

These results indicate that the accumulation of tryptophan, which is the precursor of indoleacetic acid (Figure 1), somehow causes the accumulation of the auxin. This precursor induction of product synthesis occurs in at least one other case as will be discussed next.

Lines of *D. carota* and *N. tabacum* have also been selected for resistance to *P*-fluorophenylalanine (PFP), a phenylalanine analog.[7] Methods similar to those used for the 5MT-resistance selection were employed, but the frequency of appearance of resistant cells was much lower. The tobacco line was about 10 times more resistant than the wild type, while the carrot line was about 1000 times more resistant to the analog. The resistance was retained by two cloned carrot lines after growth for over 250 generations away from PFP. The resistant carrot line shows a sixfold higher level of free phenylalanine which may account for the resistance. The resistant tobacco line did not accumulate free phenylalanine, even though the control enzyme in the pathway (chorismate mutase, Figure 1) showed lessened feedback-control properties and higher activity, which should lead to phenylalanine oversynthesis.[7] Instead, these cells accumulated about six times the normal level of soluble polyphenols. This was apparently due to a greatly increased level of phenylalanine ammonia lyase found in the resistant cells.[38] When ^{14}C-phenylalanine is fed to the cell lines, the PFP-resistant tobacco line incorporates much more label into the polyphenols than the wild type, indicating a more rapid flux through the pathway leading to polyphenols (Figure 1).[39]

Gathercole and Street[6] described a PFP-resistant *Acer pseudoplatanus* suspension-culture line which had characteristics similar to the *N. tabacum* line selected by Palmer and Widholm. The line did not contain increased levels of free phenylalanine, but did contain elevated levels of both phenylalanine ammonia lyase and soluble polyphenols.

It then appears that all three of the PFP-resistant cell lines studied[6,7] oversynthesize phenylalanine, but only the *D. carota* line accumulates the amino acid. The *N. tabacum* and *A. pseudoplatanus* lines have increased phenylalanine ammonia lyase levels which convert the excess phenylalanine into polyphenols which do accumulate. Thus, the accumulation of an amino acid again appears to be capable of triggering secondary product biosynthesis. Whether phenylalanine ammonia lyase will be turned on in most species and how this is accomplished must await further study.

Lines resistant to lysine, methionine, and proline analogs have also been selected which accumulate the corresponding natural amino acid (reviewed by Widholm[2]). We have recently selected a carrot line by sequential selection for resistance to pheylalanine, methionine, lysine, and tryptophan analogs, and the resulting line accumulated these free amino acids to levels 7, 6, 5, and 31 times those of the wild type, respectively (unpublished). The total free-amino-acid concentration was doubled.

In one case, the selection for resistance to a nucleotide analog also appears to have resulted in a line which oversynthesizes a related compound. Ohyama[15] selected a *Glycine max* line resistant to 5-bromodeoxyuridine (BUdR) by plating cells in BUdR and incubating under fluorescent light. A line isolated in this manner was extremely resistant to BUdR, and the resistance was stable for 15 generations away from the inhibitor. Unlike previously selected BUdR-resistant lines, this line did not incorporate the analog into its DNA. The line was also resistant to growth inhibition by aminopterin and 5-fluorodeoxyuridine (FUdR). Resistance to aminopterin may be due to a 50-fold increase in dihydrofolate reductase, and the FUdR resistance may be due to a threefold increase in deoxythymidine monophosphate synthetase. These two compounds should be the respective inhibitors of the two enzymes. Thymidine synthetase was also significantly increased in the resistant line. These alterations in enzyme levels which have been described may result in the increased synthesis of deoxythymidine monophosphate, which should dilute the BUdR, resulting in less incorporation of the toxic compound into DNA. The information available fits this conclusion, but the actual levels of the nucleotides in question have not been reported.

Mastrangelo and Smith[13] have selected aminopterin-resistant *Datura innoxia* lines which may have similar characteristics as the above *G. max* line. Further biochemical characterization has not been reported, however.

Systems which select for resistance give one the ability to screen very large populations. Often, however, the compound which is desired is not directly related to the primary mechanism of resistance which was selected for. Thus, the likelihood of success is diminished. However, the preliminary results give one a feeling of optimism, and only with additional work can the success or failure of such ideas be determined.

VII. AUXOTROPH SELECTION

The area of auxotrophic mutants in plants is a sparse one at present and may not be obviously relevant to the present discussion about the production of compounds by tissue cultures. Auxotrophs are defined as mutants which lack a necessary function. Thus, auxotrophs grow only if supplemented with the missing component. Often, pathways are rendered inoperable due to the lack of a functional enzyme. This block might cause a buildup of some intermediate which itself could be desirable, or this buildup might increase the flow into a branch pathway which could be useful. Other unknown interactions between pathways may exist which could result in compound production.

In general, auxotrophic selection is based on procedures where dividing nonauxotrophic (autotrophic or prototrophic) cells are killed while the nongrowing auxotrophs are spared. The auxotrophs are then rescued by adding supplements which include that required for growth. Testing of the various lines which grow is required to determine if there is actually a deficiency and to determine the exact compound required. Replica plating is ideal for this testing.

The classical system used with bacteria involves the use of penicillin. It is used by growing cells to make a defective cell wall, resulting in death. Early work with animal cells utilized the thymidine analog 5-bromodeoxyuridine (BUdR), which is incorporated into the DNA of growing cells. DNA containing BUdR is susceptible to damage by visible light which is used to destroy the cells which have incorporated BUdR into their DNA.

Carlson[40] used the BudR system with *N. tabacum* cells initiated from anther-derived haploid plants. Suspended cells were treated with the mutagen ethylmethane sulfonate and incubated in minimal medium for 4 days in order to deplete the reserves in the auxotrophs. BudR was added for 36 hr, followed by rinsing and plating in a medium containing thymidine, casein hydrolysate, and yeast extract. The plates were illuminated with fluorescent light to kill the cells with BUdR in their DNA. From 1.75×10^6 cells plated, 119 calli grew, and six were found to show a partial requirement for some compound. Growth of the lines was stimulated from two- to sixfold by added hypoxanthine, biotin, *p*-aminobenzoic acid, arginine, lysine, or proline.

The fact that only leaky mutants were obtained in these experiments was explained by Carlson as being due to the amphidiploidy of *N. tabacum* which results in a polyhaploid genome after halving the chromosome number. This points out the need to use true haploid lines in auxotrophic-selection experiments.

Other work with *N. tabacum* haploid lines has shown that complete deficiencies can apparently be found, however. Müller and Grafe[41] plated mutagenized cells in chlorate-containing medium and isolated resistant colonies. This system should select for lines which lack nitrate reductase since this enzyme is responsible for converting non-toxic chlorate to toxic chlorite. Nitrate reductase deficient lines should survive the treatment. Many lines were selected which did have very low levels of, or in some cases no, nitrate reductase activity. These lines cannot grow with nitrate, as the nitrogen source and the trait appears to be stable.

Zea mays plants which lack alcohol dehydrogenase have been selected using allyl alcohol which kills the pollen containing the enzyme.[42] The alcohol dehydrogenase can convert allyl alcohol to the highly toxic compound acrylaldehyde. Plants lacking this enzyme grow normally except when grown under anaerobic conditions. Then death occurs.[43]

The value of auxotrophic mutants in biochemical production remains to be determined. As with the other methods discussed, however, the possibilities should not be overlooked.

VIII. THE USE OF MUTAGENS

The treatment of cell populations with mutagens prior to mutant selection may be beneficial since the mutagen treatment should increase the occurrence of the desired altered trait. Of the successful selection studies reviewed by Widholm,[2] many were done with previously mutagenized cells, while in other cases this was not found to be necessary. Many resistant lines were selected at frequencies of about 10^{-6} to 10^{-7} from untreated cells. This is not surprising since spontaneous mutation rates in this range or even higher have been reported with whole-plant systems. Stadler[44] found that several dominant *Z. mays* endosperm traits would revert to the recessive at rates of 10^{-4} to 10^{-6}.

Most of the mutagen studies done with tissue cultures did not compare mutation frequencies found with both treated and untreated cells. Recently, however, information is beginning to accumulate which shows that mutagens can be effective with plant cells. Lescure and Peaud-Lenoel[45] were able to select auxin-autotrophic *A. pseudoplatanus* lines only from *N*-methyl, *N*'-nitro, *N*-nitrosoguanidine (NG) treated cells. The mutagen treatment increased the frequency of autotrophic cells from 0 to about 10^{-6}. The autotrophy was stable and might have been due to the presence of an IAA oxidase with altered kinetics.[46] Nishi et al.[27] reported that NG treatment of *D. carota* cells significantly increased the occurrence of colonies with carotene pigment alterations. They reported the selection of four stable variant lines only after NG treatment.

Sung[47] used both NG and ethylmethane sulfonate (EMS) with suspension cultured *G. max* and *D. carota* cell lines. Treated carrot cells were plated in inhibitory levels of cyclohexamide or 5-fluorouracil, and in several experiments, the frequency of resistant colonies which formed was determined. The increases found with mutagen treatment were from 1 to 140-fold with 10-fold being average. The nature of the resistance was not determined, but the resistance was stable in some cases when retested.

Müller and Grafe[41] treated haploid *N. tabacum* suspension cultures with *N*-ethyl-*N*-nitrosourea, and in one experiment, nine chlorate-resistant colonies formed from about 2×10^7 treated cells (frequency of 4.5×10^{-7}). No resistant colonies were found from 8×10^7 untreated cells in the same experiment. The spontaneous frequency of chlorate resistance found in several other experiments was about 7×10^{-9}.

About 10^5 haploid *Datura innoxia* mesophyll protoplasts were irradiated with X-rays at a dose (1000 R) which caused about 25% survival as 2.5×10^4 calli formed.[48] Following plating in a medium which stimulates greening, plants or leaves were allowed to regenerate from callus which was white or light green. Of the 10 plant strains selected in this way, five were light green, two were yellow, one pale yellow, one white, and one lacked the normal amount of anthocyanin. No white or light green callus was found in 10^5 calli formed from untreated protoplasts.

We have done some mutation-induction work with suspension-cultured *D. carota* cells.[49] Cells were treated with EMS in flasks or with UV light in open petri dishes. The EMS was rinsed away following the treatment period. Twenty-four hr after treatment, the cell viability was determined using phenosafranine, which stains dead cells.[50] The treatments used were those which reduced viability to 30 to 50% of the control level of about 95%. The cultures were incubated until the cell mass had increased about four- to eightfold to dilute out dead cells and to allow recovery from the treatment. Then 1.8×10^5 cells were inoculated into 10 mℓ of liquid medium containing an inhibitory concentration of 5MT in each flask. After 2 months incubation, growth was noted in 2 of the 63 flasks containing unmutagenized cells, a resistance frequency of about 1.7×10^{-7}. The EMS-treated cells grew in 42 of 70 flasks for a frequency of 3.3×10^{-6}, 20-fold that of the untreated cells. The UV- light-treated cells grew in 22 of 70 flasks for an 1.7×10^{-6} resistance frequency, which is 10-fold that of the untreated cells.

Most of these studies used mutagenic treatments which reduced viability to 25 to 50% followed by a recovery period of up to four cell divisions. Whether these treatments and procedures are optimal cannot be determined at present since no complete study has been done to evaluate these parameters. We have found, however, that if the cell viability is reduced to below about 30% within 24 hr of the treatment, then the cells will not recover. This is work done with suspension-cultured *D. carota* and *N. tabacum* cell lines.

While it appears that mutagens are capable of increasing the frequency of variant cells in culture, some caution is advised. The mutagens are very dangerous to work with, so must be handled carefully. Usually, several different treatment levels are needed to find the correct dose. Mutations will be induced in many genes, not just the desired ones, so they may render the treated cells less capable of rapid growth or plant regeneration. A given mutagen may not be capable of inducing the desired alteration since mutagens occasionally can have specific mutagenic effects.

IX. GENETIC BASIS FOR COMPOUND ACCUMULATION

If lines are selected which produce large amounts of desired compounds, it would be desirable to know the genetic basis of the phenotype. In other words, what basic mechanism controls the phenotypic expression? The possibilities would appear to be mutation (genetic) or differentiation, either relatively permanent (epigenetic) or short term.

A mutation or genetic change can be defined as a sudden, permanent alteration in a gene caused by a change in the DNA sequence. Epigenetic changes were defined by Meins[51] as heritable alterations in the expression of genes. Short-term differentiation refers to transitory states which do not persist.

The most desirable changes may be genetic since a gene should be permanently altered by a base change or deletion which would make the trait relatively stable. Many base change mutations are, however, able to revert back to the wild type, but this is usually at a very low rate. Periodic cloning and testing might then be necessary to retain genetic purity.

Epigenetic alterations may or may not be stable enough to be desirable. Many traits which appear to be epigenetic in nature are very stable in culture, as in the case of hormone autotrophy. Most wild-type tissue cultures require an exogenous supply of auxin or auxin and cytokinin for growth. Lines can be selected at high frequency which are hormone-autotrophic and have no hormone requirements. Cytokinin-independent *N. tabacum* cells were selected by Binns and Meins[52] at the rate of 10^{-3} per cell generation, while Syono and Furuya[53] induced auxin-autotrophy in *N. tabacum* callus at the rate of 10^{-4} or greater. This autotrophy can be reversed by various treatments[52,53,54] and be lost after plant regeneration and reinitiation of cultures. Thus, this auxin-autotrophy would be under epigenetic rather than under mutational control. The traits are stable in culture, however, so could be very useful.

Differences in pigmentation in cell lines have been discussed in Section IV. Most of these alterations seem to be stable in the cell line, but the work of Mok et al.[29] shows that the alterations were not carried back to the plant.

Since epigenetically controlled events can arise in higher frequency than mutational events, it may be easier to select for epigenetically controlled traits.

Short-term differentiated states may be valuable in compound production if the condition can be reproducibly controlled and if selection procedures can detect the condition in the first place. This situation falls more under the classical approach where entire cultures are to be turned on, but it may be possible that variants can be selected which can be turned on for short times more efficiently than the wild type. This may be the case with the alkaloid production by the selected *Catharanthus* lines which cannot be maintained for many passages in the production medium.[1]

Most of the variants found so far in cultured cells cannot be classified as being due to mutation or nonmutation. In a few cases, an altered gene product can be identified which is evidence for a mutational basis. The 5MT-resistant and PFP-resistant lines have control enzymes in the affected pathways which show altered feedback-control properties.[2] The auxin-autotrophic lines of Lescure and Peaud-Lenoel contained an IAA oxidase with kinetics different from that from the wild type.[46] The presence of an altered product is not proof of a mutation, however. Many traits have been shown to be carried to regenerated plants and/or back into cultures (reviewed by Widholm[2]). These traits include resistance to streptomycin,[4] BUdR,[3] 5MT,[10] methionine sulfoximine,[14] and *Helminthosporium maydis* Race T pathotoxin.[5] Thus, many selected traits appear to be under genetic control.

There is other evidence to indicate that genetic changes may also cause other secondary alterations. A good example is the case of the PFP-resistant lines of *N. tabacum* and *A. pseudoplatanus* which apparently overproduce phenylalanine. This induces high phenylalanine ammonia lyase activity, which in turn synthesizes high levels of polyphenols. In contrast, the PFP-resistant *D. carota* line accumulates phenylalanine and does not have high phenylalanine ammonia lyase or polyphenol levels.[6,7,38,39]

A similar case is found with 5MT-resistant *D. carota* cell lines which have an altered anthranilate synthetase and accumulate high levels of free tryptophan. Five of the 10 lines studied were found to be auxin-autotrophic.[37] The connection between high tryptophan and autotrophy is clear since tryptophan is the precursor of IAA, the natural auxin (Figure 1), but why are only half of the lines turned on? This and many other questions about these effects cannot be answered with our present knowledge.

Since we do not know much about the underlying controls, it would appear that one should use the best methods available to select lines which accumulate compounds and not worry about the underlying causes. Studies of these causes can perhaps best be done after such lines are selected.

X. CONCLUSIONS

This chapter has put forth the idea that cells able to produce certain desired compounds should be present in large cell populations or should be inducible by mutagenic treatment. These variant cells can then be selected from the population using some carefully devised scheme. Once selected, the cell line should continue to produce the compound.

The selection schemes and cell lines to be used must be tailored to the compounds desired. The culture systems which are available are much less amenable to manipulation than the microbial systems we are trying to emulate, but progress should be possible even if it is slower and more difficult.

Several successful selections for high pigmentation using visual selection have been carried out. Stable lines were obtained which had scientific, but not economic, value. A chemical-analysis selection scheme has yielded lines which produce much higher than normal levels of valuable alkaloids. The amounts produced are not quite sufficient to make the process commercially usable, however.[56]

Selection for resistance to certain analogs has produced lines which accumulate higher than normal levels of the corresponding natural compounds. This, in turn, can in some cases lead to the accumulation of compounds derived from the originally overproduced biochemical. These secondary accumulation systems are empirical and relatively undirected, but should continue to be explored because of the possibilities.

That auxotrophs can accumulate desirable biochemicals is likewise problematical, especially since the selection process itself seems to be very difficult in plants. The initial hope is that the selection schemes can be improved in order to select auxotrophs easily. Then, studies on compound accumulation can be carried out.

Mutagens will probably find a place in selection schemes as the knowledge of cell-culture mutation induction and selection systems improve. If the desired traits are found to not have a genetic basis, then mutagens may be unnecessary in these instances.

Thus, certain selection schemes have already been used successfully to select lines which accumulate certain primary and secondary compounds. With a certain amount of ingenuity, it should be possible to use the present methods as well as to devise additional ones which can select lines which produce almost any desired compound.

The reason for optimism is that after only a few attempts there is evidence of some progress. In contrast, the classical methods have made little progress after many years of effort.

REFERENCES

1. **Zenk, M. H., El-Shagi, H., Arens, H., Stöckigt, J., Weiler, E. W., and Deus, B.,** Formation of the indole alkaloids serpentine and ajmalicine in cell suspension cultures of *Catharanthus roseus,* in *Plant Tissue Culture and Its Bio-technological Application,* Barz, W., Reinhard, E., and Zenk, M. H., Eds., Springer-Verlag, Berlin, 1977, 27.
2. **Widholm, J. M.,** Selection and characterization of biochemical mutants, in *Plant Tissue Culture and Its Bio-technological Application,* Barz, W., Reinhard, E., and Zenk, M. H., Eds., Springer-Verlag, Berlin, 1977, 112.
3. **Maliga, P., Marton, L., and Sz.-Breznovits, A.,** 5-Bromodeoxyuridine-resistant cell lines from haploid tobacco, *Plant Sci. Lett.,* 1, 119, 1973.
4. **Maliga, P., Sz.-Breznovits, A., and Marton, L.,** Streptomycin-resistant plants from callus culture of haploid tobacco, *Nature (London) New Biol.,* 244, 29, 1973.

5. **Gengenbach, B. G. and Green, C. E.,** Selection of T-cytoplasm maize callus cultures resistant to *Helminthosporium maydis* race T pathotoxin, *Crop Sci.*, 15, 645, 1975.
6. **Gathercole, R. W. E. and Street, H. E.,** Isolation stability and biochemistry of a P-fluorophenylalanine-resistant cell line of *Acer pseudoplatanus* L., *New Phytol.*, 77, 29, 1976.
7. **Palmer, J. E. and Widholm, J.,** Characterization of carrot and tobacco cell cultures resistant to P-fluorophenylalanine, *Plant Physiol.*, 56, 233, 1975.
8. **Widholm, J. M.,** Cultured *Nicotiana tabacum* cells with an altered anthranilate synthetase which is less sensitive to feedback inhibition, *Biochim. Biophys. Acta*, 261, 52, 1972.
9. **Widholm, J. M.,** Anthranilate synthetase from 5-methyltryptophan-susceptible and -resistant cultured *Daucus carota* cells, *Biochim. Biophys. Acta*, 279, 48, 1972.
10. **Widholm, J. M.,** Cultured carrot cell mutants: 5-methyltryptophan-resistance trait carried from cell to plant and back, *Plant Sci. Lett.*, 3, 323, 1974.
11. **Nabors, M. W., Daniels, A., Nadolny, L., and Brown, C.,** Sodium chloride tolerant lines of tobacco cells, *Plant Sci. Lett.*, 4, 155, 1975.
12. **Dix, P. J. and Street, H. E.,** Sodium chloride-resistant cultured cell lines from *Nicotiana sylvestris* and *Capsicum annuum*, *Plant Sci. Lett.*, 5, 231, 1975.
13. **Mastrangelo, I. A. and Smith, H. H.,** Selection and differentiation of aminopterin resistant cells of *Datura innoxia*, *Plant Sci. Lett.*, 10, 171, 1977.
14. **Carlson, P. S.,** Methione sulfoximine-resistant mutants of tobacco, *Science*, 180, 1366, 1973.
15. **Ohyama, K.,** The basis for bromodeoxyuridine-resistance in plant cells, *Environ. Exp. Bot.*, 16, 209, 1976.
16. **Ravah, D., Huberman, E., and Galun, E.,** In vitro culture of tobacco protoplasts: use of feeder techniques to support division of cells plated at low densities, *In Vitro*, 9, 216, 1973.
17. **Muir, W. H., Hildebrandt, A. C., and Riker, A. J.,** Plant tissue cultures produced from single isolated cells, *Science*, 119, 877, 1954.
18. **Schulte, U. and Zenk, M. H.,** A replica plating method for plant cells, *Physiol. Plant.*, 39, 139, 1977.
19. **Nitsh, C.,** Culture of isolated microspores, in *Applied and Fundamental Aspects of Plant Cell, Tissue, and Organ Culture*, Reinert, J. and Bajaj, Y. P. S., Eds., Springer-Verlag, Berlin, 1977, 268.
20. **Eichenberger, M. E.,** Sur une mutation survenue dans une culture de tissus de carotte, *C. R. Acad. Sci.*, 145, 239, 1951.
21. **Naef, J. and Turian, G.,** Sur les carotinoides du tissu cambial de racine de carotte cultive *in vitro*, *Phytochemistry*, 2, 173, 1963.
22. **Strauss, J.,** Spontaneous changes in corn endosperm tissue culture, *Science*, 128, 537, 1958.
23. **Blakely, L. W. and Steward, F. C.,** Growth and organized development of cultured cells. VII. Cellular variation, *Am. J. Bot.*, 51, 809, 1964.
24. **Constable, F.,** Pigmentbildung in Kalluskulturen aus Beta-Rüben, *Naturwissenschaften*, 54, 175, 1967.
25. **Koblitz, H., Shumann, U., Böhm, H., and Franke, J.,** Gewebekulturen aus alkaloid-pflanzen. IV. *Macleaya microcarpa* (Maxim.) Fedde, *Experientia*, 31, 768, 1975.
26. **Davey, M. R., Fowler, M. W., and Street, H. E.,** Cell clones contrasted in growth, morphology and pigmentation isolated from a callus culture of *Atropa belladonna* var *lutea*, *Phytochemistry*, 10, 2559, 1971.
27. **Nishi, A., Yoshida, A., Mori, M., and Sugano, N.,** Isolation of variant carrot cell lines with altered pigmentation, *Phytochemistry*, 13, 1653, 1974.
28. **Alfermann, A. W., Merz, D., and Reinhard, E.,** Induktion der anthocyanbiosynthese in kalluskulturen von *Daucus carota*, *Planta Med.*, Suppl., 70, 1975.
29. **Mok, M. T., Gabelman, W. H., and Skoog, F.,** Carotenoid synthesis in tissue cultures of *Daucus carota* L., *J. Am. Soc. Hortic. Sci.*, 101, 442, 1976.
30. **Linsmaier, E. M. and Skoog, F.,** Organic growth factor requirements of tobacco tissue cultures, *Physiol. Plant.*, 18, 100, 1965.
31. **Alexander, D. E., Silvela, L., Collins, F. I., and Rodgers, R. C.,** Analysis of oil content of maize by wide-line NMR, *J. Am. Oil Chem. Soc.*, 44, 555, 1967.
32. **Chu, M. and Widholm, J. M.,** Control of the biosynthesis of phenylalanine and tyrosine in plant tissue cultures: lack of repression of chorismate mutase, *Physiol. Plant.*, 26, 24, 1972.
33. **Widholm, J. M.,** Control of tryptophan biosynthesis in plant tissue cultures: lack of repression of anthranilate and tryptophan synthetases by tryptophan, *Physiol. Plant.*, 25, 75, 1971.
34. **Moyed, H. S.,** False feedback inhibition: inhibition of tryptophan biosynthesis by 5-methyltryptophan, *J. Biol. Chem.*, 235, 1098, 1960.
35. **Sommerville, R. L. and Yanofsky, C.,** Studies on the regulation of tryptophan biosynthesis in *E. coli*, *J. Mol. Biol.*, 11, 747, 1965.

36. **Widholm, J. M.,** Tryptophan biosynthesis in *Nicotiana tabacum* and *Daucus carota* cell cultures: site of action of inhibitory tryptophan analogs, *Biochim. Biophys. Acta,* 261, 44, 1972.
37. **Widholm, J. M.,** Relation between auxin-autotrophy and tryptophan accumulation in cultured plant cells, *Planta,* 134, 103, 1977.
38. **Berlin, J. and Widholm, J. M.,** Correlation between phenylalanine ammonia lyase activity and phenolic biosynthesis in *P*-fluorophenylalanine-sensitive and -resistant tobacco and carrot tissue cultures, *Plant Physiol.,* 59, 550, 1977.
39. **Berlin, J. and Widholm, J. M.,** Metabolism of phenylalanine and tyrosine in tobacco cell lines resistant and sensitive to *P*-fluorophenylalanine, *Phytochemistry,* 17, 65, 1978.
40. **Carlson, P. S.,** Induction and isolation of auxotrophic mutants in somatic cell cultures of *Nicotiana tabacum, Science,* 168, 487, 1970.
41. **Müller, A. J. and Grafe, R.,** Mutant cell lines of *Nicotiana tabacum* deficient in nitrate reductase, *Int. Bot. Congr. Abstr.,* 12, 304, 1975.
42. **Schwartz, D. and Osterman, J.,** A pollen selection system for alcohol-dehydrogenase-negative mutants in plants, *Genetics,* 83, 63, 1976.
43. **Schwartz, D.,** An example of gene fixation resulting from selective advantage in suboptimal conditions, *Am. Nat.,* 103, 749, 1969.
44. **Stadler, L. J.,** Spontaneous mutation rates of several endosperm genes in mays, *Spragg Mem. Lect. Michigan State Univ.,* 3, 3, 1942.
45. **Lescure, A. M. and Peaud-Lenoel, C.,** Production par traitement mutagêne de lignêes cellulaires d' *Acer pseudoplatanus* L. Anergiies â l'auxin, *C. R. Acad. Sci.,* 265, 1803, 1967.
46. **Lescure, A. M.,** Preparation de clones mutants de cellules vegetales. Recherche de l'impact moleculaire de la mutation chez une lignee mutante d'acer pseudoplatanus L. independante de l'auxin, *Bull. Soc. Chim. Biol.,* 52, 953, 1970.
47. **Sung, Z. R.,** Mutagenesis of cultured plant cells, *Genetics,* 84, 51, 1976.
48. **Schieder, O.,** Isolation of mutants with altered pigments after irradiating haploid protoplasts from *Datura innoxia* Mill. with X-rays, *Mol. Gen. Genet.* 149, 251, 1976.
49. **Widholm, J. M.,** Isolation of biochemical mutants of cultured plant cells, in *Molecular Genetic Modification of Eucaryotes,* Rubenstein, I., Phillips, R. L., Green, C. E., and Desnick, R., Eds., Academic Press, New York, 1977, 57.
50. **Widholm, J. M.,** The use of fluorescein disacetate and phenosafranine for determining viability of cultured plant cells, *Stain Technol.,* 47, 189, 1972.
51. **Meins, F., Jr.,** Mechanisms underlying the persistence of tumor autonomy in crown-gall disease, in *Tissue Culture and Plant Science 1974,* Street, H. E., Ed., Academic Press, New York, 1974, 233.
52. **Binns, A. and Meins, F., Jr.,** Habituation of tobacco pith cells for factors promoting cell division is heritable and potentially reversible, *Proc. Natl. Acad. Sci. U.S.A.,* 70, 2660, 1973.
53. **Syono, K. and Furuya, T.,** Induction of auxin-nonrequiring tobacco calluses and its reversal by treatment with auxins, *Plant Cell Physiol.,* 15, 7, 1974.
54. **Meins, F., Jr.,** Temperature-sensitive expression of auxin-autotrophy by crown-gall teratoma cells of tobacco, *Planta,* 122, 1, 1975.
55. **Sacristan, M. D. and Wendt-Gallitelli, M. F.,** Transformation to auxin-autotrophy and its reversibility in a mutant line of *Crepis capillaris* callus culture, *Mol. Gen. Genet.,* 110, 355, 1971.
56. **Zenk, M. H.,** personal communication, 1978.

Chapter 5

STORAGE OF PLANT CELL LINES

Donald K. Dougall

TABLE OF CONTENTS

I. INTRODUCTION

A widespread practice in plant tissue culture is to maintain cultures by serial passage. This practice makes specific lines of cells or tissue vulnerable to loss due to failure of equipment. It is expensive in terms of labor and wasteful of cells in that a large proportion of tissue is discarded at each subculture. In addition, changes in the characteristics of cultures occur with prolonged subculture. With increased information accumulated as a result of studies, the cell lines used become more valuable. Cell lines developed for specific purposes, particularly commercial use, will be very valuable and will need protection from change or destruction. This discussion is focused on the available information on the protection of plant cell lines by some form of storage. At the onset, it must be noted that the available information is limited. Further, storage of plant cell cultures will rapidly become a pressing problem.

Two classes of methods have been considered. The first is aimed at extending the interval between subcultures, and the second is storage at super-low temperatures (cryogenic storage).

II. METHODS OF EXTENDING THE INTERVAL BETWEEN SUBCULTURES

A. Mineral-Oil Overlay

Caplin[1] examined the effects of mineral-oil overlays on the growth of carrot cultures on agar medium. He showed that with layers of oil from 5 to 40 mm deep, the growth rate of the tissue was constant and reduced substantially from that in cultures without oil. Caplin provides experimental evidence to suggest that the factors responsible for the effect of the mineral oil are reduced dessication and reduced oxygen availability to the tissue. The addition of mineral oil to cultures decreases the growth rate by at least a factor of four, thus extending the subculture interval from weeks to months.

B. Storage at 0 to 4°C

Increases in the interval between the transfer of cultures by storage of cultures in refrigerators have been used.[26] However, very little data on such storage systems is available. Bannier and Steponkus,[2] using *chrysanthemum* callus tissue in studies of cold acclimatization, maintained cultures at 4.5°C for up to 6 weeks and showed that the cultures would grow when transferred to 27°C. Sakai and Sugawara[3] studied cold acclimatizaion of *Populus euroamericana* callus. They used 8 hr at 15°C alternating with 16 hr at 0°C for 60 days followed by 20 days at 0°C and showed that the tissue would grow. McCown et al.[4] showed that callus cultures of *Dianthus* would grow slowly at 0 to 5°C over 4 weeks. Because of the objectives of these studies, the maximum length of time the tissues would survive at 0 to 4°C were not examined. Rose and Martin[5] studied the growth of suspension cultures of *Ipomoea* at temperatures from 17 to 30°C. They transferred tissue which had been grown at 17°C to fresh medium at 26°C and found that it did not grow. Tissue previously grown at 20°C showed delay in resuming growth at 26°C. Rose and Martin[5] concluded that growth at suboptimal temperatures was not a satisfactory method for prolonging the subculture interval. It is possible that these reports may be reconciled by the differences between suspension and callus cultures, growth in light or dark, differences due to the species of origin, or the differences in the lowest temperatures used.

Methods which increase the interval between subculture achieve principally a reduction in cost of maintenance. They do not remove the possibility of loss due to mechanical failure or the possibility of changes in the characteristics of cultures.

III. CRYOGENIC STORAGE

The effect of temperature on chemical reactions (i.e., rate decreases by 50% for each 10°C decrease in temperature) and the chemical basis of biological systems leads to the idea that very low temperatures would be preferable for cell storage because cellular reactions would be extremely slow. The temperatures which are used for the cryogenic storage of cells and tissues are either the temperature of liquid nitrogen (−196°C) or that of the vapor over liquid nitrogen (−140°C and lower). This is probably dictated by three pragmatic considerations.

1. The temperatures are suitable for prolonged storage of cells.
2. Liquid nitrogen and suitable storage containers are available commercially.
3. The relative nonreactivity of liquid nitrogen (compared with liquid oxygen).

At this point in time, cryogenic storage of plant cells, tissues, and organs has been the subject of very limited study. The available information should increase rapidly in response to the need to protect valuable cultures and plants.

A. Species of Plants to Which Cryogenic Storage has been Successfully Applied

It is current practice in plant tissue culture to refer cultures back to the species of origin. This has validity because, in some cases, cultures are totipotent so that plants can be regenerated and because the species is the basic unit of distinction between plants at a genetic level.

To decide whether or not a study has achieved successful cryogenic storage, the author has applied two criteria. These are

1. That the temperature achieved is lower than −140°C.
2. The cells or tissue were shown to grow after recovery from low temperatures.

These criteria do not include the retention of capacities other than growth by the cells or tissue after storage. They also do not include any evaluation of the time in storage because experience not only with plant cells, but also with animal cells, etc., indicates that the achievement of survival during the transition to and from temperatures below −140°C is much more difficult than maintaining viability at these low temperatures.

The species of origin and the nature of the cultures successfully recovered after storage at −140°C or lower are shown in Table 1. Cultures from a total of six species have been successfully frozen to −140°C or lower and thawed. Two of those, namely *D. carota* and *D. caryophyllus*, have been shown to retain morphogenetic capacities.

In Table 2, six additional species for which there is evidence of partial success during freezing and thawing are shown. These examples are separated from those in Table 1 because viability was not demonstrated by growth after thawing or because the lowest temperature reached was not −140°C or lower. Nag and Street[6] comment that on storage of carrot suspension cultures at −78°C there is a measurable, time-dependent loss of viability, while at −196°C there was no loss of viability during 100 days. We have observed no loss of viability in *D. carota* suspension cultures over 3 years storage at −140°C.[27] In some of the examples shown in Table 2, viability was estimated by staining techniques rather than growth. Staining techniques for assessing viability of plant tissue cultures have been evaluated by Widholm[7] and Towill and Mazur.[8] In studies of freezing and thawing, two staining methods have been used for rapid and convenient assessment of the extent of damage to cells. Fluorescein diacetate[7] requires only a few minutes incubation, while triphenyltetrazolium chloride (TTC) reduction[8] requires an

TABLE 1

Tissue Cultures Frozen to −140° or −196°C and Recovered

Culture type Suspension cultures	Additional characteristics shown after storage	Ref.
Daucus carota	—	19
Daucus carota	Embryogenesis	6, 16, 21
Daucus carota	Embryogensis	17
Daucus carota	Embryogenesis	18
Daucus carota	Embryogenesis	10
Acer pseudoplatanus	—	9
Ruta graveolens	—	9
Nicotiana tabacum (haploid)	—	18
Callus cultures		
Populus euramericana	—	3
Organ cultures		
Dianthus caryophyllus (shoot apices)	Plants regenerated	22

Note: Viability was assessed by the ability of the thawed tissue to grow.

TABLE 2

Tissue Cultures of the Species Which Have Been Frozen and Thawed

Culture Type Suspension cultures	Lowest temperature (°C)	Criterion of viability	Ref.
Linum usitatissimum	−50°	Growth	20
Atropa belladonna	−196°	Staining	21
Datura strammonium	−196°	Staining	18
Broussonetia razinoki	−30°	Growth	9
Nicotiana tabacum	−30°	Growth	9
Nicotiana tabacum (haploid)	−20°	Growth (plants regenerated)	18
Capsicum annuum	−30°	Growth	10
Ipomoea sp.	−40°	Growth	19
Callus cultures			
Chrysanthemum morifolium	−16°	Growth	2

overnight incubation. Several authors have commented on the correlation between staining methods and subsequent growth of frozen and thawed cultures. Sugawara and Sakai[9], using TTC, suggested that staining is a reliable estimate of survival. Bannier and Steponkus[2] concluded that there was a poor correlation. Nag and Street,[6] using fluorescein diacetate, concluded that viability by staining had to equal or exceed 35% before regrowth would occur. Withers and Street[10] concluded that viability as judged by fluorescein diacetate staining was not a reliable indicator of capacity to grow in culture after freezing and thawing. The relationship between viability determined by a staining method and the ability of cultures to grow after freezing and thawing is not clear at this time. It may be influenced by the length of time which has elapsed between thawing and the assessment of viability since some freeze-thaw injury may be repaired and some may become progressively worse. Progressive repair or damage after freezing and thawing has been demonstrated in onion bulb scales by Palta et al.[11]

B. Conditions Which have been Successfully Used

The extent of survival after freezing and thawing is affected by the type of cell being used, the nature and concentration of the cryoprotectant, the freezing rate, the thawing rate, and the method of estimating viability. These five aspects of the procedure interact with one another and they must be considered together.[12-14] Many aspects of the freezing and thawing of biological systems and possible mechanisms of injury have been discussed at length by Mazur.[13,15]

From the studies that are listed in Table 1, there appear to be some common features of successful cryogenic storage. This is particularly true for suspension cultures where more data is available than for callus or organ cultures.

1. Protective Agents

Cryoprotectants are required in all cases except for *Populus euramericana*[3] where a period of cold acclimatization was used. The cryoprotectants used are 5 to 10% dimethyl sulfoxide[6,9,10,16-21,22] or 5 to 10% glycerol, alone[16,18,19,21] or in combination with dimethyl sulfoxide.[10,19] Sugawara and Sakai[9] used dimethyl sulfoxide in combination with glucose.

Cryoprotectants are usually added as an equal volume of 2 × concentrated sterile solution in culture medium. The work of Sugawara and Sakai[9] is an exception. Some authors have concluded that slow addition to cells or tissue at 0 to 4°C is advantageous.[21] Seibert and Wetherbee[22] and Nag and Street[16,21] concluded that a period of time of approximately 1 to 1½ hr in cryoprotectant solution was necessary for maximum protection.

2. Freezing Rate

For suspension cultures, freezing rates 1 to 2°C/min have been most successful.[6,16,17,19,21] However, Sugawara and Sakai[9] decreased the temperature of *P. euramericana* callus in 5° steps each day from −5° to −30°C. Seibert and Wetherbee[22] used cooling rates of 100°C/min or greater.

Various freezing rates are achieved either with commercially available controlled-rate freezers and/or different physical arrangements which allow various rates of heat loss from the vials.[14,23]

3. Thawing Rates

Rapid thawing has been most widely used. Sakai and Sugawara[3] used relatively slow-thawing conditions. Where the effects of thawing rates have been examined, higher rates are clearly advantageous.[6,9,16,17,21,22]

Different thawing rates are achieved by using different physical conditions. The highest rates are achieved by immersing the vials of frozen material directly into water at 35 to 40°C. The high rates are achieved here by the intimate contact between the vial and water and the capacity of the water to provide heat to the vial. Lower rates of warming are achieved by standing vials in air.

4. Removal of the Protective Agent

Dimethyl sulfoxide and, to a lesser extent, glycerol are inhibitory to growth of plant tissue cultures. Their removal from the cells before culture is necessary. This is achieved by several washes in fresh medium, often with periods of time between, to allow equilibration between the tissue and the wash medium. The tissue is then evaluated for viability.

5. Estimation of Viability

The difficulties which have been experienced with the estimation of viability by staining methods have been discussed previously. Estimation of viability by the capacity of the tissue to grow is straightforward if the effects of inoculum size on growth are taken into account. There are many observations in the literature to show that with progressively smaller inocula there is an increasing lag in growth.[24,25] Growth may not be observed after freezing and thawing if the viability of tissue is sufficiently low so that the effective inoculum size is at a level where a long lag occurs before growth is evident. To avoid this problem, the effect of inoculum size on growth of tissue should be examined before freezing and thawing, and the size of the samples of tissue frozen and thawed should be chosen so that regrowth can be observed at anticipated survival rates.

6. Physiological State of the Tissue Prior to Freezing

In addition to the effects associated with the freezing-thawing-evaluation process, there are a number of suggestions that the physiological state of the tissue is important in freezing to −140°C or lower and successful recovery.

Seibert and Wetherbee[22] showed that the growth of *D. caryophyllus* plants at 4°C with 8 hr light/day for 3 days prior to excision, freezing and thawing of the shoot tips, gave a six- to sevenfold increase in the number which formed new leaf primordia or shoots. Sakai and Sugawara[3] showed that *P. euramericana* callus which had been subjected to 15°C for 8 hr alternating with 0°C for 16 hr for 60 days and then held at 0°C for 20 days could be successfully recovered from freezing to −196°C. Withers and Street[10] concluded that growth of *Acer pseudoplatanus* in 3.3% mannitol or *Capsicum annum* in 5.2% mannitol enhanced the ability of the cells to survive freezing and thawing.

In addition to the culture conditions, the point in the growth curve at which cells are taken for freezing and thawing affects the survival. Sugawara and Sakai[9] concluded that *A. pseudoplatanus* cells grown for 5 to 6 days, and which were in the late-lag or early cell-division phase, gave the greatest survival on freezing and thawing. Withers and Street[10] concluded for carrot cell cultures that cells taken from late-lag to the mid point of exponential growth gave the best regrowth after freezing to −196°C and subsequent thawing.

IV. SUMMARY

The current state of knowledge leads to the conclusion that cryogenic storage is a possible method of preservation of plant cell, tissue, and organ cultures. The available knowledge is limited, but suggests a starting point for the development of procedures for freezing to −140°C or lower and successful recovery of the cultures. Systematic study of the conditions of growth and the point in the growth curve at which tissue is taken, together with the effects of cryoprotectant (both type and concentration), freezing rate, and thawing rate on the survival of a wide variety of plant cell cultures, is needed before any firm conclusions about the general possibility of cryogenic storage can be drawn. Clearly, where cell lines have unique characteristics, the retention of these characteristics after recovery from cryogenic storage needs evaluation.

V. ADDENDUM

At the 4th Int. Congr. of Plant Tissue Culture, the proceedings of which are published, Withers reviewed all aspects of cryogenic storage of cell cultures and provided data from her own work, which involves mechanisms of injury. This allows extension of the range of materials being successfully frozen and thawed. In addition, six contributed papers dealt with storage of potato cultures at or near 0°C (Henshaw et al., Wang), the toxicity of cryoprotectants and successful freezing to liquid nitrogen temperatures of sugar cane (Finkle and Ulrich), and variations in the freezing protocol to allow successful storage of rice (Nielsen et al.), potato (Grout and Henshaw), and *Marchantia polymorpha* (Takuchi). Activity in this area is increasing rapidly, and signs of its successful extension in several directions are apparent.

REFERENCES

1. **Caplin, S. M.,** Mineral oil overlay for conservation of plant tissue cultures, *Am. J. Bot.,* 46, 324, 1959.
2. **Bannier, L. J. and Steponkus, P. L.,** Cold acclimation of chrysanthemum callus cultures, *J. Am. Soc. Hortic. Sci.,* 101, 409, 1976.
3. **Sakai, A. and Sugawara, Y.,** Survival of poplar callus at super-low temperatures after cold acclimation, *Plant Cell Physiol.,* 14, 1201, 1973.
4. **McCown, B. H., McCown, D. D., Beck, G. E., and Hall, T. C.,** Isoenzyme complements of *Dianthus* callus cultures: influence of light and temperature, *Am. J. Bot.,* 57, 148, 1970.
5. **Rose, D. and Martin, S. M.,** Growth of suspension cultures of plant cells (*Ipomoea* sp.) at various temperatures, *Can. J. Bot.,* 53, 315, 1975.
6. **Nag, K. K. and Street, H. E.,** Carrot embryogenesis from frozen cultured cells, *Nature, (London),* 245, 270, 1973.
7. **Widholm, J. M.,** The use of fluorescein diacetate and phenosafranine for determining viability of cultured plant cells, *Stain Technol.,* 47, 189, 1972.
8. **Towill, L. E. and Mazur P.,** Studies on the reduction of 2,3,4-triphenyltetrazolium chloride as a viability assay for plant tissue cultures, *Can. J. Bot.,* 53, 1097, 1975.
9. **Sugawara, Y. and Sakai, A.,** Survival of suspension-cultured sycamore cells cooled to the temperature of liquid nitrogen, *Plant Physiol.,* 54, 722, 1974.
10. **Withers, L. A. and Street, H. E.,** Freeze preservation of cultured plant cells. III. The pregrowth phase, *Physiol. Plant.,* 39, 171, 1977.
11. **Palta, J. P., Levitt, J., and Stadelmann, E. J.,** Freezing injury in onion bulb cells. II. Post-thawing injury or recovery, *Plant Physiol.,* 60, 398, 1977.
12. **Morris, G. J.,** The cryopreservation of *Chlorella.* I. Interactions of rate of cooling, protective additive and warming rate, *Arch. Microbiol.,* 107, 57, 1976.
13. **Mazur, P.** Cryobiology: the freezing of biological systems, *Science,* 168, 939, 1970.
14. **Leibo, S. P., Farrant, J., Mazur, P., Hanna, M. G., Jr., and Smith, L. H.,** Effects of freezing on marrow stem cell suspensions: interactions of cooling and warming rates in the presence of PVP, sucrose, or glycerol, *Cryobiology,* 6, 315, 1970.
15. **Mazur, P.,** Freezing injury in plants, *Annu. Rev. Plant Physiol.,* 20, 419, 1969.
16. **Nag, K. K. and Street, H. E.,** Freeze preservation of cultured plant cells. I. The pretreatment phase, *Physiol. Plant.* 34, 254, 1975.
17. **Dougall, D. K. and Wetherell, D. F.,** Storage of wild carrot cultures in the frozen state, *Cryobiology,* 11, 410, 1974.
18. **Bajaj, Y. P. S.,** Regeneration of plants from cell suspensions frozen at −20, −70 and −196°C, *Physiol. Plant,* 37, 263, 1976.
19. **Latta, R.,** Preservation of suspension cultures of plant cells by freezing, *Can. J. Bot.,* 49, 1253, 1971.
20. **Quatrano, R. S.,** Freeze-preservation of cultured flax cells utilizing dimethyl sulfoxide, *Plant Physiol.,* 43, 2057, 1968.

21. **Nag, K. K. and Street, H. E.,** Freeze preservation of cultured plant cells. II. The freezing and thawing phases, *Physiol. Plant.,* 34, 261, 1975.
22. **Seibert, M. and Wetherbee, P. J.,** Increased survival and differentiation of frozen herbaceous plant organ cultures through cold treatment, *Plant Physiol.,* 59, 1043, 1977.
23. **Morris, G. J. and Farrant, J.,** Interactions of cooling rate and protective additive on the survival of washed human erythrocytes frozen to −196°C, *Cryobiology,* 9, 173, 1972.
24. **Lescure, A. M.,** Relationship between the density of plant cells and their growth kinetics in submerged medium, *Exp. Cell. Res.,* 44, 620, 1966.
25. **Stuart, R. and Street, H. E.,** Studies on the growth in culture of plant cells. IV. The initiation of division in suspensions of stationary-phase cells of *Acer pseudoplatanus* L., *J. Exp. Bot.,* 20, 556, 1969.
26. **Nickell, L. G. and Carmichael, J. W.,** private communication, 1978.
27. **Dougall, D. K.,** unpublished, 1978.

Chapter 6

ENVIRONMENTAL FACTORS

A. LIGHT

Michael Seibert and Prakash G. Kadkade

TABLE OF CONTENTS

I. INTRODUCTION

Until about 25 years ago, biologists paid little attention to the role of light in the growth and development of plant tissue cultures. The normal practice at that time was to store sample tubes in the laboratory under prevailing light conditions, periodic exposures to an illuminance of about 100 fc. Fortuitously, this level was adequate for sustaining growth, although below the 350 fc optimal value (light source not reported) found by de Capite[1] for callus growth in *Helianthus annuus, Parthenocissus tricuspidata* and *Daucus carota*. More recently as interest in tissue culture research increased, particularly from the applications aspect, investigators began to recognize the basic role which light played in both the growth and development of the cultures.[2]

The purpose of this chapter, then, is to briefly introduce the reader to the properties of light which affect tissue cultures, to demonstrate that light does indeed influence the growth, development, and biochemical patterns of cultured plant tissue, and to discuss the cellular and molecular interactions by which light can regulate these patterns.

II. PHYSICAL ASPECTS OF LIGHT

A. What is Light?

From a simplistic point of view, light is merely the form of radiant energy to which the human eye is sensitive. More precisely, it is a propagating, orthogonal electric and magnetic field (electromagnetic radiation) characterized by specific wavelength (λ) properties. In vacuum, it travels at a constant rate of 2.998×10^8 m/sec, commonly termed the speed of light (c). The entire spectrum of electromagnetic radiation has been divided into different regions from short-wavelength cosmic rays to long-wavelength power-transmission waves. It is represented in Figure 1. Visible light as we perceive it is located in the rather narrow wavelength region of this spectrum between 380 nm and 760 nm. Ultraviolet (UV) light occupies the 200 nm region to the left of visible light, and near-infrared light (near-IR) occupies the several hundred nanometer region to the right.

Light has a dual character, displaying both wave properties (refraction, diffraction, interference, and polarization phenomena) and particle properties (light is radiated in discrete amounts of energy or photons).[3] In accordance with Planck's Law, the quantum energy of a photon is related to its wavelength (a wave property) by:

$$E = \frac{hc}{\lambda} \tag{1}$$

where h is 6.63×10^{-34} joule·sec (Planck's constant), c is in m/sec, and λ is in meters. It is the quantum energy (the particle property) that is imparted to an electron in a photoreceptor molecule (a phenomenon called absorption or excitation depending upon the point of view) which is responsible for photochemical change, and photochemical change at the molecular level is the basis for the influence of light on metabolism and morphogenesis which we will described in later sections.

B. Tissue Culture Light Requirements

The characteristics of radiation which influence plant development in general[3,4] are also those which affect plant tissue in culture. These aspects are generally classified as intensity, spectral quality, and length of the daily exposure period.[2]

Intensity, although in common usage, is a generic term. One should define this prop-

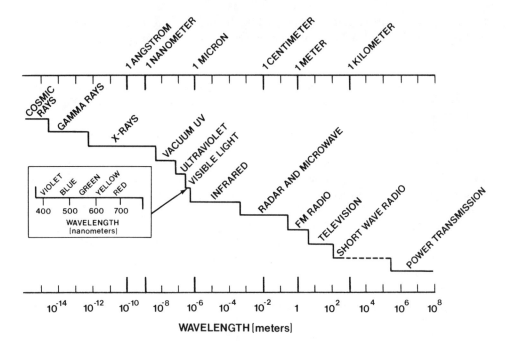

FIGURE 1. Spectrum of electromagnetic radiation plotted in meters on a logarithmic scale. The inset is an enlargement of the visible portion of the spectrum and is plotted in nanometers (10^{-9} meters) on a linear scale.

erty more precisely as either an irradiance (a radiometric term defined as the radiant flux intercepted per unit area) or an illuminance (a photometric term defined as the luminous flux intercepted per unit area).[5] An example of an irradiance unit is a W/m^2 and that of an illuminance unit is a lux. However, for the purpose of this paper, the English footcandle (fc) unit will be used rather than the lux. One fc = 10.76 lux. It is important to note that an irradiance measurement is not spectrally defined, whereas an illuminance measurement indicates the level of visible light as the human eye would see it (see Section II.D).

The peak solar irradiance at sea level in temperate regions is about 1000 W/m^2 (of which 50% is in the 380 to 760 nm region[6]). This level more than saturates the photosynthetic apparatus of most field crops,[7] but under suitable growing conditions is not high enough to damage the plants. Tissue cultures, on the other hand, normally do not grow autotrophically (except in special cases[8]) and, thus, do not require high irradiancies.[2] In fact, high light levels can be detrimental to tissue culture development.[9,10] These quantitative results explain why some plant tissue cultures fail to grow in plant growth chambers which supply high light levels necessary to support photosynthetic growth. However, it should be mentioned that when tissue-culture-derived plants are reestablished in soil, higher light levels are required.[2] The explanation is simply that in this case photosynthesis must supply the new plant with the carbon which the growth medium was supplying previously.

Spectral quality is simply the color of the light impinging on a culture. As seen in the last section, light is characterized by wavelength. Different types of light sources (see Section II.C) emit light of different wavelengths in different ratios. Tissue cultures generally require red or blue light. Thus, light sources which emit in these spectral regions will be effective in eliciting morphogenic responses (see Section III.).

Plants are also sensitive to the number of hours of light to which they are exposed each day.[11] So are tissue cultures.[9] As will be discussed later, as little as 5 min of light per day can profoundly influence morphogenesis in tissue culture systems.[12]

C. Light Sources

Besides the sun and fire, there are three general classes of light sources which are available for use in tissue culture applications. These are thermal, electrical discharge, and fluorescent.[3]

Thermal or blackbody-type sources normally operate by resistive heating of a wire filament (passing an electric current through tungsten wire enclosed in a glass envelope) to very high temperature. The white-hot filament emits visible light. Incandescent and tungsten-halogen lamps are examples of this class of light source. Electrical-discharge sources function when an electric current is passed through a gas or a metallic vapor located in a short-arc tube. The electrically excited gas or vapor subsequently emits specific wavelengths of light depending on the type of atom in the gas or vapor. Mercury, metal halide, and high-pressure sodium street lamps are examples of this second class. Fluorescent sources generate UV light (253.7 nm) in a long-arc tube by the excitation of low-pressure mercury gas using the same process described above for electrical discharge sources. The UV light then excites a phosphor material which coats the inner surface of the arc tube or tubular glass envelope. The phosphor subsequently emits specific wavelengths of fluorescent light (λ >253.7 nm), depending upon the phosphor. Many types of fluorescent lamps with different spectral emission characteristics (qualities) are readily available. Klein[13] and Seibert et al.[10] have reported inexpensive fluorescent lamp/color filter combinations for producing narrow-band light in various regions of the near-UV, visible, and near-IR spectrum. Suitable fluorescent lamps can be obtained from General Electric, GTE Sylvania, or Westinghouse. Filters are available from Strand Century (Cinemoid) or Rosco (Roscolux).

Of the three classes of artificial light sources, fluorescent sources have been used almost exclusively for tissue culture research and applications because they are more efficient at producing broadband visible light than incandescent sources and are available in much lower output wattages than electrical-discharge lamps. For these reasons, fluorescent lamps can be used in culture chambers more cost-effectively than the other classes of light sources.

D. Light Measurements

Since plant tissue is not sensitive to light in the same manner as the human eye, light should be measured in radiometric units rather than photometric units (see Section II.B.). Unfortunately, most work in the literature has been reported in the latter units, probably because light sources are rated in photometric terms and because radiometers are more expensive, less available, and harder to operate than photometers (footcandle meters). An example of how one might be misled in this respect is that it is possible for two different light sources to expose a culture to the same number of footcandles, but a vastly different number of W/m². Thus, one might not be able to explain differences in the effect of the two light sources from only footcandle measurements.

If results must be reported in photometric units, then it is absolutely necessary to describe fully the light source by name (i.e., "cool-white fluorescent," "warm-white fluorescent," etc., not "fluorescent" or "white fluorescent"). With this information, one can reproduce experimental or culture conditions from one laboratory to another and even convert the given photometric units into radiometric units using conversion factors obtainable from the literature.[14] Optimally, one should also report the spectral energy distribution (SPD) or irradiance in $W \cdot m^{-2} \cdot nm^{-1}$ as a function of wavelength for the light source and the rating of the source in lumens.

III. INFLUENCE OF LIGHT ON GROWTH AND ORGANOGENESIS

As was discussed in Section II, tissue cultures require only low levels of light to regulate morphogenic processes. This section will discuss the influence of light on plant cultures at the cell, tissue, and organ levels. The literature which has specified spectral and irradiance information about the light sources employed (or reported illuminance values in combination with a complete description of the light sources used for experimental work) has been emphasized in this section because sufficient information is available for the results to be replicated.

A. Callus Cultures

Since the time light was first reported to increase callus growth,[1] many investigators have sought to determine whether different wavelengths have differential effects on growth and development of callus cultures. Unfortunately, the early results were conflicting and did not lead to any consistent picture.[10] For example, blue light was reported to enhance callus growth in *Pelargonium zonale*,[15] but to inhibit it in *D. carota*[16] and *P. tricuspidata*.[17] The situation with *Nicotiana tabacum* was even more confusing since some authors reported that blue light enhanced callus growth,[18,19] and others reported that it inhibited callus growth.[20] Seibert et al.[10] resolved the discrepancies by pointing out that the above reported work had employed different wavelengths in the blue spectral region and different irradiances. Callus growth and shoot initiation can, in fact, be either enhanced (see also Weis and Jaffe[19]) or inhibited, depending on the wavelength and irradiance as has been demonstrated in tobacco.[10] Action spectra for the enhancement of both phenomena have been reported in tobacco and are quite similar.[10]

Other wavelengths also affect callus growth. For example, Klein[21] reported that *P. tricuspidata* crown-gall cultures were inhibited by near-UV light ($\sim$ 360 nm) and green light (550 nm). Near-UV (371 nm) also inhibits tobacco callus growth and shoot initiation, but only at irradiances higher than 3.7 W/m^2 (see Figure 2).[10] The inhibitive effects of high near-UV and blue light may involve low IAA oxidase activity,[17] destruction of vitamin B_{12},[21] photoinactivation of IAA,[22] destruction of cytochrome oxidase,[23] or increases in the amount of phenolic compounds in the tissue.[24] Darkness,[21] 6-(3-methyl-2-buten-1-ylamino)-purine (2iP),[22] and (2-chloroethyl)-trimethylammonium chloride (CCC)[22] have all been reported to reverse the inhibitive effects of near-UV light on callus cultures to various extents.

In addition to the short-wavelength effects, long wavelengths can influence callus-culture growth in some cases. Both enhancement[15] and inhibitive[16] effects of red light have been reported in various species. The enhancement effect in *P. zonale* was attributed[15] to the high-energy phytochrome reaction.[25] However, due to a lack of evidence in the near-IR spectral region, the conclusion must be considered preliminary. On the other hand, the enhancement of growth in *Crepis capillaris* cultures[26] by red light is accompanied by increases in protein synthesis and cell division. Kinetin can replace the effects of red light in cultures exposed to either far-red light or darkness, but not in cultures exposed to blue light. Green cultures of *C. capillaris* maintained for 4½ years recovered their capacity to form organs only if they were exposed to blue light in the presence of gibberellic acid.[26] Chlorophyll-free callus did not form organs in the presence of red light or darkness.

Inhibitive effects, at least in *Helianthus tuberosus* callus cultures, may be the result of decreases in cell division. Davidson and Yeoman[27] have presented evidence consistent with an hypothesis which postulates that a phytochrome-mediated reaction, activated by 665 nm light, initiates a series of events which depletes an essential metabolite

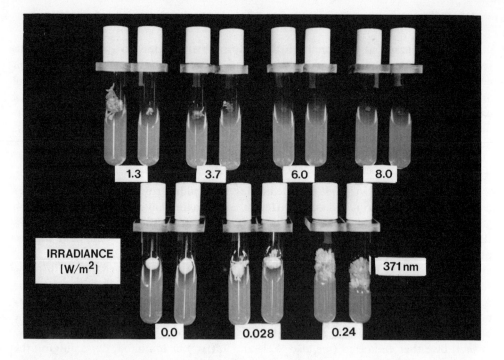

FIGURE 2.   Representative tobacco callus cultures exposed to the indicated incident near-UV (371 nm, 16 hr/day) irradiance levels for 35 days. Note that very low levels of UV light promote organogenesis while higher levels are inhibitive. (From Seibert, M., Wetherbee, P. J., and Job, D. D., *Plant Physiol.*, 56, 130, 1975. With permission.)

(probably L-phenylalanine) below a critical level required for cell division. However, James and Davidson[28] showed that the relationship between phytochrome and cell division cannot be a simple one. On the other hand, red light (660 nm) has no effect on tobacco callus growth and development[10,18-20] (at least up to irradiancies of about 20 W/m²)[10] or on *P. tricuspidata* callus growth.[17] Moreover, near-IR (700 to 800 nm) has no influence on tobacco callus growth[10,19,20] or shoot initiation.[10,19]

Tobacco callus cultures exposed to blue light during the first 2 weeks of culture and darkness,[19,29] red light,[19,29] or near-IR (far-red) light[19] for three more weeks had fewer shoots and weighed less than cultures exposed to blue light for the entire 5 weeks. Thus, these cultures require blue light throughout the culture period for optimal development and, under the above conditions, cannot distinguish between red light, near-IR, and darkness.

A rather curious and unexplained effect of light on plants regenerated from anther-derived callus cultures of *Digitalis purpurea* L. was reported by Corduan and Spix.[30] During the regeneration process, if the anthers were exposed to light, the resultant plants were tetraploid. If they were not exposed to light, the plants were diploid. Nitsch and Norreel,[31] furthermore, demonstrated that red light enhanced microspore and embryo development in tobacco anther cultures, while blue light had no effect.

Under normal tissue culture conditions, callus cultures are known to develop chloroplasts in the light,[18,32,33] carry out photosynthesis,[18,32,34] and evolve oxygen.[35] However, the presence of sucrose in the culture medium inhibits both chlorophyll synthesis and photosynthetic carbon fixation in tissue cultures.[34] Thus, what photosynthesis does occur cannot support the growth and development in callus cultures.[18] Therefore, the observations discussed above are due to the photomorphogenic rather than photosynthetic effects of light. (The situation may be different for habituated cultures and autotrophic cultures exposed to enhanced CO_2 and high-light conditions.)

For the most part, photomorphogenic studies with callus cultures have employed continuous-lighting conditions. However, Murashige and Nakano[2,36] have reported that the optimal daily photoperiod for differentiation in tobacco callus was 16 hr, while Margara[37] found that the optimal value for cauliflower was 9 hr/day.

B. Cell and Protoplast Cultures

Results similar to those reported for callus cultures have also been observed in cell cultures. Both increases and decreases in cell concentration and dry-weight production have been observed in cell cultures of several species as a result of exposure to various wavelengths of near-UV and visible light.[38-40] Increases in dry weight due to red light have been reported in *Populus* hybrids and two species of tobacco.[39] On the other hand, blue light causes the transformation of plastids to photosynthetically active chloroplasts in *N. tabacum* var. "Samsum" cultures.[41] Both red and blue light influence the development of chloroplasts in leaves, but dark-grown leaves do not contain the prolamellar bodies characteristic of the plastids observed in the cell cultures.[41]

Light increases the plating efficiency of single cells isolated from green tobacco callus, whereas it inhibits the growth of cells isolated from chlorophyll-free callus cultures.[42] The plating efficiency,[43,44] growth, and development[45,46] of protoplast cultures are dependent on the level of light to which they are exposed. Too much light can be inhibitive.[44]

C. Organ Cultures

1. Shoot-Tip Cultures

Until recently, there has been very little quantitative information about the light requirements of organ cultures. The general "rule of thumb" has been to expose shoot-tip or lateral-bud explants to about 100 fc of Gro-Lux® or cool-white fluorescent light for 16 hr/day.[2] This has proven adequate for *Asparagus officinalis, Gerbera jamesonii, Saxifraga* sp., and a number of bromeliads.[2,9] In the absence of additional information, these conditions can be used as a starting point in optimizing organ multiplication for plant propagation applications. On the basis of results with tobacco callus cultures,[10] though, it might be wise to test several different types of broadband-emitting fluorescent lamps with each new species, since the results with different types of lamps can be similar, and the costs of different fluorescent lamps vary widely.

It should be mentioned that narrow-band light may be sufficient to cause increases in callus production and axillary shoot initiation since Rolinson and Vince-Prue[47] demonstrated that short periods of exposure (16 hr) to extremely low irradiances of red light or longer exposures to far-red light led to increased rates of cell division in *Oryza sativa* shoot apices.

2. Cotyledon and Embryo Cultures

Recent results with *Lactuca sativa* cotyledons[12,48] and *Pseudotsuga menziesii* (Mirb.) Franco (Douglas fir) embryos[49] have also demonstrated that red (660 nm) light can have a profound influence on both callus growth and organogenesis in organ cultures. Adventitious shoot formation in lettuce is regulated by the low-energy phytochrome mechanism.[12] Daily exposures to as little as 5 min of 660 nm light (2.5 W/m^2) during either the second week of a 5-week culture period or during the entire culture period is sufficient to double the number of shoots differentiated in comparison with unlighted, control, cotyledon cultures.[48] The increased number of shoots were correlated with an increased number of buds which formed after 15 days of culture.[12] Adventitious bud formation in Douglas-fir-embryo cultures is also most sensitive to red light during the middle few weeks of an 8-week culture period.[49]

3. Root and Rhizome Cultures

Light also promoted the initiation of roots in cultures of *Pisum sativum* L. and *H. tuberosus*.[50-52] Letouze and Beauchesne,[51] moreover, demonstrated that red light (660 nm) and, to a lesser extent, blue light caused both root initiation and elongation in *H. tuberosus*. Gautheret reported that 12 hr of light per day was optimal.[52] We have also observed that red light enhances root initiation, although in lettuce cotyledon cultures.[48] These results are thus consistent with those of Fletcher et al.[53] who observed that red light promoted root initiation in *Phaseolus* seedlings, apparently in a phytochrome-related phenomenon (the phytochrome system is known to be active in isolated pea roots[54]).

Finally, Bonnett[55] demonstrated that red light also induces the elongation of endogenous buds in cultured root segments of *Convolvulus arvensis* L., and that the process is regulated by phytochrome.

4. Leaf Cultures

Leaf cultures of *Cichorium intybus* L.[56] require initial exposures to either darkness or daylight-fluorescent light (150 fc) for maximal adventitious shoot formation. The number of shoots formed is proportional to the initial exposure period to light and inversely proportional to initial exposure to darkness. Continuous exposure to light elicits twice the response observed in dark controls.

IV. INFLUENCE OF LIGHT ON PLANT PRODUCTS

Light, in addition to its effects on in vitro plant growth and development, also influences the production of plant metabolites. The latter observation will be examined in this section.

A. Primary Products

1. Enzymes

Plant cell cultures have yielded much information about the influence of light on the enzymatic reactions of secondary metabolism. Many of the enzymes involved in the pathways of certain secondary products such as cinnamic acids, coumarins, lignins, flavones, flavanols, chalcones, and anthocyanins have been identified. The activity of these enzymes, as well as secondary product accumulation, increases dramatically upon illumination of the cultures.[57]

Light exerts an influence on all enzymes of the flavanoid pathway.[58-62] The enzymes involved in the synthesis of flavanoids in *Petroselinum hortense* (parsley) are comprised of two different groups based on their mode of action.[61] Group 1 includes L-phenylalanine ammonia-lyase (PAL), cinnamic acid 4-hydroxylase, and *p*-coumarate: CoA ligase. Group 2 includes flavonone synthetase, glucosyltransferase, apiosyltransferase, UDP-apiose synthetase, chalcone flavonone isomerase, and others. The first group of enzymes catalyzes the formation of phenylpropane derivatives, while the enzymes of the second group are engaged exclusively in flavone glycoside synthesis. The activities of all enzymes of Groups 1 and 2 show an increase after exposure to light for 2 and 4 hr, respectively. While the activities of most of these enzymes are very low in dark-grown (for 10 days) parsley cells, cinnamic acid 4-hydroxylase and *p*-coumarate: CoA ligase activities are as much as 30 to 40% of those observed in the light.[58] Upon exposure of parsley cells to continuous irradiation, the first group of enzymes reach their maximum activities after 15 to 23 hr, while those of the second group attain their maximum activities after 24 to 37 hr. Hahlbrock et al.[58] have suggested that the group of enzymes involved in the synthesis of phenylpropanoids are regulated by a different mechanism from those which are specific to flavone biosynthesis. This view is supported by experiments employing transcription and translation inhibitors.[63] When such inhibitors are added to parsley-cell cultures before exposure to light, the increase of PAL activity is inhibited up to 100%, compared with untreated cultures. Under these conditions, the activities of all other Group 1 enzymes and chalcone flavanone isomerase are also much lower than in untreated cultures.[63] The enzyme activities of the remaining enzymes of the second group, however, are unaffected by the addition of these inhibitors. Light-induced increases in PAL activity are thus due to *de novo* synthesis and not to activation of a preexisting, inactive form of the enzyme.[64,65] In addition, PAL activity is strongly influenced by the addition of inhibitors to *P. hortense* cell cultures at different times after exposure to light.[64] The inhibitory effect of actinomycin D on PAL activity decreases linearly with time, while that of cycloheximide remains constant throughout the lag phase and diminishes thereafter. These results demonstrate that RNA and protein synthesis are required during *de novo* formation on PAL.

In addition to the effects of light and inhibitors, the activities of Group 1 enzymes are also enhanced when 10-day-old dark-grown parsley cells are transferred to fresh medium.[66] With the exception of cinnamic acid 4-hydroxylase, maximal enzyme activities are observed 17 hr after subculturing. Similar results have been observed in the cell cultures of citrus species[67] and *Haplopappus gracilis*,[68] although the timescales were longer.

A large increase in Group 1-enzyme activities also occurs after transfer of dark-grown parsley cells into distilled water.[69] The cause is a dilution of at least one compound arising from the cells. The extent of the PAL-activity change depends on the degree of cell dilution. A second increase is observed 5 hr after dilution, and it is inducible by light. The dilution effects are inhibited by both actinomycin D and cycloheximide. Similar results have been reported in *Glycine max*[70] and Paul's Scarlet Rose cell cultures.[71] Cinnamic acid 4-hydroxylase and p-coumarate: CoA ligase in cell cultures of *G. max* exhibit the same behavior as PAL. These results demonstrated that increases in Group 1-enzyme activities are possible in the absence of light induction.

In determining the active spectral region, several investigators have shown that blue light increases PAL activity and subsequent anthocyanin production in callus and cell cultures of *H. gracilis*.[68,72,73] Maximum sensitivity occurs 3 weeks after subculturing.[68,72] Subsequent irradiation for 48 hr results in a 400% rise in PAL activity followed by a gradual decline.[68] Irradiation with red and far-red light alone or after induction with blue light had no effect on PAL activity.[68] Actinomycin D and puromycin treatments inhibit blue-light-induced enzyme activity.[68] Stark et al.[74] however, were unable to show a correlation between PAL activity and anthocyanin formation in certain cell lines of *Daucus carota* cultures. In three cell lines of carrot which produce anthocyanins in the dark, PAL activity was not enhanced by light. However, in cell lines which do not produce anthocyanins in the dark, PAL activity was enhanced by light. Stark et al.[74] suggested that, in the former cell lines, anthocyanin biosynthesis is not regulated by PAL, but by an enzyme which is located later on in the biosynthetic pathway. However, the interpretation of these experiments is difficult since the enzyme activities change during the cell cycle even in dark-grown cultures. Furthermore, light-induced PAL activity varies considerably with the age of culture.[75]

2. Carbohydrates

Thorpe and Meir[76] have studied starch metabolism in tobacco callus. Conditions favoring meristemoid and shoot primordia development greatly enhance both the synthesis and breakdown of starch. Cultures maintained under 16 hr of light per day (Gro-lux® fluorescent, 270 fc) accumulate starch earlier than dark-grown tissue. Maximal starch accumulation in light-grown cultures coincides with the emergence of organized structures (thereafter, starch levels decrease).

3. Lipids

Cell-suspension cultures of *Chenopodium rubrum* grown under photoautotrophic conditions display relatively large amounts of the lipid classes typically found in photosynthetic tissues.[77] Monogalactosyldiacylglycerols, digalactosyldiacylglycerols, glycerolphosphoglycerides, and some sulfoquinovosyldiacylglycerols are examples of such lipid classes. Heterotrophic cultures, on the other hand, contain at most 1 to 2% of the two galactolipids and only traces of the glycerophosphoglycerides and sulfolipids. The fatty acid patterns of the lipids in photoautotrophic cultures resemble those of green leaves of *C. rubrum*. Linolenic acid constitutes about 30% of the total fatty acids in the photoautotrophic cultures, whereas the heterotrophic cultures contain only 15% of this acid.

4. Amino Acids

A few investigators have shown that light can affect amino acid concentrations and compositions in cell-suspension cultures.[78-81] In peanut cells, light treatment increases glutamine formation while darkness causes the accumulation of asparagine.[78] Durzan et al.[79] reported that the acceleration of *Pinus banksiana* cell-suspension culture growth by light correlated directly with total nitrogen content. On the other hand, these cells lost free amino nitrogen in the dark. Continuous light also optimized final cell size and bound nitrogen. These results somehow involve the ability of cells to maintain higher levels of soluble nitrogen both internally and externally in the medium.[25]

3,4-Dihydroxyphenylalanine (L-Dopa) accumulation in cell-suspension cultures of *Vicia faba* and *Mucuna holtonii* is influenced by both light and hormones.[80] Although continuous exposure to cool-white fluorescent light increases the growth of cell cultures, it decreases L-Dopa accumulation in both the cells and the medium. L-Dopa levels are higher in dark-grown suspension cells, and most of it accumulates in the medium. Similar results are observed in static cultures derived from *Mucuna pruriens* seeds.[81]

5. Other Products

Matsumoto et al.[82] reported that riboflavin enhanced anthocyanin production in light-grown, but not dark-grown, *Populus* cell-suspension cultures. They suggested that riboflavin or one of its photochemical derivatives might function as a photoreceptor.

Cultural conditions, viz., light vs. darkness, affect the amount of hormones found in plant tissue cultures.[83-85] Dark-grown tobacco cultures produce higher levels of endogenous gibberellins than light-grown cultures.[83] Under conditions where tobacco cells grow more rapidly in the dark than in light, the dark-grown cells metabolize (^{3}H) GA$_{20}$ more effectively.[84] The slow growth rate and the low levels of endogenous GA found in light-grown tissue may be due to reduced synthesis of certain growth-promoting gibberellins (see also Section III.A). The presence or absence of light is also an important factor in modulating somatic embryo development in cultured cells of caraway.[85] In light, zeatin eliminates abscisic acid (ABA) growth inhibition, whereas gibberellic acid partially reverses the ABA effect.[85]

B. Secondary Products

The secondary products described in this section will be confined to those compounds for which no definite function has been assigned and which are considered to be nonessential metabolites.[86]

1. Flavones and Flavonols

As long as *P. hortense* cultures are kept in the dark, they multiply, but do not form flavanoids. Once they are exposed to light, the glycoside, apiin, can be detected in appreciable amounts. Similarly, more than 20 flavone and flavonol glycosides are produced when the cultures are grown under continuous cool-white fluorescent light.[61,87] The formation of flavone glycosides begins after a lag phase of 4 to 6 hr and reaches a constant level 3 to 4 days after the onset of light.

Flavone glycoside synthesis is most sensitive to UV light below 320 nm.[88] Red light alone is ineffective. However, after UV preirradiation, red light does influence flavone glycoside synthesis and the red/far red phytochrome system is involved.[89,90] Presumably, phytochrome changes from an inactive to an active form after preirradiation with UV light. Triggering of apigenin synthesis by light has also been observed in *Glycine max.*[91]

2. Anthocyanins

Triggering of anthocyanin synthesis by light has been demonstrated in callus and cell-suspension cultures from several plant species.[68,82,91-95] Reinert et al.[92] reported that blue light stimulated anthocyanin synthesis in *H. gracilis* callus, while red light was ineffective. Lachmann[96] confirmed this observation and reported an action spectrum with peaks at 438 nm and 372 nm.

Alfermann et al.,[94] working with carrot-cell cultures, were able to replace the light requirement of anthocyanin biosynthesis with auxin. The time dependence of light-induced and auxin-induced anthocyanin synthesis, however, was quite different.[95] Anthocyanins were detectable 3 days after exposure to light, but 6 days after addition of auxin. Cycloheximide and 2-thiouracil[71] inhibited auxin-induced anthocyanin formation, but promoted anthocyanin synthesis in light-grown cultures. These results suggest that there are at least two different mechanisms involved in anthocyanin accumulation in carrot-cell cultures.[95] Gibberellic acid, moreover, inhibits both light-induced[97,98] and auxin-induced anthocyanin production[98] in cell cultures of *H. gracilis* and *D. carota*. Maximum anthocyanin synthesis depends upon the developmental stage of *H. gracilis* suspension cultures at the time of light exposure.[99] Cultures left in the dark for 3 days prior to light exposure accumulate more anthocyanin compared to the cultures kept in the dark for only the day prior to light exposure.[99] Anthocyanin synthesis was also influenced by the growth period of cultures.[93] Initially, the ratio of cyanidin-3-glucoside to cyanidin-3-rutinoside was 5:1, but changed to 1:1 during the growth period of *H. gracilis* cell cultures grown under blue light.

3. Naphthoquinones and Polyphenols

The biosynthesis of naphthoquinones in callus cultures of *Lithospermum erythrorhizon* is inhibited by cool-white fluorescent light (530 fc). Studies using monochromatic light revealed that the inhibition is caused by blue light and not by red or green. Tabata et al.[100] suggested that blue light represses either the induction of a common precursor or the conversion of an intermediate involved in the synthetic pathways.

Polyphenol synthesis in plant tissue cultures is stimulated by light.[101,102] Upon illumination, callus cultures derived from *Camellia sinensis* show a severalfold increase in catechin, epicatechin, and leucoanthocyanin concentration. Light, however, has no effect on polymerization of leucoanthocyanins.[101] Davis[102] reported that the initial rate of polyphenol synthesis in cell-suspension cultures of Paul's Scarlet Rose was influenced by several factors, including auxin concentration in the medium and light intensity. High light intensities partially reversed the inhibition of polyphenol synthesis caused by 5×10^{-5} M 2,4-D and stimulated accumulation at 5×10^{-7} M 2,4-D.[102]

4. Volatile Oils and Terpenes

The synthesis and composition of volatile oils in stem tissue cultures of *Ruta grav-eolens* depend on both light intensity and quality.[103-105] Volatile-oil composition of cultures grown under continuous cool-white light (250 fc) resembles that of green plants. The major components are undecanone, undecylacetate, and undecanol, and the minor components are nonanone, nonylacetate, and nonanol. Traces of geijerene and pregeijerene are also present in the callus cultures.[103,104] Cell cultures derived from root tissue synthesize geijerene and pregeijerene exclusively, both in the light as well as in the dark. Light also stimulates the formation of specialized oil passages.[105] Vola-tile oils are secreted into these passages, and the anatomical features of the passages resemble those found in parts of the intact plant.

Cell cultures grown under continuous red or far-red light (1.25 W/m^2) produce the same major oil components (geijerene and pregeijerene) as those found in the dark-grown cultures. In contrast, cultures grown under blue light produce an oil composi-tion similar to those grown under cool-white fluorescent light (250 fc) for 15 or 24 hr/ day. Cultures grown under short-day (6 hr) conditions produced oil compositions half-way between those obtained under continuous light and dark conditions.[105] Butcher et al.[106] reported an alteration in the pattern of sesquiterpenes in callus and suspension culturxs derived from *Andrographis paniculata* after exposure to light.

5. Other Products

Light also affects the yield of other secondary metabolites in plant tissue cultures. Hasegawa et al.[107] reported stimulation of lignin formation in callus cultures of *Pinus strobus* while Haddon and Northcote[108] found that increased lignin biosynthesis cor-related with the appearance of PAL activity. Callus and suspension cultures of *R. graveolens* undergo a severalfold increase in coumarin production when exposed to cool-white fluorescent light.[109] Glycoalkaloid levels in tissue cultures of *Solanum xan-thocarpum*[110] and *Solanum acculeatissimum*[111,112] are influenced both by growth regu-lators and light. Callus cultures derived from seeds of *S. acculeatissimum*[112] produce significant amounts of total glycoalkaloids when grown under Gro-lux® fluorescent light (16-hr days). It is noteworthy that free solasodine and solamargine were not de-tected in dark-grown cultures.[112]

Steroidal sapogenin production in cultures of *Dioscorea* species is also enhanced by growth hormones[113,114] and light.[114] Although light does not significantly affect the callus growth, it does stimulate diosgenin biosynthesis in both callus and cell-suspen-sion cultures obtained from tubers of *D. nelsonii*, *D. composita*, and *D. bernoul-liana*.[114] During the first 8 days after initiation of the cultures, the amount of diosgenin formed in light- and dark-grown tissue cultures is about the same.[114] However, after 8 days, diosgenin production in light-grown cultures (400 fc of continuous cool-white fluorescent light) is significantly higher than that in dark-grown cultures.[114] These ob-servations clearly indicated that light can substantially improve the yield of certain primary and secondary metabolites in tissue cultures.

V. INFLUENCE OF LIGHT ON UPTAKE OF MOLECULES AND BIOTRANSFORMATION

The importance of light in stimulation of anion accumulation in excised leaf tissue of *Vallisneria spiralis* was recognized as early as 1953.[115] However, it was not until

1961 that Derbyshire and Street[116] showed that glucose assimilation and nitrate absorption by excised wheat roots could be promoted by light. Excised wheat roots grown under a mixture of fluorescent and incandescent light (80 fc) absorb nitrates from the culture medium and convert organic nitrogen to protein faster than dark-grown excised roots.[116]

Subsequent studies by other investigators[117-119] have demonstrated that enhanced uptake of ^{14}C-sugar into terminal buds can be stimulated by red light. Etiolated pea epicotyls, excised above the cotyledon and dipped basally into a ^{14}C-sucrose solution, served as the experimental material. Enhanced uptake of ^{14}C-sucrose can be detected within 60 min after the onset of light exposure,[117] and the effect is under phytochrome control.[118] Furthermore, transport of sucrose requires oxygen and is inhibited by both low temperature and 2,4-dinitrophenol.[119] Jones et al.[120] demonstrated that increased uptake of nitrate and increases in nitrate reductase activity are also regulated by the low-energy phytochrome system. Jaffe and Thoma[121] reported similar results for the uptake of ^{14}C-sodium acetate in bean roots. Thus, increases in the uptake of sucrose, nitrate, and sodium acetate stimulated by red light can be explained at least in part by a phytochrome-dependent increase in the intracellular ATP[122,123] which stimulates active uptake.

Furthermore, Bergman[124] found that uptake of 3-O-methylglucose in aerobic, mixotropically grown cells of tobacco is nearly two times higher in the light than in the dark. Since uptake is inhibited by 3-(3,4-dichlorophenyl)-1,1-dimethylurea (DCMU), energy is probably required for the active transport of 3-O-methylglucose.

The accumulation of chlorogenic acid in *H. gracilis* callus cultures[93] and potato tuber discs[125] is enhanced by exposure to cool-white fluorescent light. Blue light is the active spectral region.[125] Exogenous supply of phenylalanine, a precursor compound, results in a severalfold increase in chlorogenic acid production. Phenylalanine plus light has a greater effect on chlorogenic acid formation than either phenylalanine or light alone.[125] On the other hand, light does not enhance chlorogenic acid formation in the presence of trans-cinnamic acid. Thus, the ability of light to increase chlorogenic acid levels over control values depends on the precursor present.

In other examples of light-enhanced biotransformation, Fritsch et al.[99] reported rapid conversion of phenylalanine, tetrahydroxychalcone, and dihydrokaempferol into cyanidin when suspension cultures of *H. gracilis* were exposed to blue light. The addition of cholesterol to suspension cultures of *D. deltoidea*[113] and *D. composita*[126] causes a doubling to tripling of diosgenin content over control levels. Larger increases in diosgenin content, however, are observed when the cultures are illuminated with continuous cool-white fluorescent light.[126]

VI. FUTURE OUTLOOK FOR THE USE OF LIGHT IN PLANT TISSUE CULTURE RESEARCH AND APPLICATION

Knowledge of the influence of light on in vitro propagation of plant tissue has increased considerably in recent years. By the proper use of artificial light and new techniques, many plant species can be regenerated from cell and tissue cultures throughout the year. However, continued research is required to understand more completely the importance of spectral quality, irradiance, length of irradiation, and the developmental period in which irradiation is most effective for the improvement of the quality and quantity of tissue culture plants. Little is known about the sequence of biochemical events involved in the initiation of photoregulated organogenesis once the photoreceptor system has been triggered by light. Light interaction with hormone levels and metabolic inhibitors could be used to probe the pathway of such events.

The production of medicinal compounds by plant cell and tissue cultures has been pursued during the last two decades, and light plays an important role in the regulation of secondary metabolism. However, more effort is needed to understand precisely how light functions in the control of key biochemical regulative mechanisms.

The biosynthesis and accumulation of secondary products in the intact plant occur in response to changes in environmental conditions or the stage of development, and in many instances, they are associated with the differentiation and development of specialized cell structures in plants. To date, however, there has not been enough emphasis on research related to the influence of light on the development of specialized structures in cell and tissue cultures.

The ability of light to stimulate biotransformation of certain substrates into more useful compounds in plant cell and tissue cultures offers an exciting area for future research. This technique has great potential for applications in modifying the chemical structure of certain compounds where modification can not be accomplished easily by conventional means. The use of specific narrow-band light may provide a means to effect the alteration in membrane permeability of cells in order to facilitate the release of cellular metabolites into the culture medium. This is especially important in preventing possible negative feedback or regression due to excess intracellular accumulation of the final product.

Dramatic progress has been made in protoplast-culture technology resulting in remarkable achievements in the genetic manipulation of cells. However, there are still major difficulties regarding the transfer of genetic information by uptake and integration of foreign DNA into plant cells. Since light quality plays an important role in controlling membrane permeability, it will be of interest to determine whether light can influence uptake and subsequent integration of DNA in plant cells and protoplasts.

Finally, the development of photoautotropic cell lines may render cell and tissue culture techniques superior to intact plants from the standpoint of biotechnological application. The decade ahead will show to what extent light can be used in the successful industrial exploitation of plant cell and tissue cultures for in vitro plant propagation and for economic production of physiologically active compounds.

VII. SUMMARY

This review described the importance of light in plant tissue culture development both at the physiological and biochemical level. Cell and tissue culture growth and organogenesis are profoundly influenced by intensity, spectral quality, and length of the daily exposure period. Light also has a marked influence on the production of certain primary and secondary plant metabolites. Effects on the activities of the enzymes involved in flavanoid synthesis, on the enzymes associated with the accumulation of flavone and flavonol glycosides, and on the formation of amino acids, coumarins, polyphenols, anthocyanins, terpenes, steroidal sapogenins, and alkaloids are discussed.

The role of light in differentiation and tissue organization is of the utmost importance from the viewpoint of synthesis and accumulation of certain metabolites associated with highly specialized cells. Biosynthesis of volatile oils in callus cultures of *R. graveolens* and lignins in callus cultures of *P. strobus* illustrate this point. Finally, uptake and biotransformation of certain compounds by a number of cell and organ cultures are significantly enhanced by light.

ACKNOWLEDGMENT

We wish to thank Dr. H. K. Mangold for kindly supplying us with some of his unpublished results.

REFERENCES

1. de Capite, L., Action of light and temperature on growth of plant tissue cultures *in vitro, Am. J. Bot.*, 42, 869, 1955.
2. Murashige, T., Plant propagation through tissue cultures, *Ann. Rev. Plant Physiol.*, 25, 135, 1974.
3. Bickford, E. D. and Dunn, S., *Lighting For Plant Growth*, Kent State University Press, Kent, Ohio, 1972, chap. 1, 2, and 4.
4. Went, F. W., *The Experimental Control of Plant Growth*, Ronald Press, New York, 1957, chap. 2, 8, and 18.
5. Nemhauser, R. I., Alexander, G., and Duda, R., Radiometry and photometry: once over lightly, *Opt. Spectra*, 10, 30, 1976.
6. Goldberg, B. and Klein, W. H., Variations in the spectral distribution of daylight at various geographical locations on the earth's surface, *Sol. Energy*, 19, 3, 1977.
7. Thomas, M. D. and Hill, G. R., in *Photosynthesis in Plants*, Franck, J. and Loomis, W. E., Eds., Iowa State University Press, Ames, 1949, 19.
8. Berlyn, M. B. and Zelitch, I., Photoautotrophic growth and photosynthesis in tobacco callus cells, *Plant Physiol.*, 56, 752, 1975.
9. Hasegawa, P. M., Murashige, T., and Takatori, F. H., Propagation of asparagus through shoot apex culture. II. Light and temperature requirements, transplantability of plants, and cyto-histological characteristics, *J. Am. Soc. Hortic. Sci.*, 98, 143, 1973.
10. Seibert, M., Wetherbee, P. J., and Job, D. D., The effects of light intensity and spectral quality on growth and shoot initiation in tobacco callus, *Plant Physiol.*, 56, 130, 1975.
11. Garner, W. W. and Allard, H. A., Effect of the relative length of day and night and other factors of the environment on growth and reproduction in plants, *J. Agric. Res. (Washington, D.C.)*, 18, 553, 1920.
12. Kadkade, P. G. and Seibert, M., Phytochrome regulated organogenesis in lettuce tissue culture, *Nature (London)*, 270, 49, 1977.
13. Klein, R. M., An inexpensive filter system for photomorphogenic research, *Photochem. Photobiol.*, 4, 625, 1965.
14. Campbell, L. E., Thimijan, R. W., and Cathey, H. M., Spectral radiant power of lamps used in horticulture, *Trans. Am. Soc. Agric. Eng.*, 18, 952, 1975.
15. Ward, H. B. and Vance, B. D., Effects of monochromatic radiations on growth of *Pelargonium* callus tissue, *J. Exp. Biol.*, 19, 119, 1968.
16. Polevaya, V. S., Effect of light of different spectral compositions on the growth of isolated carrot tissue cultures (trans.), *Fiziol. Rast.*, 14, 48, 1967.
17. Butenko, R. G., Yakovleva, Z. M., and Dmitrieva, N. N., Effect of gibberellic acid on the growth and auxin metabolism of isolated tissue cultures grown under different light conditions, *Dokl. Akad. Nauk S.S.S.R.*, 139, 1246, 1961 (English trans., Bot. Sci. Sect., 139, 147, 1962).
18. Bergmann, L. and Bälz, A., Der Einfluss von Farblicht auf Wachstum und zusammensetzung pflanzlicher Gewebekulturen. I. Mitteilung *Nicotiana tabacum* var. 'samsun', *Planta*, 70, 285, 1966.
19. Weis, J. S. and Jaffe, M. J., Photoenhancement by blue light of organogenesis in tobacco pith cultures, *Physiol. Plant.*, 22, 171, 1969.
20. Beauchesne, G. and Poulain, M. C., Influence des eclairements approximativement monochromatiques sur le developpement des tissus de moelle de tabac cultivés *in vitro* en presênce d'auxine et de kinetine, *Photochem. Photobiol.*, 5, 157, 1966.
21. Klein, R. M., Repression of tissue culture growth by visible and near visible radiation, *Plant. Physiol.*, 39, 536, 1964.
22. Fridborg, G. and Eriksson, T., Partial reversal by cytokinin and (2-chloroethyl)-trimethylammonium chloride of near-ultraviolet inhibited growth and morphogenesis in callus cultures, *Physiol. Plant.*, 34, 162, 1975.
23. El-Mansy, H. E. and Salisbury, F. B., Biochemical responses of *Xanthium* leaves to UV radiation, *Radiat. Bot.*, 11, 325, 1971.
24. Andersen, R. A. and Kasperbauer, M. J., Effects of near-ultraviolet radiation and temperature on soluble phenols in *Nicotiana tabacum*, *Phytochemistry*, 10, 1229, 1971.
25. Mohr, H., *Lectures in Photomorphogenesis*, Springer-Verlag, New York, 1972, chap. 4.
26. Hüsemann, W. and Reinert, J., Steuerung des Wachstums und der Morphogenese von Zellkulturen aus *Crepis capillaris* durch Licht and Phytohormone, *Protoplasma*, 90, 353, 1976.
27. Davidson, A. W. and Yeoman, M. M., A phytochrome-mediated sequence of reactions regulating cell division in developing callus cultures, *Ann. Bot. (London)*, 38, 545, 1974.
28. James, D. J. and Davidson, A. W., Phytochrome control of PAL levels and the regulation of cell division in artichoke callus cultures, *Ann. Bot. (London)*, 41, 873, 1977.

29. **Seibert, M. and Kadkade, P. G.**, unpublished data, 1977.

30. **Corduan, G. and Spix, C.**, Haploid callus and regeneration of plants from anthers of *Digitalis purpurea* L., *Planta*, 124, 1, 1975.

31. **Nitsch, C. and Norreel, B.**, Factors favoring the formation of androgenetic embryos in anther culture, in *Genes, Enzymes and Populations*, Vol. 2, Srb, A. M., Ed., Plenum Press, New York, 1972, 129.

32. **Neumann, K.-H.**, Untersuchungen über den linfluss essentieller Schwermetalle auf das Wachstum und den Proteinstoffwechsel von Karottengewebedulturen, Ph. D. dissertation, J. Liebig-Universitat, Giessen, West Germany, 1962.

33. **Isreal, H. W. and Steward, F. C.**, The fine structure of quiescent and growing carrot cells: Its relation to growth induction, *Ann. Bot. (London)*, 30, 63, 1966.

34. **Neumann, K.-H. and Raafat, A.**, Further studies on photosynthesis of carrot tissue cultures, *Plant Physiol.*, 51, 685, 1973.

35. **Neumann, K.-H., Cireli, E., and Cireli, B.**, Untersuchungen über beziehungen zurischen Zellteilung und Morphogenese bei Gewebekulturen von *D. carota*, *Physiol. Plant.*, 22, 787, 1969.

36. **Murashige, T. and Nakano, R. T.**, The light requirements for shoot initiation in tobacco callus culture, *Am. J. Bot.*, 55, 710, 1969.

37. **Margara, J.**, Étude des facteurs de la néoformation de bourgeons en culture *in vitro* chez le choufleur (*Brassica oleracea* l., var. Botrytis), *Ann. Physiol. Veg.*, 11, 95, 1969.

38. **Klein, R. M. and Edsall, P. C.**, Interference by near ultraviolet and green light with growth of animal and plant cell cultures, *Photochem. Photobiol.*, 6, 841, 1967.

39. **Matsumoto, T., Okunishi, K., Nishida, K., and Noguchi, M.**, Effects of physical factors and antibiotics on the growth of higher plant cells in suspension culture, *Agric. Biol. Chem.*, 36, 2177, 1972.

40. **Ohta, Y., Katoh, K., and Miyake, K.**, Establishment and growth characteristics of a cell suspension culture of *Marchantia polymorpha* L. with high chlorophyll contents, *Planta*, 139, 229, 1977.

41. **Bergmann, L. and Berger, Ch.**, Light-color and differentiation of plastids in cell cultures of *Nicotiana tabacum* var. "samsun", *Planta*, 69, 58, 1966.

42. **Logemann, H. and Bergmann, L.**, Influence of light and medium on the plating efficiency of isolated cells from callus cultures of *Nicotiana tabacum* var. "samsum", *Planta*, 121, 283, 1974.

43. **Enzmann-Becker, G.**, Plating efficiency of protoplasts of tobacco in different light conditions, *Z. Naturforsch. Teil C*, 28, 470, 1973.

44. **Binding, H.**, Regeneration of haploid and diploid plants from protoplasts of *Petunia hybrida* L., *Z. Pflanzenphysiol.*, 74, 327, 1974.

45. **Shepard, J. F. and Totten, R. E.**, Mesophyll cell protoplasts of potato. Isolation, proliferation and plant regeneration, *Plant Physiol.*, 60, 313, 1977.

46. **Kohno, H. and Yoshida, F.**, Culture of chlorophyllous tobacco cells not requiring any organic additives except sucrose in the medium, *Plant Cell Physiol.*, 18, 907, 1977.

47. **Rolinson, A. E. and Vince-Prue, D.**, Responses of the rice shoot apex to irradiation with red and far-red light, *Planta*, 132, 215, 1976.

48. **Kadkade, P. G. and Seibert, M.**, unpublished data, 1976.

49. **Kadkade, P. G. and O'Connor, H. J.**, Influence of light quality on organogenesis in Douglas fir tissue cultures, in *Proceedings of the Forest Biology and Wood Chemistry Conference*, Technical Association of the Pulp and Paper Industry, Atlanta, 1977, 71.

50. **Leroux, M. R.**, Action de l'acide gibberéllique sur la rhizogenesè de fragments de tiges de pois (*Pisum sativum* L.) cultivés *in vitro* en pré-sence d'auxine à l'obscurité ou a la lumière, *C. R. Acad. Sci. Ser D.*, 266, 106, 1968.

51. **Letouzé, R. and Beauchesne, G.**, Action d'éclairements monochromatiques sur la rhizogenese de tissus de topinambour, *C. R. Acad. Sci. Ser. D*, 269, 1528, 1969.

52. **Gautheret, R. J.**, Investigations on the root formation in the tissues of *Helianthus tuberosus* cultured *in vitro*, *Am. J. Bot.*, 56, 702, 1969.

53. **Fletcher, R. A., Peterson, R. L., and Zalik, S.**, Effect of light quality on elongation, adventitious root production and the relation of cell number and cell size to bean seedling elongation, *Plant Physiol.*, 40, 541, 1965.

54. **Furuya, M. and Torrey, J. G.**, The reversible inhibition by red and far-red light of auxin induced lateral root initiation in isolated pea roots, *Plant Physiol.*, 39, 987, 1964.

55. **Bonnett, H. T.**, Phytochrome regulation of endogenous bud development in root cultures of *Convolvulus arvensis*, *Planta*, 106, 325, 1972.

56. **Legrand, B.**, Influence des conditions initiales d'éclairement sur le bourgeonnement et la polarite de tissus de feuilles d'endive cultivés *in vitro*, *C. R. Acad. Sci. Ser. D*, 275, 31, 1972.

57. **Butcher, D. N.**, Secondary products in tissue cultures, in *Plant Cell Tissue and Organ Culture*, Reinert, J. and Bajaj, Y. P. S., Eds., Springer-Verlag, Berlin, 1977.

58. **Hahlbrock, K., Ebel, J., Ortmann, R., Sutter, A., Wellmann, E., and Grisebach, H.**, Regulation of enzyme activities related to the biosynthesis of flavone glycoside in cell suspension cultures of *Petroselinum hortense, Biochim. Biophys. Acta*, 244, 7, 1977.

59. **Sutter, A. and Griseback, H.**, UDP-glucose: flavonol 3-O-glucosyltransferase from cell suspension cultures of parsley, *Biochim. Biophys. Acta*, 309, 289, 1973.

60. **Ortmann, R., Sutter, A., and Grisebach, H.**, Purification and properties of UDP-apiose: 7-Oβ-D-glucosyl-flavone apiotransferase from cell suspension cultures of parsley, *Biochim. Biophys. Acta*, 258, 293, 1972.

61. **Grisebach, H. and Hahlbrock, K.**, Enzymology and regulation of flavanoid and lignin biosynthesis in plants and plant cell suspension cultures, in *Metabolism and Regulation of Secondary Plant Products*, Runeckles, V. C. and Conn, E. E., Eds., Academic Press, New York, 1974.

62. **Hahlbrock, K., Knobloch, K. H., Kreuzaler, F., Potts, J. R. M., and Wellmann, E.**, Coordinated induction and subsequent activity changes of two groups of metabolically interrelated enzymes. Light-induced synthesis of flavanoid glycosides in cell suspension cultures of *Petroselinum hortense, Eur. J. Biochem.*, 61, 199, 1976.

63. **Hahlbrock, K. and Ragg, H.**, Light-induced changes of enzyme activities in parsley cell suspension cultures. Effects of inhibitors of RNA and protein synthesis, *Arch. Biochem. Biophys.*, 166, 41, 1975.

64. **Hahlbrock, K. and Schroder, J.**, Light-induced changes of enzyme activities in parsley cell suspension cultures. Increased rate of synthesis of phenylalanine ammonia-lyase, *Arch. Biochem. Biophys.*, 166, 47, 1975.

65. **Wellmann, E. and Schoffer, P.**, Phytochrome-mediated *de novo* synthesis of phenylalanine ammonia-lyase in cell suspension cultures of parsley, *Plant Physiol.*, 55, 822, 1975.

66. **Hahlbrock, K. and Wellmann, E.**, Light-induced flavone biosynthesis and activity of phenylalanine ammonia-lyase and UDP-synthetase in cell suspension cultures of *Petroselinum hortense, Planta*, 94, 236, 1970.

67. **Thorpe, T. A., Maier, V. P., and Hasegawa, S.**, Phenylalanine ammonia-lyase activity in citrus fruit tissue cultured *in vitro, Phytochemistry*, 10, 711, 1971.

68. **Gregor, H. D. and Reinert, J.**, Induktion der Phenylalanin Ammoniumlyase in Gewebekulturen von *Haplopappus gracilis, Protoplasma*, 74, 307, 1972.

69. **Hahlbrock, K. and Schroder, J.**, Specific effects on enzyme activities upon dilution of *Petroselinum hortense* cell cultures into water, *Arch. Biochem. Biophys.*, 171, 500, 1975.

69. **Hahlbrock, K. and Schroder, J.**, Specific effects on enzyme activities upon dilution of *Petroselinum hortense* call cultures into water, *Arch. Biochem. Biophys.*, 171, 500, 1975.

70. **Hahlbrock, K., Kuhlen, E., and Lindl, T.**, Anderungen von enzymaktivitaten Wahrend des Wachstums von Zellsuspensionskulturen von *Glycine max:* Phenylalanin Ammoniumlyase und P-cumarat: CoA ligase, *Planta*, 99, 311, 1971.

71. **Davies, M. E.**, Effects of auxin on polyphenol accumulation and the development of phenylalanine ammonia-lyase activity in dark-grown suspension cultures, *Biochim. Biophys. Acta.*, 362, 417, 1974.

72. **Strickland, R. G. and Sunderland, N.**, Production of anthocyanins, flavonols and chlorogenic acids by cultured callus tissues of *Haplopappus gracilis, Ann. Bot. (London)*, 36, 443, 1972.

73. **Constabel, F., Shyluk, J. P., and Gamborg, O. L.**, The effect of hormones on anthocyanin accumulation in cell cultures of *Haplopappus gracilis, Planta*, 96, 306, 1971.

74. **Zimmermann, A. and Hahlbrock, K.**, Light induced changes in enzyme activities in parsley cell suspension cultures. Purification and some properties of phenylalanine ammonia-lyase, *Arch. Biochem. Biophys.*, 166, 54, 1975.

75. **Stark, V., Alfermann, A. W., and Reinhard, E.**, Verlauf von Phenylalanin Ammoniumlyase-Activität Anthocyan und Chlorogensaürebildung in erschiedenen Zellstammen von *Daucus carota, Planta Med.*, 30, 104, 1976.

76. **Thorpe, T. A. and Meir, D. D.**, Starch metabolism, respiration and shoot formation in tobacco callus cultures, *Physiol. Plat.*, 27, 365, 1972.

77. **Husemann, W., Radman, S. S., Mangold, H. K., and Barz, W.**, The lipids in heterotrophic and photo-autotrophic cell suspension cultures, *Chem. Phys. Lipids*, in press, 1978.

78. **Krikorian, A. D. and Steward, F. C.**, Biochemicals differentiation: the biosynthetic potentialities of growing and quiescent tissue, in *Plant Physiology: A Treatise*, Vol. 5B, Steward, F. C., Ed., Academic Press, New York, 1969.

79. **Durzan, D. J. and Chalupa, V.**, Growth and metabolism of cells and tissue of jack pine (*Pinus banksiana*). Free nitrogenous compounds in cell suspension compounds in cell suspension cultures of jack pine as affected by light and darkness, *Can. J. Bot.*, 54, 496, 1976.

80. **Kadkade, P. G., Micheo, F. P., and Lujan, C.**, L-Dopa in plant tissue cultures, in *Informé de Actividades Programa Multinacional de Extractos Vegetales*, Rolz, C., Ed., Instituto Centro Americano Investigacion Technologia Industrial, Guatemala City, 1972.

81. **Brain, K. R.**, Accumulation of L-Dopa in cultures from *Mucuna pruriens, Plant Sci. Lett.*, 7, 157, 1976.
82. **Matsumoto, T., Nishida, K., Noguchi, M., and Tamaki, E.**, Some factors affecting anthocyanin formation by *Populus* cells in suspension cultures, *Agric. Biol. Chem.*, 37, 561, 1973.
83. **Lance, B., Reid, D. M., and Thorpe, T. A.**, Endogenous gibberellins and growth of tobacco callus cultures, *Physiol. Plant.*, 36, 287, 1976.
84. **Lance, B., Durley, R. C., Reid, D. M., Thorpe, T. A., and Pharis, R. P.**, Metabolism of ^{3}H-gibberellin A_{20} in light and dark-grown tobacco callus cultures, *Plant Physiol.*, 58, 387, 1976.
85. **Ammirato, P. V.**, Hormonal control of somatic embryo development from cultured cells of caraway, *Plant Physiol.*, 59, 579, 1977.
86. **Nickell, L. G.**, Submerged growth of plant cells, *Adv. Appl. Microbiol.*, 4, 213, 1962.
87. **Brunet, G. and Ibrahim, R. K.**, Tissue culture of citrus peel and its potential for flavanoid synthesis, *Z. Pflanzenphysiol.*, 69, 152, 1973.
88. **Wellmann, E.**, Phytochrome-mediated flavone glycoside synthesis in cell suspension cultures of *Petroselinum hortense* after preirradiation with ultraviolet light, *Planta*, 101, 283, 1971.
89. **Wellmann, E. and Boron, D.**, Durch Phytochrom kontrollierte Enzyme der Flavonoidsynthese in Zellsuspensionskulturen von Petersilie (*Petroselinum hortense* Hoffm.,), *Planta*, 119, 161, 1974.
90. **Wellmann, E.**, UV dose dependent induction of enzyme related to flavanoid biosynthesis in cell suspension cultures of parsley, *FEBS Lett.*, 51, 105, 1975.
91. **Hahlbrock, K.**, Isolation of apigenin from illuminated cell suspension cultures of soybean, *Glycine max, Phytochemistry*, 11, 165, 1972.
92. **Reinert, J., Glauss, H., and von Ardenne, R.**, Anthocyanbildung in Gewebeculturen von *Haplopappus gracilis* in Licht verschiedener Qualität, *Naturwissenschaften*, 51, 87, 1964.
93. **Strickland, R. G. and Sunderland, N.**, Photocontrol of growth, and of anthocyanin and chlorogenic acid production in cultured callus tissues of *Haplopappus gracilis, Ann. Bot. (London)*, 36, 671, 1972.
94. **Alfermann, W. and Reinhard, E.**, Isolierung anthocyanhaltiger und anthocyanfreier Gewebestamme von *Daucus carota*. Einfluss von Auxinen auf die Anthocyanbildung, *Experientia*, 27, 353, 1971.
95. **Alfermann, A. W.**, Untersuchungen zur Anthocyansynthese in Calluskulturen von *Daucus carota* L., Ph.D. dissertation, Eberhard-Karls Universität, Tübingen, West Germany, 1973.
96. **Lackmann, I.**, Wirkungsspektren der Anthocyansynthese in Gewebekulturen und Keimlingen von *Haplopappus gracilis, Planta*, 98, 258, 1971.
97. **Gregor, H. D.**, Effect of gibberillic acid (GA$_3$) on phenylalanine-ammonia lyase activity and on the synthesis of phenylpropanoid compounds in cell suspension cultures of *Haplopappus gracilis, Protoplasma*, 80, 273, 1974.
98. **Schmitz, M. and Seitz, U.**, Hemmung der Anthocyansynthese durch Gibberellinsaure A$_3$ bei Kalluskulturen von *Daucus carota, Z. Pflanzenzeucht.*, 68, 259, 1972.
99. **Fritsch, H., Hahlbrock, K., and Grisebach, H.**, Biosynthese von Cyanidin in Zellsuspensionskulturen von *Haplopappus gracilis, Z. Naturforsch.*, 26б, 581, 1971.
100. **Tabata, M., Mizukami, H., Hiraoka, N., and Konoshima, M.**, Pigment formation in callus cultures of *Lithospermum erythrorhizon, Phytochemistry*, 13, 927, 1973.
101. **Forrest, G. E.**, Studies of polyphenol metabolism of tissue cultures derived from the tea plant *(Camellia sinensis* L.), *Biochem. J.*, 113, 765, 1969.
102. **Davis, M. E.**, Polyphenol synthesis in cell suspension cultures of Paul's Scarlet Rose, *Planta*, 104, 50, 1972.
103. **Reinhard, E., Corduan, G., and von Brocke, W.**, Untersuchungen über das atherische Öl und die Cumarine in Gewebekulturen von *Ruta graveolens, Herba Hung.*, 10, 9, 1971.
104. **Corduan, G. and Reinhard, E.**, Synthesis of volatile oils in tissue cultures of *Ruta graveolens, Phytochemistry*, 11, 917, 1972.
105. **Nagel, M. and Reinhard, E.**, Das atherische Öl der Calluskulturen von *Ruta graveolens*. II. Physiologie zur Bildung des atherischen Öles, *Planta Med.*, 27, 264, 1975.
106. **Butcher, D. N. and Connolly, J. D.**, An investigation of factors which influence the production of abnormal terpenoids by callus cultures of *Andrographis paniculata* Nees., *J. Exp. Bot.*, 22, 314, 1971.
107. **Hasegawa, M., Higuchi, T., and Ishikawa, H.**, Formation of lignin in tissue cultures of *Pinus strobus, Plant Cell Physiol.*, 1, 173, 1960.
108. **Haddon, L. E. and Northcote, D. H.**, Quantitative measurement of bean callus differentiation, *J. Cell Sci.*, 17, 11, 1975.
109. **Brocke, W., Reinhard, E., Nicholson, G., and Konig, W. A.**, Über das Vorkomnen von *Ruta graveolens, Z. Naturforsch.*, 22б, 1252, 1971.
110. **Heble, M. R., Narayanaswami, S., and Chadha, M. S.**, Hormonal control of steroid synthesis in *Solanum xanthocarpum* tissue cultures, *Phytochemistry*, 10, 2393, 1971.

111. **Kadkade, P. G. and Madrid, T. R.**, Glycoalkaloids in tissue cultures of *Solanum acculeatissimum, Naturwissenschaften,* 64, 147, 1977.

112. **Kadkade, P. G. and Madrid, T. R.**, Influence of some factors on steroidal alkaloid production by *Solanum acculeatissimum* tissue cultures, unpublished data, 1978.

113. **Kaul, B., Stochs, S. J., and Staba, E. J.**, Dioscorea tissue cultures. III. Influence of various factors on diosgenin production by *Dioscorea deltoidea* callus and suspension cultures, *Lloydia,* 32, 347, 1969.

114. **Kadkade, P. G. and Andrade, J. E.**, Production of diosgenin by *Dioscorea* sps. tissue cultures, in *Informé de Actividades Programa Multinacional de Extractos Vegetales,* Rolz, C., Ed., Instituto Centro Americano Investigacion Technologia Industrial, Guatemala City, 1971.

115. **Arisz, W. H.**, Active uptake, vacuole secretion, and plasmatic transport of chloride ions in leaves of *Vallisneria spiralis, Acta Bot. Neerl.,* 1, 506, 1953.

116. **Derbyshire, E. and Street, H. E.**, Studies of the growth in culture of excised wheat roots. V. The influence of light on nitrate uptake and assimilation, *Physiol. Plant.,* 17, 107, 1964.

117. **Gordon, S. A.**, The intracellular distribution of phytochrome in corn seedlings, in *Progress in Photobiology,* Christensen, B. C. and Buchman, B., Eds., Elsevier, Amsterdam, 1961, 441.

118. **Goren, R. and Galston, A. W.**, Control by phytochrome of ^{14}C-sucrose incorporated into buds of etiolated pea seedlings, *Plant Physiol.,* 41, 1055, 1966.

119. **Anand, R. and Galston, A. W.**, Further investigations on phytochrome-controlled sucrose uptake into apical buds of etiolated peas, *Am. J. Bot.,* 59, 327, 1972.

120. **Jones, R. W. and Sheard, R. W.**, Phytochrome, nitrate movement, and induction of nitrate reductase in etiolated pea terminal buds, *Plant Physiol.,* 55, 954, 1975.

121. **Jaffe, M. J. and Thoma, L.**, Rapid phytochrome-mediated changes in the uptake by bean roots of sodium acetate ($1-^{14}$C) and their modification by cholinergic drugs, *Planta,* 113, 283, 1973.

122. **White, J. M. and Pike, C. S.**, Rapid phytochrome-mediated changes in adenosine 5'-triphosphate content of etiolated bean buds, *Plant Physiol.,* 53, 76, 1974.

123. **Kirshner, R. L., White, J. M., and Pike, C. S.**, Control of bean bud ATP levels by regulatory molecules and phytochrome, *Physiol. Plant.,* 34, 373, 1975.

124. **Bergmann, L.**, Plating of plant cells, in *Plant Tissue Culture and its Biotechnological Application,* Barz, W., Reinhard, E., and Zenk, M. H, Eds., Springer-Verlag, Berlin, 1977, 213.

125. **Lamb, C. J. and Rubery, P. H.**, Photocontrol of chlorogenic acid biosynthesis in potato tuber discs, *Phytochemistry,* 15, 661, 1976.

126. **Kadkade, P. G., Andrade, J. E., and Madrid, T. R.**, unpublished data, 1973.

Chapter 6

ENVIRONMENTAL FACTORS

B. TEMPERATURE, AERATION, AND pH*

S. M. Martin

TABLE OF CONTENTS

*   N.R.C.C. No. 17955.

I. INTRODUCTION

Techniques for plant cell culture have advanced to the point where it seems entirely logical to set as a goal the biosynthesis of a vast array of useful plant metabolites on a commercial basis. Before such a goal can be reached, however, much must still be done to reduce cost factors. Increased productivity, hence, lower costs, can be achieved through judicious selection of the cell lines used and the chemical and physical environment under which the cells are cultivated. It is the purpose of this report to see how temperature, aeration, and pH bear upon this problem.

II. TEMPERATURE

Studies on the in vitro growth of plant cells have indicated that the optimum temperature is generally within the range 25 to 30°C, but that species could differ considerably.[1,2] Tulecke and Nickell[3] examined the effect of temperature on five suspension cultures. The extreme optima were 20 to 21°C (*Solium*) and 31 to 32°C (*Rosa*). Erikson[4] found that *Haplopappus gracilis* cell-suspension cultures grew several times faster at 30 than at 25°C. Matsumoto,[5] using cultures of *Populus* and *Nicotiana*, observed that growth was better at 32°C than at either 28 or 24°C. Rose and Martin[6] made an extensive study of the growth of *Ipomoea* cells at temperatures in the range 15 to 34°C. Maximum growth occurred between 25 and 32°C, with temperature variations within this range having little effect on growth rates based on dry cell yields. On either side of this range, the growth rate declined dramatically. It was also observed that the rate of sucrose and amino nitrogen utilization was maximal between 30 and 32°C. Both of these parameters declined by about 25% from 30 to 25°C, whereas the growth rate declined very little. At temperatures below 25°C, nitrogen utilization was reduced to a greater extent than was sucrose utilization, indicating temperature-dependent shifts in metabolism. Little if anything seems to have been reported on temperature optima for growth vs. those for metabolite production.

III. AERATION

A. Oxygen

Givan and Collin[7] using shake-flask cultures of sycamore found that oxygen uptake rose sharply (from 3.8 $\mu\ell$ O_2/mg dry cells/hr at day one to 7.8 at day six) and then declined. A similar early rise and then decline was also observed by Nash and Davies[8] using rose cells. Here the maximum rate was 6.8 $\mu\ell$ O_2/g fresh weight/min. Rajasekhar et al.[9] studied the effect of shaking rate on the growth of belladonna and sycamore cells and concluded that reduced growth at suboptimum shaking speeds was not due to oxygen deficiency or accumulation of CO_2. They suggested that the effect was due either to retention of a volatile toxic factor or to restricted nutrient uptake resulting from a stationary liquid-phase boundary to the cells. The reported oxygen uptake rates ranged from 20 to 47 nmol O_2/10^6 cells/min for belladonna and from 18 to 27 for sycamore. Matsumoto et al.[5] examined the effect of shaking rate (reciprocal shaker, 25 mℓ medium in 100 mℓ flasks) on cells of *Populus* hybrid, *Nicotiana glutinosa*, and *N. tabacum*. Although 90 reciprocations per minute was optimum, the growth was not greatly different at 80 and 110.

In a study of density-inhibited cultures of *Arachis*, Verma and Marcus[10] observed an oxygen uptake rate of 0.6 $\mu\ell$ O_2/10^6 cells/min in the stationary phase (undiluted) and 1.6 immediately after dilution. The increased respiratory rate was thought to be the result of increased oxygen availability. Fowler[11] reported uptake rates ranging from about 0.18 to 0.62 μmol O_2/10^6 cells/min for *Acer pseudoplatanus* cells growing in a chemostat at specific growth rates ranging from 0.05 to 0.19, respectively. Kessell and Carr[12] examined the effect of dissolved oxygen concentration (DO) on growth and differentiation of carrot cells in agitated/aerated culture and observed that there was a critical oxygen level (1300 $\mu\ell$ O_2/ℓ or 16% saturation) above which growth was unaffected by increasing DO. Above the critical level, growth as judged by dry weight or cell numbers was exponential. Below this level, dry weight increase was linear, while cell numbers increased exponentially. Low DO favored embryogenesis, and high DO favored rhizogenesis. They also observed a DO-related effect on nutrient uptake.

Using large-scale equipment, Yasuda et al.[13] found the optimum operating conditions for a suspension culture of tobacco cells to be in the range K_d 1.3 × 10⁻⁶ mol O_2/min·mℓ·atm. These workers progressively increased the aeration rate during the growth period: 0.3 vvm, 0 to 2 days; 0.5 vvm, 2 to 5 days; 1.0 vvm, last 5 days. Kato et al. [14] observed that, with tobacco cells growing in a 30-ℓ fermentor, the dissolved oxygen content of the medium had dropped essentially to zero by the third day. From this point onward, the culture seems to have suffered an oxygen deficiency as judged by a better than 50% decrease in growth rate. We have examined (unpublished) the effect of a decreased aeration rate on the growth of morning glory cells in 7.5-ℓ fermentors. In fermentors aerated at 0.3 vvm, the cultures increased in weight exponentially for 7 days (t_d = 54 hr), and throughout the growth period, we were unable to detect a significant oxygen uptake or carbon dioxide evolution in the effluent gas stream. In cultures aerated at 0.03 vvm, growth at t_d = 54 hr was maintained for the first 3 to 4 days. Then, a new exponential growth rate (t_d = 98 hr) was established. In cultures under low aeration, the oxygen content of the effluent gas dropped to a minimum of 19.5% and the carbon dioxide rose to 1%. It was established that this was a true oxygen effect. Increasing the PO_2 while maintaining the low flow of input gas resulted in normal growth. Increasing the flow rate with nitrogen while maintaining the low air flow was without effect. Increasing the PCO_2 in the high air flow was without effect until a level of 5% was reached. Increasing the rate of agitation from 200 to 400 rpm increased the growth rate to some extent.

Kato et al.[15] examined the effect of the initial volumetric oxygen-transfer coefficient (K_{La}) on the growth of tobacco cells in batch cultures in a 15-ℓ flat-blade turbine fermentor. In the 15-ℓ fermentor, aeration rates from 0.25 to 1.0 vvm and agitation rates from 0 to 200 rpm were used. Data are presented which show that when K_{La} values of 5.3 and 12.1 hr⁻¹ were used in the 15-ℓ fermentor, the growth rate was nearly the same for the first 70 hr. After 70 hr. growth markedly decreased at K_{La} 5.3 hr⁻¹, whereas the cells continued to grow well at K_{La} 12.1 hr⁻¹. Another experiment indicated that K_{La} values of from 10 to 25 hr⁻¹ gave the same final cell yield at 144 hr (about 14.9 g/ℓ). The growth yield was 0.43 g cells/g sucrose, and the maximum specific growth rate was about 0.68 day⁻¹. The effect of agitation, independent of K_{La}, was also examined. When the agitation speed was set at 150 or 200 rpm, bulking, foaming, and attaching of cells to the wall and shaft of the fermentor occurred. This resulted in data scattering and lower yields. An agitation speed of 50 to 100 rpm was recommended. Kato et al.,[16] using a 15-ℓ flat-blade turbine fermentor and a 1500-ℓ bubble fermentor for cultivation of tobacco cells, observed maximum specific growth rates of 0.69 and 0.62 day⁻¹, respectively. This was despite the fact that K_{La} was 12 hr⁻¹ for the stirred jar as opposed to 15 hr⁻¹ for the bubble fermentor. The difference was attributed to lack of adequate mixing of the culture.

Wagner and Vogelman[17] examined several types of fermentors [flat-blade turbine, draft tube with turbine, and draft tube with air lift (see Martin[18])] with respect to growth and metabolite production. They found the air-lift fermentor to be superior to the other two because of its ability to provide good macromixing and oxygen transfer while subjecting the cells to a minimum of mechanical damage.

B. Carbon Dioxide

There is little evidence in the literature that exogenously supplied CO_2 is a significant factor in terms of the growth of plant cell cultures, although Nesius and Fletcher[19] did show that during the first 5 days of cultivation growth of rose cells was reduced in the presence of a CO_2 absorber. Berlyn and Zelitch[20] cultured tobacco cells photoautrophically with CO_2 as the sole source of carbon. Nesius and Fletcher[21] have shown extensive $^{14}CO_2$ incorporation into rose cells. We noted above that increasing the CO_2 content of the input air had no effect on growth of morning-glory cells in fermentors until a level of 5% was reached.

IV. pH

In general, the most favorable pH for the growth of plant cell suspensions is in the range pH 5 to 6, and most media are so adjusted prior to autoclaving. Undefined media containing relatively large amounts of ingredients, such as coconut milk, yeast hydrolysate, or casein hydrolysate, and defined media containing amino acids, such as glutamic or aspartic acids, may be fairly well buffered, and the pH shifts relatively little during the course of culture development. On the other hand, many media are poorly buffered, and the pH shifts dramatically. Cultures go acid because of the production of organic acids or the utilization of ammonium ions from nitrogen sources such as ammonium sulphate and chloride. Conversely, cultures go alkaline when nitrate ions from sodium or potassium nitrate are utilized by the cells or when ammonium ions are released into the medium by deamination of amino acids or by the reduction of nitrate by nitrate and nitrite reductases.

Matsumoto et al.[5] examined growth of *Populus* hybrid, *Nicotiana glutinosa*, and *N. tabacum* under conditions of differing initial pH (5.0, 5.5, 6.8, and 7.5 after autoclaving) and found that, when examined after 3 days, all cultures had a pH within the range 5.0 to 5.3. There was little to suggest that under these conditions initial pH had any effect on subsequent growth of the cultures. Rose and Martin[22] grew morning-glory cells in a defined medium containing ammonium and nitrate as the nitrogen sources. The medium was autoclaved at pH 5.0, but because of the high pH of the inoculum and the low buffer capacity of the medium, the pH rose to about 6.4 on inoculation. It then fell to about pH 5.0 and finally rose to about pH 7.0 during periods corresponding with utilization of ammonium and nitrate, respectively.

Nesius and Fletcher[19] used 2-(N-morpholino)ethane sulphonic acid (MES) to buffer Paul's Scarlet Rose cell cultures and found the optimum pH for growth to be 5.2 to 5.4. Martin and Rose[23] grew cells of *Ipomoea* in defined medium at controlled pH levels (pH-stat) of 4.8, 5.6, 6.4, and 7.1 with ammonium and nitrate as the nitrogen sources. Although the cells grew at all pH's, the yield was reduced at the extremes, and the data suggested that pH influenced development through its effect on the utilization of ammonium and nitrate. The ability of the cells to use ammonium increased with increasing pH, whereas the ability to use nitrate decreased (essentially to zero at pH 7.1). At pH 4.8, ammonium accumulated in the medium during part of the growth cycle, indicating that the rate of nitrate (and nitrite) reduction exceeded the rate of uptake of ammonium thus formed. Martin et al.[24] demonstrated that under pH-stat conditions it was possible to grow morning glory and soybean cells with ammonium as the sole source of nitrogen. Since these cultures produced little if any organic acids during cultivation, it also was possible, by using ammonium hydroxide as the titrant, to maintain constant the ammonium level in the medium (combined pH-state/ammonium-stat).

In a study of nitrogen assimilation and nitrate and nitrite reductases in *Ipomoea* cultures, Zink and Veliky[25] found that cells grown on nitrate and maintained at pH

4.8 released ammonium into the medium, whereas at pH 6.5 they secreted nitrite. Veliky et al.[26] observed that the uptake of magnesium increased with increasing pH. Veliky[27] has shown that cell cultures of *Ipomoea* transform tryptophan into a variety of indole metabolites, one of which was identified as tryptophol. When cultures were grown at pH 6.3 in a pH-stat, the yield of tryptophol was nearly double that found in cultures in which the pH was allowed to run free. At pH 4.8 tryptophol formation was inhibited.

V. CONCLUSION

There are still many problems associated with plant cell culture under submerged conditions which must be resolved before the economic production of useful metabolites can be achieved. In general, it may be stated that most often in the past, rapid growth has been the criterion for selection of cell lines, media, and environmental conditions. This has resulted in impressive growth rates and yields, but has provided little basis on which to optimize biosynthetic capabilities. Fortunately, this situation is changing, and it is to be expected that the next few years will see a much greater effort being made toward defining the effects of environmental factors on metabolite production.

REFERENCES

1. **Carew, D. P. and Staba, E. J.**, Plant tissue culture: its fundamentals, applications and relation to medicinal plant studies, *Lloydia*, 28, 1, 1965.
2. **Puchan, Z. and Martin, S. M.**, The industrial potential of plant cell culture, *Prog. Ind. Microbiol.*, 9, 13, 1971.
3. **Tulecke, W. and Nickell, L. G.**, Methods, problems and results of growing plant cells under submerged conditions, *Trans. N.Y. Acad. Sci.*, 22, 196, 1960.
4. **Eriksson, T.**, Studies on the growth requirements and growth measurements of *Haplopappus gracilis*, *Physiol. Plant.*, 18, 976, 1965.
5. **Matsumoto, T., Ohunishi, K., Nishida, K., and Noguchi, M.**, Effect of physical factors and antibiotics on the growth of higher plant cells in suspension culture, *Agric. Biol. Chem.*, 36, 2177, 1972.
6. **Rose, D. and Martin, S. M.**, Growth of suspension cultures of plant cells (*Ipomoea* sp.) at various temperatures, *Can. J. Bot.*, 53, 315, 1975.
7. **Givan, C. V. and Collin, H. A.**, Studies on the growth in culture of plant cells. II. Changes in respiration rate and nitrogen content associated with the growth of *Acer pseudoplatanus* L. cells in suspension culture, *J. Exp. Bot.*, 18, 321, 1967.
8. **Nash, D. T. and Davies, M. E.**, Some aspects of growth and metabolism of Paul's Scarlet Rose cell suspensions, *J. Exp. Bot.*, 23, 75, 1972.
9. **Rajasekhar, E. W., Edwards, M., Wilson, S. B., and Street, H. E.**, Studies on the growth in culture of plant cells. XI. The influence of shaking rate on the growth of suspension cultures, *J. Exp. Bot.*, 22, 107, 1971.
10. **Verma, D. P. S. and Marcus, A.**, Oxygen availability as a control factor in the density-dependent regulation of protein synthesis in cell cultures, *J. Cell Sci.*, 41, 331, 1974.
11. **Fowler, M. W.**, Growth of cell cultures under chemostat conditions, in *Plant Tissue Culture and its Bio-technological Applications*, Barz, W., Reinhard, E., and Zenk, M. H., Eds., Springer-Verlag, Berlin, 1977.
12. **Kessell, R. H. J. and Carr, A. H.**, The effect of dissolved oxygen concentrations on growth and differentiation of carrot (*Daucus carota*) tissue, *J. Exp. Bot.*, 23, 996, 1972.
13. **Yasuda, S., Satoh, K., Ishii, T., and Furuya, T.**, Studies on the cultural conditions of plant cell suspension culture. *Proc. IV IFS: Ferment. Technol. Today*, Terui, G., Ed., Society Fermentation Technology, Osaka, Japan, 1972.
14. **Kato, K., Shiozawa, Y., Yamada, A., Nishida, K., and Noguchi, M.**, A jar fermentor culture of *Nicotiana tabacum* L. cell suspensions. *Agric. Biol. Chem.*, 36, 899, 1972.

15. **Kato, A., Shimizu, Y., and Nagai, S.,** Effect of initial K_{La} on the growth of tobacco cells in batch culture, *J. Ferment. Technol.,* 53, 744, 1975.

16. **Kato, A., Kawazoe, S., Iijima, M., and Shimizu, Y.,** Continuous culture of tobacco cells, *J. Ferment. Technol.,* 54, 82, 1976.

17. **Wagner, F. and Vogelmann, H.,** Cultivation of plant tissue cultures in bioreactors and formation of secondary metabolites, in *Plant Tissue Culture and its Bio-technological Applications,* Barz, W., Reinhard, E., and Zenk, M. H., Eds., Springer-Verlag, Berlin, 1977.

18. **Martin, S. M.,** Mass culture systems for plant cell suspensions, in *Plant Tissue Culture as a Source of Biochemicals,* Staba, J., Ed., CRC Press, Boca Raton, Fla., 1980.

19. **Nesius, K. K. and Fletcher, J. S.,** Carbon dioxide and pH requirements of non-photosynthetic tissue culture cells. *Physiol. Plant.,* 28, 259, 1973.

20. **Berlyn, M. B. and Zelitch, I.,** Photoautotrophic growth and photosynthesis in tobacco callus cells, *Plant Physiol.,* 56, 752, 1975.

21. **Nesius, K. K. and Fletcher, J. S.,** Contribution of nonautotrophic carbon dioxide fixation to protein synthesis in suspension cultures of Paul's Scarlet Rose, *Plant Physiol.,* 55, 643, 1975.

22. **Rose, D. and Martin, S. M.,** Effect of ammonium on growth of plant cells (*Ipomoea* sp.) in suspension cultures, *Can. J. Bot.,* 53, 1942, 1975.

23. **Martin, S. M. and Rose, D.,** Growth of plant cell (*Ipomoea*) suspension cultures at controlled pH levels, *Can. J. Bot.,* 54, 1264, 1975.

24. **Martin, S. M., Rose, D., and Hui, V.,** Growth of plant cell suspension cultures with ammonium as the sole source of nitrogen, *Can. J. Bot.,* 55, 2838, 1977.

25. **Zink, M. W. and Veliky, I. A.,** Nitrogen assimilation and regulation of nitrate and nitrite reductases in cultured *Ipomoea* cells, *Can. J. Bot.,* 55, 1557, 1977.

26. **Veliky, I. A., Rose, D., and Zink, M. W.,** Uptake of magnesium by suspension cultures of plant cells (*Ipomoea* sp.), *Can. J. Bot.,* 55, 1143, 1977.

27. **Veliky, I. A.,** Effect of pH on tryptophol formation by cultured *Ipomoea* sp. plant cells, *Lloydia,* 40, 482, 1977.

Chapter 7

MASS CULTURE SYSTEMS FOR PLANT CELL SUSPENSIONS*

S. M. Martin

TABLE OF CONTENTS

I. Introduction 150

II. Mass Culture Systems 150
- A. Batch Culture Systems 150
- B. Batch Culture Scale-up 156
- C. Semicontinuous Culture Systems 161
- D. Continuous Culture Systems 161

III. Conclusion 164

References 165

* N.R.C.C. No. 17956.

I. INTRODUCTION

Recent advances in plant tissue culture have made the production of metabolites of considerable contemporary interest. It thus seems appropriate to review the development of mass culture systems used for plant cell suspensions. Because our interest is focused on potential for industrial application, we will limit our discussion essentially to those systems which have a scale-up potential. Furthermore, equipment will not be described in detail; rather, schematics will be used to illustrate design and operating principles. Unfortunately, this approach does not do justice to many rather elegant pieces of equipment which have been designed for growing plant cells. It should also be noted that no attempt has been made to examine all systems used for mass culture of plant cells or to provide details of auxiliary equipment such as sample receivers, aeration control systems, etc.

Large-scale cultivation of plant cells has been fraught with many difficulties, perhaps the least of which has turned out in the long run to be equipment design. The pioneers in the field, of course, did not have the advantage of hindsight that current workers have and often attempted to solve their problems by designing new culture systems. Some of these truly advanced the cause of mass culture, whereas others were simply at a dead end. Regardless of this, all have served a purpose.

II. MASS CULTURE SYSTEMS

A. Batch Culture Systems

In 1959, Tulecke and Nickell[1] described the first truly large-scale culture system for plant cells (Figure 1). This simple system consisted of a rubber-stoppered 20-ℓ carboy fitted with four tubes — "air in", "air out", "medium in", and "sample out". Filtered compressed air supplied both aeration and agitation. With this system, they successfully grew cell lines derived from a number of different plants, e.g., ginkgo, holly, *Lolium*, and rose. Perhaps even more important than the equipment in the success achieved was the fact that they used as inoculum a large volume of a fast-growing culture. Cultures were carried in liquid medium (100 mℓ/300 mℓ shake flask). For inoculum build-up, one of these cultures, 1 week old, was transferred to 900 mℓ of medium in a 3-ℓ Fernbach shake flask which, after cultivation for 1 week, was used to inoculate 9 ℓ of medium in the carboy. These workers[2] also reported that they had used successfully 30- and 134-ℓ stainless steel tanks as culture vessels.

Wang and Staba[3] in 1963 used a dual carboy system (Figure 2) for the cultivation of spearmint cells. One half of the unit, i.e., carboy unit, was similar to the apparatus of Tulecke and Nickell[1] in that a rubber-stoppered bottle was used as the growth vessel. However, a fritted aeration disc, a stirrer, and a condenser on the exhaust line were added. They used a 5-day-old, 15% (v/v) inoculum. Stirring was a step in the right direction, but the use of such a stirring bar could be faulted as being inefficient in heavy suspensions and as having a tendency to grind cells between the bar and the bottom of the carboy. The exhaust condenser served the useful purpose of reducing evaporation from the culture. The advantages of having the second growth vessel in parallel with the first is not apparent and indeed seems to have been rather unsuccessful, since carboy 2 routinely performed poorly. Apparently the problem of poor growth in carboy 2 was not solved, but the authors did suggest that it might have been an effect of the quality of the stainless steel spargers.

In 1964, Lamport[4] described a roller-bottle system based on the use of a 10-ℓ flask with an aseptic sampling device inserted through a cotton plug (Figure 3). Short et al.[5] used a similar but slightly more elaborate system employing two 10-ℓ bottles rotating

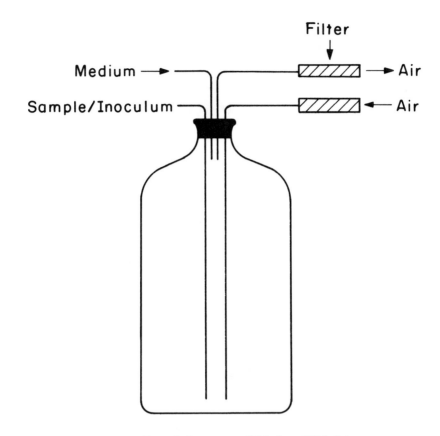

FIGURE 1.   Carboy system of Tulecke and Nickell.[1]

on a single shaft. Although without much scale-up potential, the system is of interest because of its simplicity.

Graebe and Novelli[6] in 1966 published the description of a rather elaborate apparatus for the large-scale cultivation of plant cells. The reason behind the development of this equipment was that "propagation involves sterile transfer of liter amounts, calling for special methods, since simple aseptic techniques do not ensure repeated success at this scale".[6] Certainly contamination has been a major problem in the plant cell culture field, and many workers have resorted to lacing their media with antibiotics to prevent it.[2,3,7,8] Plant cell cultures grow slowly in media which also support the growth of bacteria, molds, and yeasts, and since these microorganisms easily outgrow the less vigorous plant cells, the risk of contamination is great. However, contamination is essentially a problem of technique rather than of equipment design. On the other hand, it is important to recognize that as the complexity of the culture apparatus increases from test tube or flask to large-scale fermentors, so also does the risk of contamination increase, regardless of the biological system being cultivated.

A schematic of the Graebe and Novelli[6] culture system is shown in Figure 4. The culture vessel was either a 6- or 12-ℓ Florence flask, the neck of which was fitted with a large standard taper joint below which was located an outlet for exhaust gas. Onto the standard taper was fitted a glass cap with transfer and aeration tubes. The transfer tube was also fitted with a standard taper joint onto which fitted either a closing cap or a connecting tube. A magnetic stirring bar, placed in the culture vessel, was used only intermittently to break up aggregates, since it was noted that continuous use eventually macerated the cells and prevented further growth. The culture was agitated and

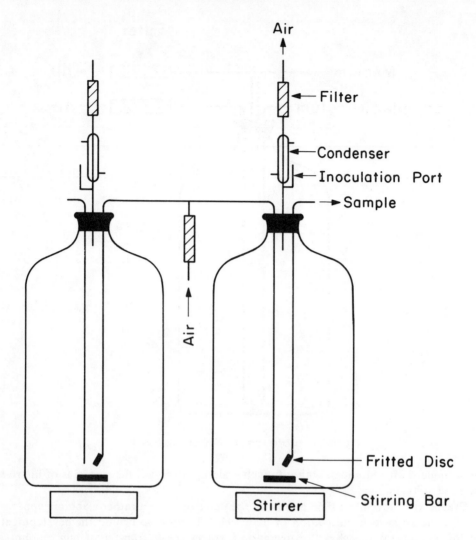

FIGURE 2.   Dual carboy system of Wang and Staba.[3]

aerated by passing sterile air through the fritted sparger, the transfer tube being closed with a closing cap. Additions of fresh medium were made by replacing the closing cap with a connecting tube attached to a medium reservoir and pushing the medium over with sterile air. Samples were taken by pushing culture back through a transfer tube to a receiving flask. Culture filtrate could be removed through the sparger and aeration line. Two growth vessels could be connected via connecting tubes and rubber tubing. In this way, one culture could be divided or an inoculum pushed over in fresh medium in the second flask. Although the system was reasonably versatile, its complexity would make operation difficult and would in the long run create more contamination problems than it would solve.

In 1971, Verma and van Huystee[9] described a culture system (Figure 5) which, according to the authors, "drastically reduced the chances of contamination during sampling of the tissue and transferring of the medium". The growth vessel was a 5-ℓ three-necked distilling flask with a sampling valve fitted into the side. One neck was used for exhaustion gas, the next carried a finger action stirrer, and the third was fitted with an F-shaped glass fitting for air and medium inlets. The sampling valve was a three-way vacuum stopcock arranged such that the valve and sampling tube could be

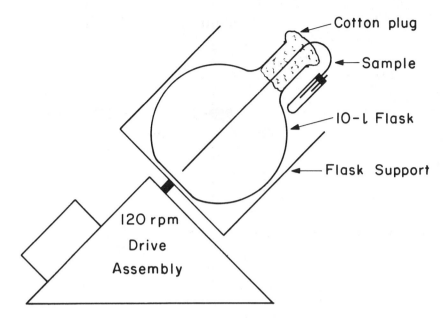

FIGURE 3.   Roller flask system of Lamport.[4]

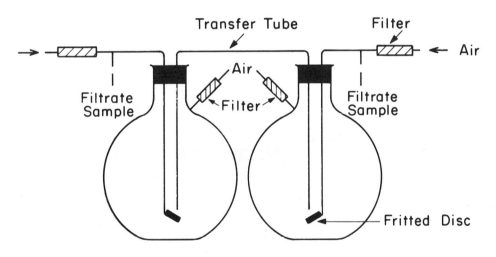

FIGURE 4.   System of Graebe and Novelli.[6]

flushed with sterile water after each use. Between samplings, the end of the tube was kept immersed in 50% ethanol. Lack of flexibility in design and complexity of operation would detract from this system, although the data presented would indicate that it was used successfully.

In 1970, Veliky and Martin[10] described a culture vessel fashioned from an inverted Erlenmeyer flask (Figure 6). On a glass pin situated at the bottom of the vessel was an arrangement carrying two teflon-coated stirring bars. A drain/sample port was also located at the bottom of the vessel. The top of the vessel was fitted with four standard taper penetrations.

It would seem that our path should be leading to a standard flat-blade turbine reactor, and indeed that is where we have ended up. In truth, however, we could almost have begun there, since as early as 1962 Byrne and co-workers[7,8] reported on the suc-

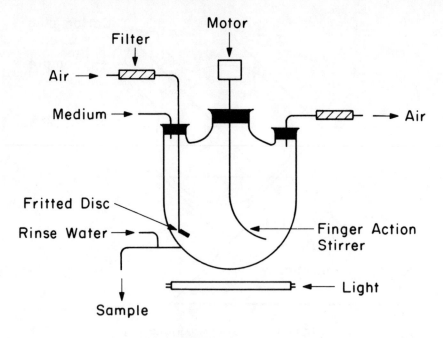

FIGURE 5.   System of Verma and van Huystee.[9]

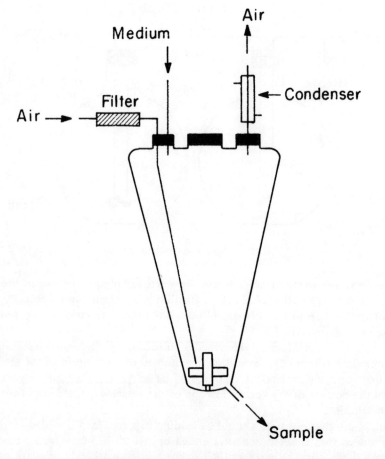

FIGURE 6.   System of Veliky and Martin.[10]

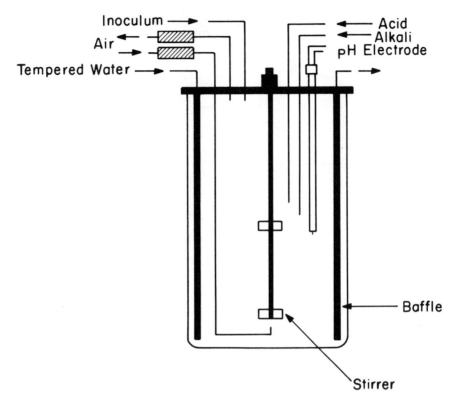

FIGURE 7. Stirrer-jar fermentor.

cessful use of New Brunswick fermentors for growing plant cells (Figure 7). Many others[11-15] have also used jar fermentors. In our own work[16-20] with 7.5-ℓ New Brunswick Microferm fermentors, we have increased the size of each impeller blade to 1 in.[2] in order to achieve complete mixing while stirring at a low rate (175 rpm). Kato et al.[15] examined the influence of agitation speed on the growth of tobacco cells in stirred-jar fermentors and suggested that an agitation speed of 50 to 100 rpm was most appropriate. It seems obvious that cell lines differ in their resistance to shear effects and that a single optimum agitation speed cannot be designated for all lines.

Several other fermentor types (bubble, draft tube with turbine, and draft tube with air lift) will be discussed in the section on batch culture scale-up.

Since we have done most of our experimental work in 7.5- or 14-ℓ stirred-jar fermentors and require a constant source of large volumes of actively growing inocula, we routinely carry our heavily used cultures in 3-ℓ glass fermentors (Figure 8.)[34] Agitation and aeration is by means of a Vibromixer, through the shaft of which is passed sterile air. The five penetrations in the vessel cover give considerable flexibility in setting up the apparatus. Temperature is controlled by means of tempered water flowing through the jacket.

Details of construction of the fermentor are shown in Figure 9. The design is based on the use of Sovirel glassware and fittings, but has been largely custom made.* The key to the flexibility of the series of culture vessels used is the 100 mm neck which is "O" ring sealed and clamped to the cover. Shown here is the 3-1 jacketed vessel, but it can be unjacketed or of any capacity and still have the 100 mm neck and cover. The

* Peqasus Industrial Specialties, Ltd., Agincourt, Ontario, Canada.

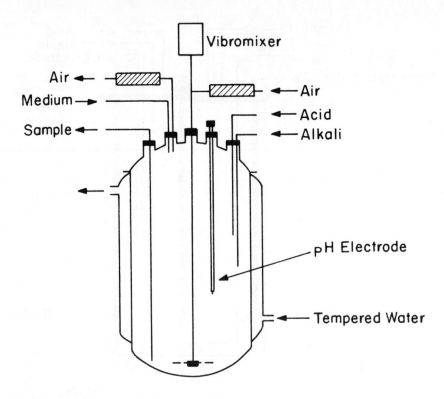

FIGURE 8.   Vibromixer fermentor.

cover has one SVL #30 threaded fitting in the center, surrounded by four SVL #22 fittings. Screw caps, bored caps, and flange fittings are used to complete the assembly of the fermentor. Through the center penetration is passed the aerator/agitator shaft of the Vibromixer, with the diaphragm seal held in place atop the glass fitting with a bored cap. Although we are rather partial to the Vibromixer method of agitation, we have used an SVL paddle stirrer, the bearing of which is attached to the SVL #30 joint. The four SVL #22 joints may be capped with screw caps, or tubes, electrodes, etc. may be inserted through silicone rubber septa held in place with bored caps. In the setup shown here, we have inserted a combination pH electrode in one penetration and tubes for acid and alkali addition in another. The third penetration carries a glass fitting which serves as a medium inlet and air outlet. Through the fourth penetration passes a ¼-in. stainless steel sample tube. The same device used for medium inlet/air outlet is fastened to the distal end of the sample tube and allows for attachment of sample receivers (tubes, flasks, or graduated cylinder equipped with SVL #22 threaded tops). If this particular setup is used, the electrode is sterilized separately and that port is used for inoculation prior to insertion of the electrode. When large samples are to be removed, it is most convenient to connect the receiver to the sampler via rubber tubing and an SVL #22 thread/tubing adaptor. A dispensing flask with the bottom take-off attached via rubber tubing to an aseptic filling bell is used to transfer inoculum from one fermentor to another. This fermentor, or an earlier version of it, has been in use for 5 years and has proven to be convenient and flexible. Neither contamination nor foaming has been a problem.

B. Batch Culture Scale-up

Many workers have a scaled-up batch culture operation. As noted earlier, Tulecke and Nickell[2] were able to scale up their carboy system to 30- and 134-*l* stainless steel

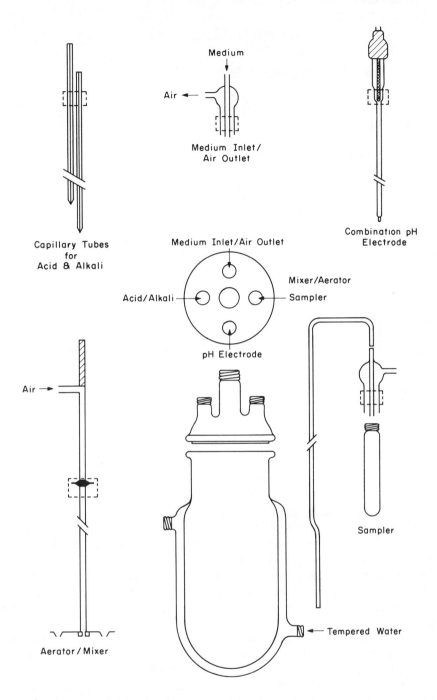

FIGURE 9.   Details of Vibromixer fermentor.

tanks. Kato et al.[11] cultured tobacco cells in a 30-ℓ jar fermentor and have reported data on changes in cell dry weight and inorganic medium constituents during the 5-day growth period. Yasuda et al.[12] used 30-ℓ jar fermentors and 130- and 600-ℓ pilot plant fermentors for the cultivation of tobacco cells. In the 600-ℓ fermentor, conditions were: operating volume, 300 ℓ; aeration, 0.3 vvm (0 to 2 days), 0.5 vvm (2 to 5 days), 1.0 vvm (last 5 days); agitaion, 100 rpm; vessel pressure, 1.0 kg/cm²; fresh medium (5% v/v) fed daily last 5 days. The first inoculum was grown in shake flasks and the

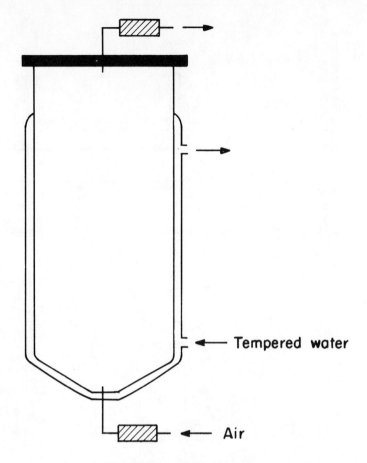

FIGURE 10.   Bubble fermentor.

second in a 130-l fermentor (operating volume, 50l, aeration, 0.5 vvm; agitation, 60 rpm; vessel pressure, 1.0 kg/cm^2). We[35] have scaled up the cultivation of morning glory cells from a 7.5-l stirred jar (operating volume, 5 l; inoculum, 10%, aeration, 0.3 vvm; agitation, 200 rpm; temperature 26°C) to a 150-l stainless steel pilot plant fermentor (operating volume, 60 l; inoculum, 10%; aeration, 0.2 vvm; agitation, 40 rpm). In both fermentors, the dry cell yield was 11.2 g/l and the mass doubling time was 53 hr. Noguchi et al.[14] mention briefly the production of tobacco cells in a 20,000-l tank.

Kato et al.[15,21] used bubble-type reactors (Figure 10) ranging in size from 65 to 1500 l in which air supplied both aeration and agitation. The air rising from a multihole ring sparger located at the bottom of the conical fermentor base provides a much more gentle agitation than is normally attainable in a flat-blade turbine reactor. However, it was noted that the specific growth rate was somewhat lower in the bubble fermentor than in the stirred jar, a fact attributed to a deficiency in the overall mixing of the culture.

In a particularly interesting paper, Wagner and Vogelmann[22] reported on growth and metabolite production in a variety of fermentor types. Included in the study were reactors with agitation based on the use of flat-blade turbines (Figure 7), draft tube with turbine (Figure 11), and draft tube with air lift (Figure 12). In the reactor with draft tube and turbine, the turbine acts in the manner of a pump forcing the culture up at high speed through the annular space between draft tube and reactor wall, and

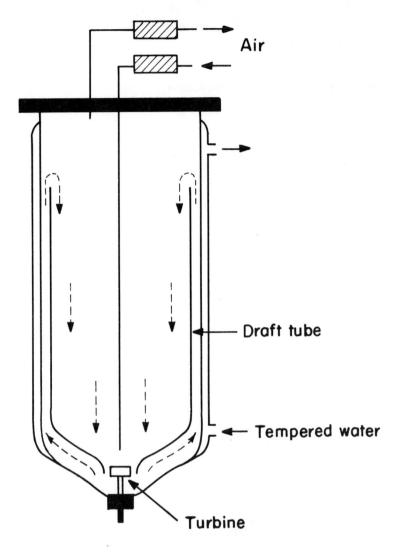

Air

Draft tube

Tempered water

Turbine

FIGURE 11. Fermentor with draft tube and turbine.

from thence it spills to the interior of the reactor. High turbine speeds are required and shear is very high in the region of the turbine. In the air lift fermentor, agitation is accomplished by the lifting action of the air rising in the draft tub. Here very good mixing is achieved under conditions of low shear. With cells of *Morinda citrifolia*, the yield of anthroquinones in the air lift fermentor was about 30% more than that in shake flasks and twice that in the other fermentors. However, cell yields were relatively unaffected by the type of reactor used. In the case of indolalkaloid production by *Catharanthus roseus,* they found reactors with mechanical agitation to be quite unsatisfactory, whereas the air lift fermentor gave yields comparable to those in shake flasks. On the basis of these findings, it would seem that the air lift fermentor will prove to be a most useful reactor for plant cell cultures. However, it is unlikely to be a panacea. Zenk et al.[23] found the air lift fermentor much less efficient than shake flasks for the production of rosmarinic acid by coleus cells.

It is generally accepted that the size of inoculum has an important bearing on the time required to initiate growth and that there is a critical minimum inoculum size below which subcultures will not grow.[24] In large-scale culture work, it is customary

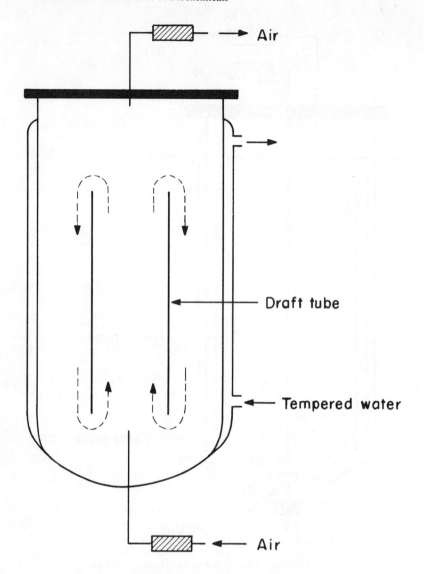

FIGURE 12.   Air lift fermentor.

to use large inocula (10 + %) well above the critical limit. Rose and Martin[18] examined the growth of *Ipomoea* cultures in 7.5-ℓ fermentors initiated with inocula ranging in size from 2.5 to 20%. The cultures grew at essentially the same rate (approximately 20 mg/g/hr), and there was no indication of a lag phase. Yasuda et al.,[12] using shake flask cultures of tobacco cells with inocula ranging from 1 to 20%, also found that the growth rates were essentially equal.

Since plant cells are aerobic, forced aeration is essential for any truly large-scale suspension, and each culture has a minimum critical level of aeration below which it cannot grow at its maximum rate. It is also important to recognize that agitation and aeration are intimately connected and that the aeration rate optimum for growth is not necessarily the same as that for the production of a specific product.

Many workers[2,3,7,8,25,26] have used antifoam agents to suppress excessive foaming in cultures grown under forced aeration and have reported that these agents are not toxic. However, Yasuda et al.[12] have noted that additions of antifoam agent have a tendency to accelerate the build-up of wall growth. We have observed a distinct reduction in growth rate[36] when the defoamer, polypropylene glycol, was used in morning glory suspension cultures. It was assumed that this was the result of a decreased oxygen transfer rate, since final yield of cells was unaffected. Although excessive foaming should be avoided, the use of antifoam agents should be viewed with caution.

C. Semicontinuous Culture Systems

A semicontinuous culture system is simply a batch system provided with the facility to remove at intervals a large volume of culture and replace it with fresh sterile medium. The usual operating procedure is to allow the culture to develop until near maximum yield is attained. Then every day or two a portion (up to 50%) of the culture is harvested and replaced with fresh medium. An attempt is made to keep the weight of cells in the culture constant by adjustment of the harvest size and frequency. In operating practice, the semicontinuous system differs only little from the continuing batch system except that the volume of culture harvested is much larger (about 90%, and the cycles are much longer. If properly operated, both systems may be operated for long periods of time. Neither system should be confused with batch systems to which fresh medium is added intermittently during the culture period without an equivalent volume of culture being harvested.[12] Furthermore, none of these is a continuous culture system in the now commonly accepted sense, since a steady state is not achieved. For example, Kato et al.[11] ran a large-scale semicontinuous culture of tobacco cells, harvesting and replacing 50% of the culture each day, commencing after the fifth day. During each cycle, the cell yield increased exponentially; the pH dropped from 5.4 to 4.8 within 2 to 3 hr and then rose to 5.4; and the dissolved oxygen content of the medium dropped sharply and became almost zero within 3 hr and remained there. One can also assume that gross changes also occurred in the concentration of nutrients.

Byrne and Koch[7,8] in 1962 reported on the use of stirred-jar fermentors in a semicontinuous culture system run for up to 38 days. Culture (3 ℓ) was harvested and replaced every 2 days. The culture produced 9 g of dry tissue per liter or a total of 492 g for the 55 ℓ of culture harvested. In 1965, Tulecke et al.[26] described a "phytostat" based on their original carboy concept, but which was much more elaborate in design. An 8-ℓ culture was used with usually 1 ℓ of culture being harvested each day from the seventh onward. The best run lasted 55 days, and 200 g dry cells were harvested. As noted earlier, Kato et al.[11] grew tobacco cells in 20-ℓ semicontinuous culture. The dry cell yield was 120 to 130 gm per day.

D. Continuous Culture Systems

In batch culture, plant cells go through a growth cycle rather analogous to that in microorganisms. The culture environment is constantly changing, and the cells pass through a succession of physiological states. In continuous culture, cell division takes place at a defined rate and in a uniform environment. The theory of continuous culture is based on the Monod formula for the dependence of growth rate on substrate concentration:

$$\mu = \mu_{max} \frac{S}{K + S}$$

where μ = specific growth rate, μ_{max} = specific maximum growth rate, K = saturation constant, and S = substrate concentration. Equilibrium is reached because one nutrient becomes limiting, the others being held constant or in excess.

A number of continuous culture systems have been devised for plant cells, some of

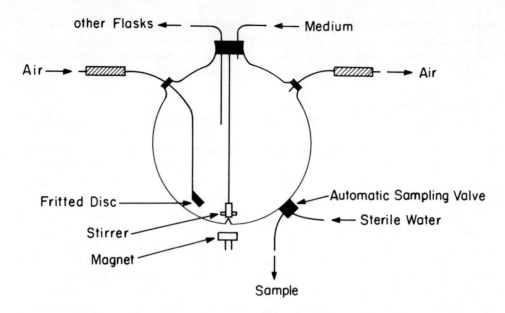

FIGURE 13.   Continuous fermentor of Miller et al.[26]

which are described below. Unfortunately, in many early papers, although the apparatus is described in great detail, very few data are furnished to confirm the actual utility of the apparatus.

In 1967, Miller et al.[27] described the continuous culture apparatus shown schematically in Figure 13. Air was supplied through a glass sparger and agitation by a magnetic stirrer located above the bottom of the vessel. The most interesting feature of the apparatus was an automatic sampling valve featuring zero dead volume and a large orifice. The valve was solenoid operated and controlled by a timer and relay. Medium was fed continuously, and samples were removed every 20 min.

The system described by Kurz[28,29] (Figure 14) was based on a novel method of agitation and aeration, which was said to prevent cells clumping together. The vessel consisted of a thin-walled glass tube. The tube at bottom center served for aeration, while the two smaller tubes were sampling and harvest ports. Ports at the top provided for inoculation, medium inlet, and air outlet. A dual peristaltic pump provided a constant and equal flow of fresh medium and harvested culture. Pulses of sterile air controlled by a magnetic valve assembly arranged to give a 0.1 sec pulse every 2 to 3 sec were shot into the vessel. Each pulse resulted in a single bubble having the same diameter as the vessel. As the bubble moved slowly upward, the entire culture passed as a thin layer between the vessel wall and the bubble surface. The flow rate of the harvest/medium pump was adjusted according to the mass doubling time (doubling time = retention time × log$_e$ 2) of the cells being cultured, which with soybean was between 25 and 35 hr.

A continuous culture apparatus which could operate in chemostat or turbidostat modes was developed by Wilson et al.[30] Figure 15 shows the chemostat mode. The 4-ℓ vessel was stirred by a magnetic stirrer held off the bottom, and temperature was controlled by tempered water flowing through a glass coil. Fresh medium was introduced into the vessel via a variable speed pump. A vessel side-arm equipped with two electrodes served as a constant level device. Two tubes located toward the bottom of the vessel were connected by a length of silicone rubber tubing through which the culture could be circulated by a peristaltic pump. Downstream of the pump was an optical

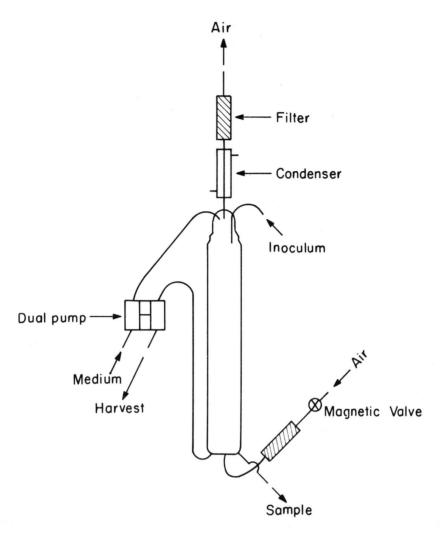

FIGURE 14.   Continuous fermentor of Kurz.[27]

density monitor, while upstream was a side-arm leading via a solenoid valve to the sample collector. In operation, the vessel was inoculated, the circulating pump started, and the fresh medium flow begun. When the medium touched the upper electrode, the solenoid valve opened, and culture flowed by gravity into the sample collector. When the medium level dropped, the solenoid closed. Thus, by using a limiting nutrient, growth was controlled by the flow rate, i.e., the system operated as a chemostat. The density monitor was not a part of the control system. In the turbidostat mode, the fresh medium outlet was connected to the circulating pump via a double-action solenoid valve. When the O.D. of the circulating culture reached the upper set-point, the circulating line was closed, the medium inlet line was opened, and fresh medium was pumped into the system. As fresh medium flowed into the density monitor, the lower set-point was passed, the medium supply was cut off, and the culture was circulated. The constant level device functioned as before to maintain the volume of the culture.

The chemostat system of Wilson et al.[30] has been used extensively for the study of *Acer* cells. This work has recently been reviewed by Fowler.[31]

Noguchi et al.[14] has used a two-stage, two-stream continuous culture system in which

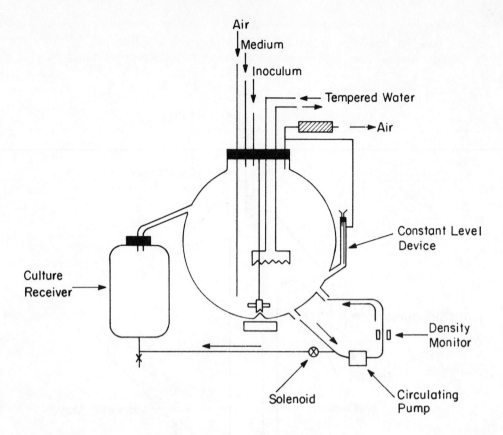

FIGURE 15.   Continuous fermentor of Wilson et al.[29]

flat-blade turbine bioreactors were employed with the objective of achieving high productivity of low-nitrogen content cells. Kato et al.[15] used large-scale bubble fermentors for continuous culture of tobacco cells.

Wilson[32] devised a chemostat of simple design and operation and established steady-state growth of *Acer pseudoplatanus* cells under phosphate limitation. Subsequently, Wilson[33] applied the same apparatus to a study of growth and anthroquinone synthesis in *Galium mollugo* cells.

III. CONCLUSION

It has been established that quite ordinary "microbiological" fermentors can be used for the mass cultivation of plant cell suspensions. Normal operating procedures can be used except that it is necessary to employ low-stirring rates or other means to reduce shear. Use of peripheral equipment for the monitoring and/or control of such parameters as pH and dissolved oxygen presents no particular problem. This is not to suggest, however, that there are still no problems associated with batch cultivation of suspension cultures. In the past few years, detailed engineering studies on growth kinetics and physical-chemical characteristics of suspension cultures have begun to make their appearance in the literature. Such studies are essential for the effective scaling-up of the production of biomass and/or metabolites in plant cell cultures.

Continuous culture techniques have been developed which should prove particularly advantageous for the study of cell growth and metabolism. As with microorganisms, it should be anticipated that, except in exceptional cases, continuous culture will not be used for the commercial production of metabolites by plant cells. The technique should, however, have a great impact on more fundamental studies of the relationship between the environment and growth and secondary metabolite production.

REFERENCES

1. **Tulecke, W. and Nickell, L. G.**, Production of large amounts of plant tissue by submerged culture, *Science,* 130, 863, 1959.
2. **Tulecke, W. and Nickell, L. G.**, Methods, problems and results of growing plant cells under submerged conditions, *Trans. N.Y. Acad. Sci.,* 22, 196, 1960.
3. **Wang, C-J. and Staba, E. J.**, Peppermint and spearmint tissue culture. II. Dual-carboy culture of spearmint tissues, *J. Pharm. Sci.,* 52, 1058, 1963.
4. **Lamport, D. T. A.**, Cell suspension cultures of higher plants: isolation and growth energetics, *Exp. Cell Res.,* 33, 195, 1964.
5. **Short, K. C., Brown, E. G., and Street, H. E.**, Studies on the growth in culture of plant cells. V. Large-scale culture of *Acer pseudoplatanus,* L. cell suspensions, *J. Exp. Bot.,* 20, 572, 1969.
6. **Graebe, J. E. and Novelli, G. D.**, A practical method for large-scale plant tissue culture, *Exp. Cell Res.,* 41, 509, 1966.
7. **Byrne, A. F.**, Food Production by Submerged Culture of Plant Tissue Cells, Acivities Report 14, Armed Forces Food and Container Institute, Chicago, 1962, 177.
8. **Byrne, A. F. and Koch, M. B.**, Food production by submerged culture of plant tissue cells, *Science,* 135, 215, 1962.
9. **Verma, D. P. S. and van Huystee, R. B.**, Derivation, characteristics and large scale cultivation of a cell line from *Arachis hypogaea,* L. cotyledons, *Exp. Cell Res.,* 69, 402, 1971.
10. **Veliky, I. and Martin, S. M.**, A fermentor for plant cell suspension cultures, *Can. J. Microbiol.,* 16, 223, 1970.
11. **Kato, K., Shiozawa, Y., Yamada, A., Nishida, K., and Noguchi, M.**, A jar fermentor culture of *Nicotiana tabacum* L. cell suspensions, *Agric. Biol. Chem.,* 36, 899, 1972.
12. **Yasuda, S., Satoh, K., Ishii, T., and Furuya, T.**, Studies on the cultural conditions of plant cell suspension culture, *Proc. IV IFS, Ferment. Technol. Today,* 697, 1972.
13. **Kato, K., Matsumoto, T., Koiwai, A., Mizusaki, S., Nishida, K., Noguchi, M., and Tamaki, E.**, Liquid suspension culture of tobacco cells, *Proc. IV IFS, Ferment. Technol. Today,* 689, 1972.
14. **Noguchi, M., Matsumoto, T., Hirata, Y., Tamamoto, K., Katsuyama, A., Kato, A., Azechi, S., and Kato, K.**, Improvement of growth rates of plant cell cultures, in *Plant Tissue Culture and its Bio-technological Applications,* Barz, W., Reinhard, E., and Zenk, M. H., Eds., Springer-Verlag, Berlin, 1977.
15. **Kato, A., Kawazoe, S., Iizima, M., and Shimizu, Y.**, Continuous culture of tobacco cells, *J. Ferment. Technol.,* 54, 82, 1976.
16. **Martin, S. M. and Rose, D.**, Growth of plant cells (*Ipomoea*) suspension cultures at controlled pH levels, *Can. J. Bot.,* 54, 1264, 1976.
17. **Martin, S. M., Rose, D., and Hui, V.**, Growth of plant cell suspension cultures with ammonium as the sole source of nitrogen, *Can. J. Bot.,* 55, 2838, 1977.
18. **Rose, D. and Martin, S. M.**, Parameters for growth measurement in suspension culture of plant cells, *Can. J. Bot.,* 52, 903, 1974.
19. **Rose, D. and Martin, S. M.**, Growth of suspension cultures of plant cells (*Ipomoea* sp.) at various temperatures, *Can. J. Bot.,* 53, 315, 1975.
20. **Rose, D., Martin, S. M., and Clay, P. P. F.**, Metabolic rates for major nutrients in suspension cultures of plant cells, *Can. J. Bot.,* 50, 1301, 1972.
21. **Kato, A., Shimizu, Y., and Nagai, S.**, Effect of initial KLa on the growth of tobacco cells in batch culture, *J. Ferment. Technol.,* 53, 744, 1975.
22. **Wagner, F. and Vogelmann, H.**, Cultivation of plant tissue cultures in bioreactors and formation of secondary metabolites, in *Plant Tissue Culture and its Bio-technological Applications,* Barz, W., Reinhard, E., and Zenk, M. H., Eds., Springer-Verlag, Berlin, 1977.
23. **Zenk, M. H., El-Shagi, H., and Ulbrich, H.**, Production of rosmarinic acid by cell-suspension cultures of *Coleus blumei, Naturwissenschaften,* 64, 585, 1977.

24. **Puhan, Z. and Martin, S. M.,** The industrial potential of plant cell culture, *Prog. Ind. Microbiol.,* 9, 13, 1971.
25. **Tulecke, W.,** Continuous culture of higher plant cells in liquid medium: the advantages and potential use of a phytostat, *Ann. N. Y. Acad. Sci.,* 139, 162, 1966.
26. **Tulecke, W., Taggart, R., and Colavito, L.,** Continuous culture of higher plant cells in liquid media, *Contrib. Boyce Thompson Inst.,* 23, 33, 1965.
27. **Miller, R. A., Shyluk, J. P., Gamborg, O. L., and Kirkpatrick, J. W.,** Phytostat for continuous culture and automatic sampling of plant-cell suspensions, *Science,* 159, 540, 1968.
28. **Kurz, W. G. W.,** A chemostat for growing higher plant cells in single cell suspension cultures, *Exp. Cell Res.,* 64, 477, 1971.
29. **Kurz, W. G. W.,** A fermentor system for the continuous culture of plant cells, in *Plant Tissue Culture Methods,* Gamborg, O. L. and Wetter, L. R., Eds., National Research Council, Saskatoon, 1975.
30. **Wilson, S. B., King, P. J., and Street, H. E.,** Studies of the growth in culture of plant cells. XII. A versatile system for the large scale batch or continuous culture of plant cell suspensions, *J. Exp. Bot.,* 22, 177, 1971.
31. **Fowler, M. W.,** Growth of cell cultures under chemostat conditions, in *Plant Tissue Culture and its Bio-technological Application,* Barz, W., Reinhard, E. and Zenk, M. H., Eds., Springer-Verlag, Berlin, 1977.
32. **Wilson, G.,** A simple and inexpensive design of chemostat enabling steady-state growth of *Acer pseudoplatanus* L. cells under phosphate-limiting conditions, *Ann. Bot.,* 40, 919, 1976.
33. **Wilson, G.,** The application of the chemostat technique to the study of growth and anthroquinone synthesis by *Galium mollugo* cells, in *Production of Natural Compounds by Cell Culture Methods,* Alfermann, A. W. and Reinhard, E., Eds., BPT-Report 1/78, Gesellschaft für Strahlen und Umweltforschung mbH, Munich, 1978.
34. **Martin, S. M.,** unpublished results.
35. **Martin, S. M.,** unpublished results.
36. **Martin, S. M.,** unpublished results.

Chapter 8

INDUSTRIAL AND GOVERNMENT RESEARCH

Masanaru Misawa

TABLE OF CONTENTS

I. INTRODUCTION

Since the pioneering works carried out at Charles Pfizer Co., Inc.,[1] the interest in the use of plant tissue cultures for industrial production of useful plant metabolites has continued.[2-5] Development of industrial fermentation techniques also stimulated these studies.

Higher plants are very useful, not only as foods, but also as a source of natural drugs or other raw materials. Therefore, it is quite advantageous if these metabolites could be produced by tissue-culture techniques. Unfortunately, these studies are still in laboratory scale at industrial and governmental laboratories and at universities. Their application in industry has not yet been achieved. *Chemical Week* in 1976[6] predicted that commercialization of the plant tissue culture would be achieved by the early 1980s and quoted the production costs estimated by Laves Chemie in West Germany. According to their estimation, a minimum producing cost was $2,000 to 3,000/lb. Therefore, the first commercial applications were suggested to be in pharmaceuticals rather than in foodstuffs. The author also believes that tissue-culture techniques should be applied to production of high-cost compounds such as drugs and perfumes from rare or inaccessible plants.

Recently, the new techniques for increasing the product level have been introduced by several groups,[7,8] and application of these techniques will advance the studies of large-scale productions in industry.

In this chapter, the author will discuss a few recent studies from industrial and government laboratories which would seem to have good industrial potential.

II. ALKALOIDS

Alkaloids are widely distributed in the plant kingdom and have been used as pharmaceuticals because of their physiological activities. More than 1000 kinds of alkaloids have already been isolated, and new ones are still being isolated, mainly from higher plants, but also from limited kinds of fungi and actinomycetes.[9]

Studies on production of alkaloids through tissue culture have been actively carried out because of shortage of alkaloid-producing plants. There are a number of papers and patents on alkaloid production with callus tissues and cultured cells, but their industrial application has not yet been realized.

A. Indole Alkaloids

Among alkaloids, the antitumor alkaloids, vincristine and vinblastine, are very expensive and already have a significant market. Therefore, their production by plant tissue culture has been extensively studied.[10] In spite of the efforts by Carew and Krueger, the accumulation of these alkaloids by cultured *Vinca rosea* cells has not been recognized.[11] On the other hand, a patent filed by Petiard and Guinebault[12] described that 540 g of *Vinca minor* cells were harvested from a 15-ℓ fermentor culture under the conditions of 1.5 ℓ/min aeration, 30°C, and 100 rpm for 21 days. From the cells, 545 mg of alkaloids were obtained, but their antitumor activity was not clearly stated.

Although these antitumor alkaloids have not been isolated from *Vinca rosea* cultured cells, ajmalicine and serpentine were found to be synthesized in high amounts with suspension-cultured cells of *Catharanthus roseus* (= *Vinca rosea*) by Zenk and his group at Ruhr University in West Germany[7] (Figure 1). This excellent study, supported by the German Government, showed many possibilities for industrial application of plant tissue cultures. Both ajmalicine and serpentine are indole alkaloids. Ajmalicine is useful in the treatment of circulatory diseases, and serpentine is easily

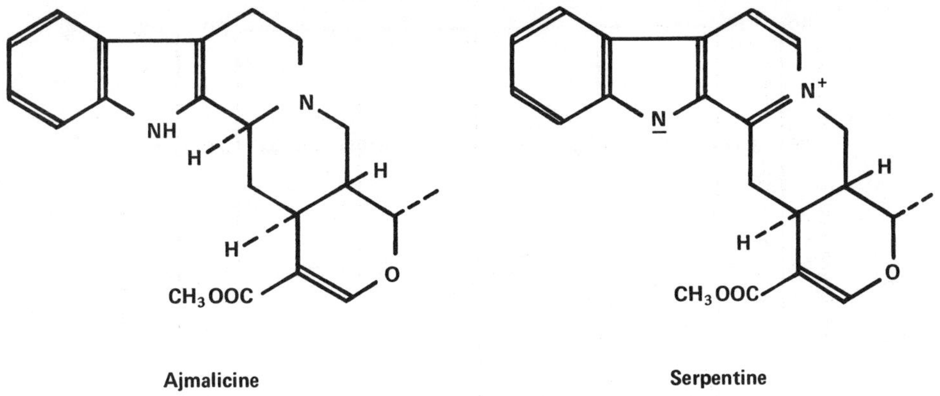

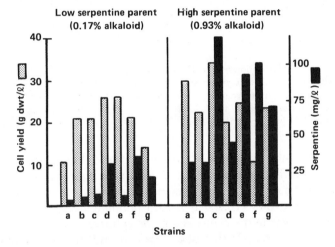

Ajmalicine

Serpentine

FIGURE 1.   Chemical structures of ajmalicine and serpentine.

FIGURE 2.   Cell yield and serpentine content of suspension-cultured *Catharanthus roseus* cells derived from seed callus of low- and high-alkaloid-containing parents. (From Zenk, M. H., el-Shagi, H., Arens, H., Stockigt, J., Weiler, E. W., and Ders, B., in *Plant Tissue Culture and Its Bio-technological Application*, Barz, W. C., Reinhard, E., and Zenk, M. H., Eds., Springer-Verlag, Berlin, 1977, 27. With permission.)

hydrated chemically to ajmalicine. To obtain the cells which have the ability to synthesize higher levels of the alkaloids, they first selected a plant which contained the highest concentration of serpentine and ajmalicine from a number of *C. roseus* plants. Callus tissues were derived from the selected plant and were cultivated in suspension. As seen in Figure 2, cells derived from the high-alkaloid-producing plants accumulated much higher level of serpentine than those from the low-producing plants, i.e., the former cells produced 70 mg of serpentine per mℓ of the medium, whereas the latter produced only 16. High-serpentine-producing cells were spread on the agar media in Petri dishes and cultivated for 2 months. The alkaloid contents of 160 colonies grown were analyzed, and the results showed the levels of serpentine to be distributed between 0 and 1.4%. and those of ajmalicine between 0 and 0.8%. A strain which produced the highest levels of the alkaloids was isolated and cultivated on both agar and liquid media successively in order to stabilize its productivity. It was shown to accumulate approxi-

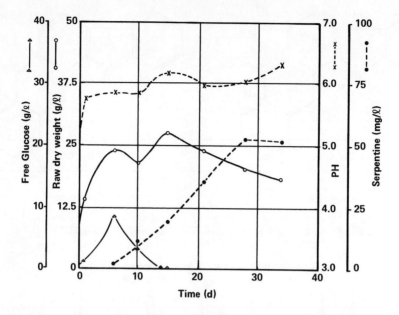

FIGURE 3.   Cultivation of *Catharanthus roseus* cells in an airlift fermentor. Reaction volume, 10 *ℓ*; temperature, 28°C; aeration rate, 0.33 vvm; inoculum size, 20%. (Data from Wagner, F. and Vogelmann, H., in *Plant Tissue Culture and Its Bio-technological Applications,* Barz, W. C., Reinhard, E., and Zenk, M. H., Eds., Springer-Verlag, Berlin, 1977, 245. With permission.)

mately 1.3% of both alkaloids on a dry cell-weight basis in suspension cultures. This corresponds to an alkaloid level about 1.5 times higher than that in the mother plant, and also about five times higher than the average alkaloid concentration in the roots.

It is noteworthy that they effectively used a radioimmunoassay method for determination of the alkaloids in the plants and in the cultured cells. This method was very helpful, particularly for the selection of a variant strain with high alkaloid-producing ability. As Weiler in the same group stated,[13] the radioimmunoassay method, which is extremely sensitive and highly specific, is a great help in determining very small amounts of metabolites accumulated in plant cells.

Using a cell line thus obtained, they established a medium suitable for alkaloid production, which consisted of Murashige-Skoog's salts, 5% sucrose, indole acetic acid, benzyladenine, and 0.05% L-tryptophan as a precursor. With this medium, one strain of *C. roseus* produced 162 mg/*ℓ* serpentine, and a second strain produced 77 mg/*ℓ* serpentine and 264 mg/*ℓ* ajmalicine simultaneously.

Wagner and Vogelmann[14] at Gesellschaft für Biotechnologische Forschung mbH in West Germany investigated the mass production of serpentine by Zenk's strain. The cells were cultivated in 10 *ℓ* of the medium using an airlift fermentor whose draft tube diameter/column-diameter value was 0.44 and column diameter/column-height volume was 0.47. The cells were cultivated for more than 30 days at 28°C, an aeration rate of 0.33 vvm, and 20% inoculum. As shown in Figure 3, cell growth and alkaloid production were partially decoupled for the cultivation, and approximately 50 mg of serpentine was accumulated after about 30 days of incubation. Since the culture period is too long for large-scale production, more rapid cultivation is necessary for industrial application. They also emphasized that the airlift type is the most suitable fermentor for plant cell-suspension cultures.

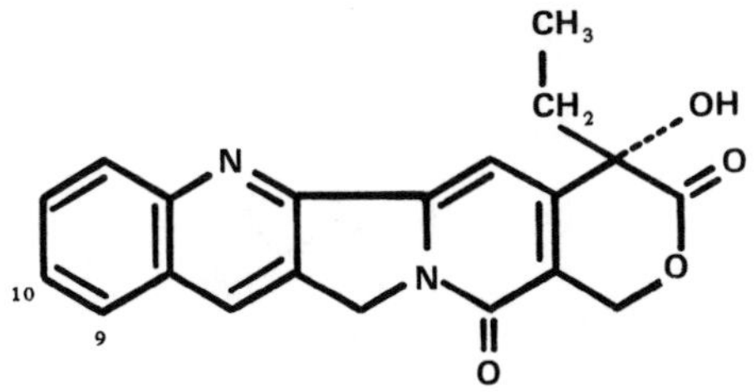

FIGURE 4. Chemical structure of camptothe-cin.

B. Nicotine

Nicotine production by plant cell culture is not of industrial interest because it is easily and inexpensively available from tobacco leaves, but some reports on production of nicotine are very suggestive for commercial production of other metabolites.

Tabata et al.[8] at Kyoto University in Japan reported the selection of higher nicotine-producing strains using *Nicotiana rustica* L. var. *brasilia* cells. They found that most of callus tissues produced 0.25 to 0.58% of nicotine in dry cell weight during a few passages subsequent to callus induction, but after that the cells lost the ability to produce nicotine. Then, they cultivated mainly single cells and a small number of 2 to 8 cell aggregates on the agar medium in a Petri dish for about 1 month. The colonies thus grown were transferred individually to the fresh medium in a test tube, and their alkaloid contents were analyzed spectrophotometrically. As a result, most of these strains lost their nicotine-producing abilities, while one of them, Strain No. 10b, was shown to produce 0.29% of nicotine even after 54 passages. The reason why the isolated cell had such ability was not clear, but this technique is similar to a microbial-mutation method.

C. Isoquinoline Alkaloids

Several patents on production of alkaloids by cell cultures and differentiated tissue cultures have been filed by industrial companies. Examples are production of berberine and palmatine with callus tissues, crown-gall cells, or plant differentiated from the cells of *Coptis japonica* and its varieties by Meiji Seika Kaisha Co., Ltd.[15] and with *Phellodendron amurense* callus by Kanebo, Ltd.[16] McCormick at American Cyanamid Co.[17] applied for a patent which covered production of a variety of alkaloids and other metabolites by the cells with primordia.

D. Camptothecin

The author and co-workers at Kyowa Hakko Kogyo Co., Ltd.[18] studied the production of an antitumor alkaloid, camptothecin (Figure 4) by cell-suspension cultures of *Camptotheca acuminata*, a plant indigenous to mainland China. This alkaloid was isolated from tree stems, and its structure was determined by Wall and his associates.[19] Camptothecin has antitumor activity in several experimental antitumor systems including L1210, P-338, L-5178Y, and K-1964 leukemias. It is also active against the Walker 256 carcinosarcoma in vivo, is cytotoxic in vitro against various leukemia cell lines and PHA-stimulated human lymphocytes, and inhibited DNA and RNA syntheses in HeLa and mouse-lymphoma-cell culture L-5178. The content of the alkaloid in the tree is low, and its growth is slow. In order to produce this alkaloid more efficiently, suspension cultures of *C. acuminata* were established. After 15 days cultivation at 30°C and 180 rpm in the dark, the cells were harvested and the alkaloid was isolated by chloroform extraction and silica-gel G-thin layer chromatography. Although the

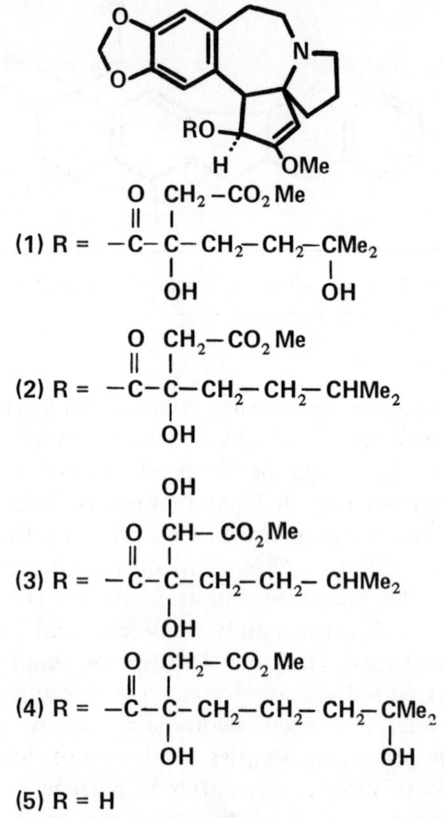

(1) R = $-\overset{\overset{\displaystyle O}{\|}}{C}-\overset{\overset{\displaystyle CH_2-CO_2Me}{|}}{\underset{\underset{\displaystyle OH}{|}}{C}}-CH_2-CH_2-\overset{}{\underset{\underset{\displaystyle OH}{|}}{C}Me_2}$

(2) R = $-\overset{\overset{\displaystyle O}{\|}}{C}-\overset{\overset{\displaystyle CH_2-CO_2Me}{|}}{\underset{\underset{\displaystyle OH}{|}}{C}}-CH_2-CH_2-CHMe_2$

(3) R = $-\overset{\overset{\displaystyle O}{\|}}{C}-\overset{\overset{\displaystyle CH-CO_2Me}{|}}{\underset{\underset{\displaystyle OH}{|}}{C}}-CH_2-CH_2-CHMe_2$ (with OH on the CH)

(4) R = $-\overset{\overset{\displaystyle O}{\|}}{C}-\overset{\overset{\displaystyle CH_2-CO_2Me}{|}}{\underset{\underset{\displaystyle OH}{|}}{C}}-CH_2-CH_2-CH_2-\overset{}{\underset{\underset{\displaystyle OH}{|}}{C}Me_2}$

(5) R = H

FIGURE 5.   Chemical structures of harringtonine and other esters of cephalotaxine. (1) Harringtonine, (2) deoxyharringtonine, (3) isoharringtonine, (4) homoharringtonine, (5) cephalotaxine.

yield was $2.54 \times 10^{-4}\%$, a level was lower than $5 \times 10^{-3}\%$ in the intact plant, the growth rate of the cultured cells is much faster than that of the intact plant. Unfortunately, it was found by the National Cancer Institute in the U.S. that camptothecin showed some side effects in clinical trial, and this study was terminated.

E. Harringtonine

Another study on the production of an antitumor alkaloid was described by Delfel and Rothfus at the U.S. Department of Agriculture.[20] The Japanese plumyew, *Cephalotaxus harringtonia* var. *harringtonia* (Forbes) K. Koch contains four interesting antitumor alkaloids: harringtonine, deoxyharringtonine, isoharringtonine, and homoharringtonine which are esters of cephalotaxine (Figure 5). Since this plant is a slow-growing tree, they investigated the production of these alkaloids by plant tissue-culture technique. The callus of *C. harringtonia* was induced on Murashige-Skoog's medium supplemented with 1 g enzymatic protein hydrolyzate, 25 mg hypoxanthine, vitamins, 10 mg NAA, and 1 mg kinetin per liter. The callus growth was so slow that the levels of alkaloids were analyzed after 3 and 6 months cultivation. As a result, cephalotaxine and its three antitumor esters were recognized in the callus and in the medium, whereas deoxyharringtonine was present in relatively large amounts only in the medium (Table 1). Since the National Cancer Institute in the U.S. is very interested in these alkaloids

9

73

TABLE 1

Antitumor Alkaloid Concentration Based on the Fresh Weight of *Cephalotaxus harringtonia* Callus and Medium

| | Concentration (μg/kg) | | | |
| | 3-Month Culture | | 6-Month Culture | |
Alkaloids	Callus	Medium	Callus	Medium
Cephalotaxine	50	13	40	144
Deoxyharring-tonine	0	18	0	25
Harringtonine	8	1	tr[a]	11
Isoharringtonine	11	4	11	48
Homoharring-tonine	15	4	0.5	27

[a] tr = Trace.

Data from Delfel, N. E. and Rothfus, J. A., *Phytochemistry*, 16, 1595, 1977.

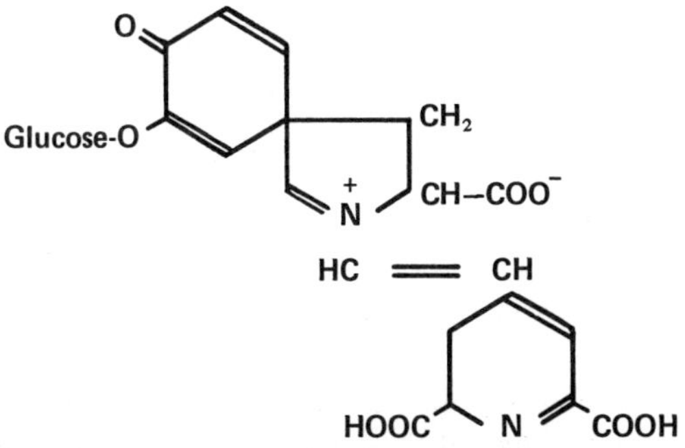

FIGURE 6.   Structure of betanin.

as new antitumor drugs,[21] this paper is very attractive, but extensive studies aimed at more rapid cultivation and an increase of alkaloid content are required for its industrial production.

F. Betacyanins

The red pigments, betacyanins (Figure 6), are alkaloids which occur in plants belonging to the Centrospermae. Recently, the need for pigments from natural sources to replace artificial ones has been raised in the food industry. The author[22] and Komatsu et al. in Kibun Co., Ltd.[23] in Japan studied the accumulation of betacyanins by cultured cells of *Phytolacca americana*, *Beta vulgaris* var. *rubra*, *Chenopodium album* L var. *cetrorubrum* and *Spinacia oleraceae*. Although the pigments could be accumulated in relatively large amounts by these cell lines in the light, there are still difficulties for economical production.

G. Furoquinoline Alkaloids

Steck and Constabel[24] at National Research Council of Canada used *Ruta graveolens* cultured cells for production of furoquinoline alkaloids by transformation from a precursor. By addition of 4-hydroxy-2-quinolone to the suspension cultures of *R. grav-*

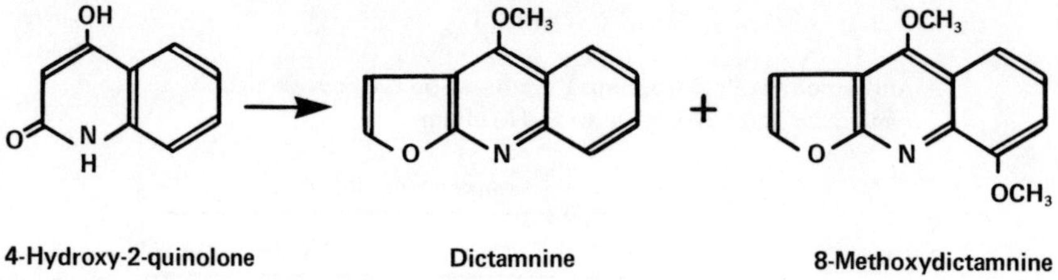

4-Hydroxy-2-quinolone   **Dictamnine**   **8-Methoxydictamnine**

FIGURE 7.   Biotransformation of furoquinoline alkaloids by *Ruta graveolens* cells.

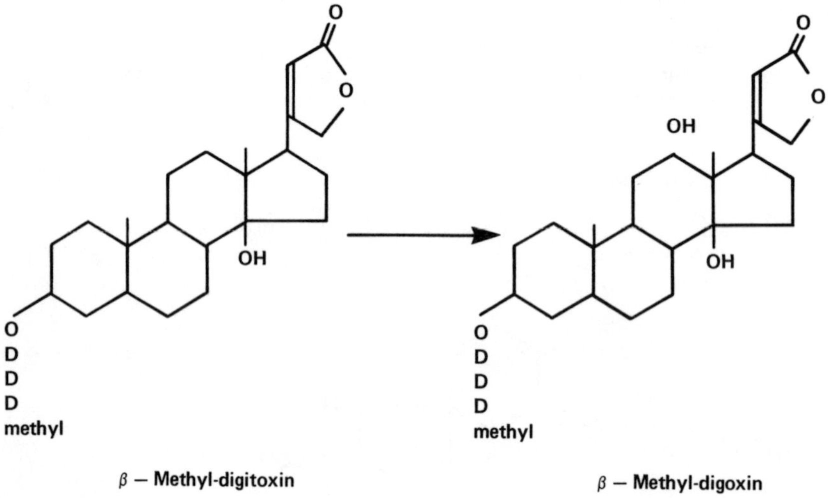

β — Methyl-digitoxin β — Methyl-digoxin

FIGURE 8.   Biotransformation of β- methyldigitoxin by the cultured cells of *Digitalis lanata*.

eolens, dictamnine and 8-methoxy dictamnine were synthesized (Figure 7), and their amounts were approximately 0.6% of the cells on a dry-weight basis.

Veliky in Canada also added tryptophan into a *Phaseolus vulgaris* cell suspension and detected the alkaloids harman and norharman.[25] In this system, 18 other amino acids failed to bring about alkaloid production.

As indicated in these papers, a biotransformation method appears to be a help to produce alkaloids.

III. STEROIDS

A. Digoxin

A number of reports on studies of steroid synthesis and their biotransformation by cultured plant cells have appeared. Most of them are fundamental researches and are far from application. However, the results by Reinhard at Lehrstuhl für Pharmazeutische Biologie der Universität Tübingen, West Germany[26] are of interest. They investigated the biotransformation of digitoxin or methyldigitoxin to digoxin or methyldigoxin with *Digitalis lanata* suspension-cultured cells (Figure 8) for which there is a growing need. In their experiments, they incubated 10 g of the fresh cells with 2 mg of methyldigitoxin at 25°C. Since this substrate is not glucosylated because of occupation by a methyl group, 12-β hydroxylation occurred very rapidly and efficiently. Thus, after 24 hr of incubation, 15% of β-methyldigoxin was found, and the maximum conversion yield, 70%, was obtained after 7 days.

Using the same systems, Alfermann et al.[27] examined the biotransformation on a large scale. When the fermentor equipped with ordinary blade or turbine stirrers was used, the reaction did not proceed. They explained that the reason must be sensitivity of the cells to stirring. Therefore, they used a 20-*l* airlift fermentor. By controlling pH at 6.1 with glucose feeding, 50% of β-methyldigitoxin was found to be converted to β-methyldigoxin.

These results indicate that the cultured plant cells might be used as enzyme sources for industrial biotransformation of useful metabolites in the near future.

B. Diosgenin

Production of diosgenin, which is a raw material of steroidal hormones, is also attractive. A high level accumulation of diosgenin occurred in *Dioscorea deltoidea* suspension cultures on feeding cholesterol.[28]

IV. TERPENES

A. Radix Ginseng

Production of radix ginseng, which contains biologically active triterpenoid saponins, appears to be one of the most interesting targets for commercial application.[29] *Panax ginseng* is a perennial herb indigenous to eastern Asia and is cultivated in China, Korea, and Japan. Ginseng root, so-called "radix ginseng", has been widely used as a tonic and natural medicine in oriental countries. Cultivation of the plant in the field requires 4 to 7 years, and it is impossible to plant consecutively for 20 to 50 years. Furuya at Kitasato University and Meiji Seika Kaisha in Japan studied the large-scale cultivation of *P. ginseng*.[30] According to their patent,[30] crown-gall cells, callus tissues, and redifferentiated roots of *P. ginseng* were able to accumulate saponins and sapogenins which have been known as the metabolites in the intact plant. The cells were cultivated for several weeks at 25 to 28°C on both Murashige-Skoog's agar and liquid media containing vitamins, sucrose, 2,4-D, and suitable natural substances such as soybean powder or beef extracts. The Rf values of the saponins accumulated in the cultured cells on thin-layer chromatography corresponded to those of ginsenosides Rb and Rg, which are biologically active saponins. The levels of crude saponins were 21.2% in the callus, 19.3% in the crown gall, and 27.4% in the redifferentiated root, much higher than the 4.1% occurring in the natural roots. Furuya et al.[31] also isolated panaxadiol, panaxatriol, and oleanoic acid, whose yields were 7 mg, 23 mg, and 15 mg from 25 g of the callus tissue, respectively.

The specific growth rate (μ, day^{-1}) of *P. ginseng* cultured cells was 0.10 in the exponential growth phase. For improvement of the growth rate, Yasuda et al. at the same company[32] selected the suitable cultural conditions in suspension. They used not only Erlenmeyer flasks, but 30-*l* jar fermentors and 130-*l* and 600-*l* tanks, but their detailed experimental results have not been published. Figure 9 shows a time course of *P. ginseng* cells in a static culture. Using agar media, they showed that addition of 0.5 mg of 2,4-D per liter of the medium gave satisfactory growth and saponin production, and that the maximum levels of cells and of saponins accumulated were obtained after 5 weeks of inoculation. In spite of their interesting results, the studies were terminated and industrial application has not been pursued.

The *Soviet Weekly*[33] in June, 1976 announced that a plant in Efremov, near Moscow, is producing ginseng 20 times faster than the growth rate of the natural plants. However, the cultural methods and the producing scale are obscure.

B. Radix Bupleuri

The dried root of *Bupleurum falcatum*, "radix bupleuri", is used as an antipyretic,

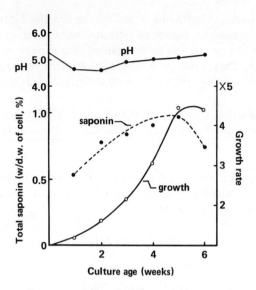

FIGURE 9.   Time course of *Panax ginseng* cells in a static culture. (From Yasuda, S., Satoh, K., Ishii, T., and Furuya, T., in *Fermentation Technology Today*, Terui, G., Ed., Society of Fermentation Technology, Osaka, Japan, 1972, 697. With permission.)

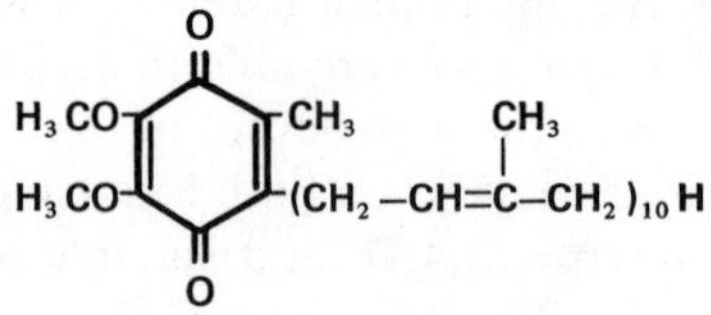

FIGURE 10.   Chemical structure of ubiquinone-10.

a tonic, and an anodyne in oriental countries. Shionogi and Co., Ltd.[34] in Japan described production of *B. falcatum* cells in their patent. The cells were cultivated in the liquid medium containing 10^{-6} M 2,4-D and 0.2 mg/ℓ kinetin for 12 days and then transferred to the medium containing 10^{-7} M 2,4-D or IAA and 0.2 mg/ℓ kinetin. A number of plantlets with roots and primordia were developed by successive transfers for several months. The roots harvested from the suspension cultured broth were recognized to contain 19.4 mg of saponins per gram of the dried material, which was the same level as had accumulated in the natural plants, 18.47 mg/g.

V. QUINONES

A. Ubiquinone-10

Some studies in this field are quite suggestive for industrial application of plant cell cultures. Ikeda et al.[35] in the Japan Tobacco and Salt Public Corporation found that *N. tabacum* cultured cells accumulated ubiquinone-10 known as Coenzyme Q (Figure 10), which is active in electron transfer systems and in oxidative phosphorylation. This compound is also used as a drug for heart disease.

The cells of *N. tabacum* were incubated in 100 mℓ of Linsmaier-Skoog's medium

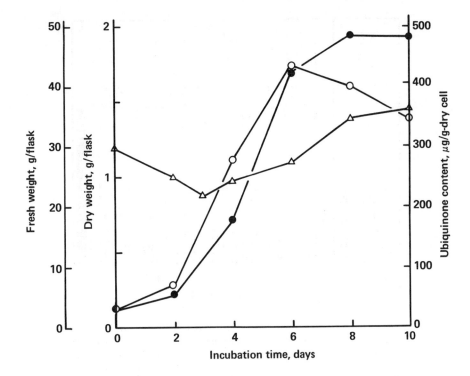

FIGURE 11.   Time course of cell growth and ubiquinone content in cultured tobacco cells. •
Cell growth (fresh weight), O, cell growth (dry weight), △, ubiquinone content. (From Ikeda,
T., Matsumoto, T., and Noguchi, M., *Phytochemistry*, 15, 568, 1976. With permission.)

supplemented with 3 g of sucrose, 0.02 mg of 2,4-D, and vitamins within a 500 mℓ
Erlenmeyer flask for 10 days at 28°C in the dark on a reciprocal shaker. As shown in
Figure 11, the highest level of ubiquinone-10, 360 μg/g of dried cells, was obtained at
the 10th day of cultivation, and the level was approximately 10 times higher than that
in the tobacco leaves. For increasing the level of ubiquinone-10 accumulated, they
indicated that lower concentrations of sugar and a higher concentration of 2,4-D in
the medium were favorable.

B. Naphthoquinones

Two examples which the author will mention below are not from studies in industry,
but these are very suggestive. One was carried out at Kyoto University[36] in Japan and
the other at Ruhr University[37] in West Germany.

Using cultured cells of *Lithospermum erythrorhizon*, Mizukami et al.[36] succeeded
in increasing naphthoquinone pigment levels. The pigments are used for the treatment
of burns, skin diseases, and hemorrhoids. Their study on the improvement of productivity showed that the content of the pigments, which consisted of shikonin derivatives,
increased to about 12% of the dry cell weight, and this was 8 times higher than that
in the perennial root used as the crude drug. They showed that the components of
these shikonin derivatives produced by the cultured cells were similar to those in the
natural roots and that their formation was inhibited by blue-light radiation and stimulated by addition of streptomycin in the medium.

C. Anthraquinones

The concentration of anthraquinones produced by *Morinda citrifolia* suspension-
cultured cells was also high,[37] namely 2.5 g/ℓ of the medium were accumulated. These

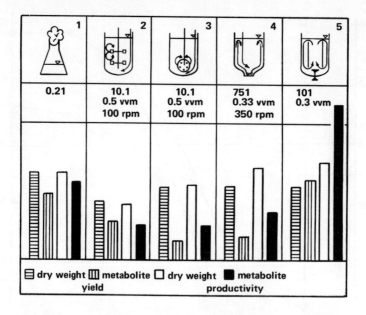

FIGURE 12.   Comparison of yield and productivity for cell mass and anthraquinones by *Morinda citrifolia* cells in various fermentor systems. 1. Shake flask. 2. Flat blade turbine. 3. Perforated-disk impeller. 4. Draft-tube fermentor with Kaplan turbine. 5. Airlift fermentor. Data from Wagner, F. and Vogelmann, H., in *Plant Tissue Culture and Its Bio-technological Applications*, Barz, W., Reinhard, E., and Zenk, M. H., Eds. , Springer-Verlag, Berlin, 1977, 245. With permission.)

levels were to 10 times higher than those in natural plants. Wagner and Vogelmann[14] examined their production on a large scale with various types of fermentors as shown in Figure 12. This figure shows that the airlift fermentor is the most suitable type for producion of anthraquinones. This is similar to the production of serpentine. They pointed out that this increased productivity was caused by the additive effects of the defined flow characteristics, low shear rates, and sufficient oxygen supply in the airlift fermentor. A typical time course of *M. citrifolia* culture in a 10-ℓ airlift fermentor is shown in Figure 13. As they indicated, the phase of cell growth is clearly separated from the second phase of anthraquinone formation. The maximum yield of products was obtained after 10 days of cultivation.

VI. OTHER PHYSIOLOGICALLY ACTIVE SUBSTANCES

Some other products of plant tissue culture which have physiological activities are also of interest because some of them are very expensive. Here, several papers and patents on the production of new or already known physiologically active substances not described above will be mentioned.

A. Antibiotics

Some higher plants are known to accumulate antibiotic substances for protecting themselves against microbial infections, and several reports describe the formation of these compounds by cultured cells. For example, Lin and Mathes[38] detected antibiotic activities in a few kinds of callus extracts, and Veliky and Latta at the National Research Council of Canada[39] also found activities against several bacteria in *Lactuca sativa, Cannabis sativa* and *Ipomoea* sp. However, they did not isolate these antibiotics. The author[40] isolated a compound from a suspension-cultured medium of *Phyto-*

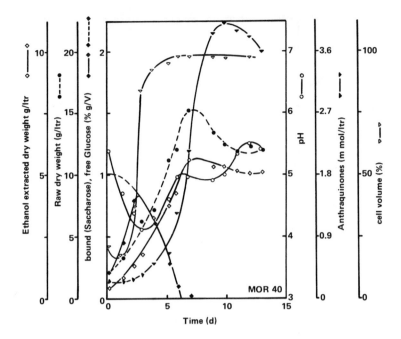

FIGURE 13. Time course of cell growth and production of anthraquinones by *Morinda citrifolia* cells in a 10-ℓ airlift fermentor. Inoculum size, 10%; temperature, 28°C; aeration rate, 0.5 vvm. (From Wagner, F. and Vogelmann, H., in *Plant Tissue Culture and Its Bio-technological Applications*, Barz, Reinhard, E., and Zenk, M. H., Eds., Springer-Verlag, Berlin, 1977, 245. With permission.)

lacca americana with ion-exchange resins. Its molecular weight was 976 and molecular formula was $C_{35}H_{80}O_{21}N_{10}$. The minimum inhibitory concentrations of the antibiotic was 5.8 μg/mℓ against *Bacillus subtilis* and 11.2 μg/mℓ against *Streptococcus faecalis*. The LD_{50} was 400 mg/kg.

B. Antitumor Substances

As seen in the reviews by Hartwell[41] and Kupchan,[42] antitumor substances from the plant kingdom are of interest, but there are some difficulties because of the low concentration in the parent materials. However, there are few studies on production of antitumor substances by tissue culture other than camptothecin and harringtonine as already described.

C. Anti-Plant Virus Substances

There is considerable practical need for nonphytotoxic plant-virus inhibitor. A large number of compounds have therefore been examined for their possible inhibitory effect on plant viruses, but none has proved practically useful. The extracts from some higher plants inhibit virus infection have been recognized by many researchers, and these active principles have been shown to be proteins, sugars, tannins, and phenolic compounds.[43]

It has been recognized that *P. americana*, pokeweed, contains a variety of biologically active substances such as antibacterial, antifungal, spermatocidal, antiinflammatory, antiplant-virus substances, and phytohemagglutinin. The author[44] found that *P. americana* callus had very strong inhibitory activity against tobacco mosaic virus (TMV) infection on tobacco leaves. Through use of a modified Murashige-Skoog's

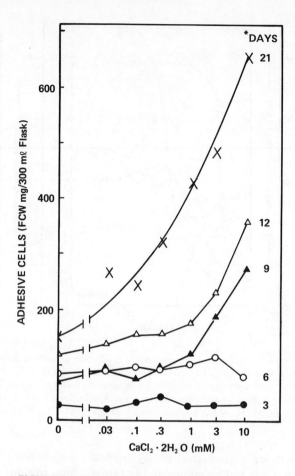

FIGURE 14.   Effect of Ca++ level on adhesion of the cells of *Agrostemma githago*, Days: culture periods; 100 m*l* - medium /300 m*l* Erlenmeyer flask. (Data from Takayama, S., Misawa, M., Ko, K., and M Misato, T., *Physiol. Plant.*, 41, 315, 1977.

medium, growth of the cells and productivity of the inhibitor were very much improved. Further study showed a cell line from *Agrostemma githago* to be a more potent producer,[45] and its cultural conditions for growth and production were examined. Thus, a suitable medium was established in which the levels of KH_2PO_4 were increased to 340 mg/l and those of $CaCl_2 \cdot 2H_2O$ were decreased to 22 mg as compared to those in ordinary Murashige-Skoog nutrients. Using this medium, the highest levels of cell growth and of antiviral substances were obtained after 5- to 6-days cultivation. It was shown that the cells of *A. githago* were very fine and pipettable when they were incubated in this medium at 28°C on a rotary shaker operated at 180 rpm. Furthermore, we found that the decreased level of Ca++ in the medium gave interesting results, i.e., when the Ca++ concentration was decreased to 0.1 m*M* from 3.0 m*M* in Murashige-Skoog's medium, growth of *A. githago* cells was not affected, but adhesion of the cells on the surface of the fermentor was prevented (Figure 14). Foaming in a low-Ca++ medium was also reduced remarkably. These qualities are very advantageous for large-scale cultivation of plant cells in suspension.

Both *P. americana* and *A. githago* cells cultivated in suspension were disrupted by a homogenizer for a couple of minutes and centrifuged. The supernatant was diluted with an appropriate volume of water and was applied on the leaves of plants. As seen

TABLE 2

Inhibition of TMV Infection on Tomato Leaves by Inhibitor from a Suspension Culture of *Phytolacca americana*

Inhibitor[a] dilution	Inhibitory activity[b] TMV-free plants/total plants
× 1	Phytotoxic
× 5	6/6
× 10	6/6
× 20	5/6
× 50	5/6
×100	4/6
Control[c]	1/6

Note: The height of the tomato plant,
Lycopersicon esculentum, was
about 15 cm. TMV (OM-strain)
was applied by a spray method.

[a] The supernatant of disrupted
whole culture of *P. americana* cultivated for 9 days in the ordinary
medium was used for the experiments. It was diluted by water as
described in this column. Application was made before 3 hr of inoculation.

[b] Determined after 16 days of TMV
inoculation.

[c] Without application of the supernatant.

From Misawa, M., Hayashi, M., Tanaka, H., Ko, K., and Misato, T., *Biotechnol. Bioeng.*, 17, 1335, 1975. With
permission.

in Table 2, the crude extract of *P. americana* thus obtained inhibited TMV infection.

Active principles were isolated from both cells with Column-Lite® chromatography and electrofocusing. From *P. americana* cells, at least four basic proteins were ob-tained whose molecular weights varied from 1.10×10^4 to 1.65×10^4. Also this cell line contained a sugar protein of 3.1×10^4. On the other hand, *A. githago* was found to contain only one basic protein, and its molecular weight was 2.5×10^4. Amino acid compositions of these principles and sugar compositions of the sugar protein are shown in Tables 3 and 4, respectively. These are different from that of an inhibitor isolated from the intact *P. americana* plant by Wyatt and Shepherd.[46]

Table 5 shows antiplant-virus activities of a purified *A. githago* inhibitor and of other antiplant-virus compounds produced by microorganisms. About 90% of TMV infection was inhibited by 1 μg of *A. githago* inhibitor per mℓ, and this activity was rather stronger than those of others. The crude extracts and purified compounds of both cells were also active when applied to the underside of leaves of tobacco and bean plants onto which TMV was inoculated on the opposite side. This suggests the inhibi-tory substance(s) or a part of the active fractions can penetrate into the leaves. Large-scale cultivation of both cell lines was examined. It was recognized that 0.5 vvm of

TABLE 3

Amino Acid Compositions and Molecular Weights of Plant-Virus Inhibitors Produced by Suspension-Cultured *Phytolacca americana* and *Agrostemma githago*

Amino Acids	P. americana				A. githago	P. americana plant[a]
	I	III	IV	V		
Lys	28	6	7	7	15	24
His	9	2	5	4	4	2
Arg	6	2	6	7	23	8
CySO₃H	0	0	2	4	—	0
Asx	30	12	12	18	17	28
Thr	15	3	9	12	15	20
Ser	24	7	9	13	40	18
Glx	19	9	9	15	27	20
Pro	17	5	11	21	8	10
Gly	19	13	13	29	36	16
Ala	11	5	8	22	16	16
Cys	5	1	0	0	—	4
Val	13	5	7	6	8	12
Met	0	0	2	0	7	6
Ile	8	5	5	8	5	12
Leu	23	7	9	8	9	18
Tyr	7	4	3	6	—	6
Phe	15	5	7	9	6	10
Trp	4	2	0	5	—	2
Total	253	93	124	194	236	232
Mol. Wt. (cultulated)	28814[b]	11750	11322	17086	24674	25726
Mol. Wt. (determined)	31000	11000	12000	16500	25000	27000

[a]   Data from Wyatt and Shepherd.[46]

[b]   Protein part.

TABLE 4

Sugar Composition of a Cultured
Phytolacca americana Plant-Virus
Inhibitor, Fraction I

Sugars	Concentration (%)
Ribose	81
Galactose	5
Mannose	7
Glucose	8

Note: Total sugar content in Fraction I is 7%.

aeration was sufficient for *A. githago* cell growth in 2 *l* of the medium with a 3-*l* bubble-column-type fermentor. On the other hand, 1.7 vvm of aeration and 300 rpm of agitation were required in 3 *l* of the medium with a 5-*l* jar fermentor. In the case

TABLE 5

Inhibition of Tobacco-Mosaic-Virus Infection by Various
Virus Inhibitors

Inhibitors	Assay Conc. (μg/ml)	Inhibition (%)
Aabomycin A	1.0	0
Blasticidin S	1.0	75
Miharamycin A,B	1.0	27
P. americana (cultured, V)	33	76
P. americana (intact)[a]	1.0	81
A. githago (cultured)	1.0	78
	7.0	91

Note: Performed by a local lesion method with TMV and
P. vulgaris.

[a] From Professor Shepherd.

of 20 l of the culture medium in a 30-l jar fermentor, 1.7 vvm and 250 rpm were the best conditions.

D. Proteinase Inhibitors

The author[47,48] also investigated the production of proteinase inhibitors in *Scopolia japonica* suspension cultures, because it has been known that proteinase inhibitors are useful for diagnosis and therapy of various diseases caused by proteinase such as inflammation, pancreatitis, shock, and emphysema. Since the over-production of plasmin, a fibrinolytic proteinase, also causes many disorders, the inhibitory activities of plasmin in a number of callus extracts were determined. Among them, *S. japonica* cells were shown to produce a potent inhibitory substance, and environmental conditions for rapid cell growth and for its production were examined with suspension cultures. As a result, 1.0 mg of 2,4-D and 0.02 mg of kinetin per liter of Murashige-Skoog's medium were chosen as growth hormones. Increase of the KNO_3 level to four times and decrease of the NH_4NO_3 level to half of that in the ordinary medium promoted the production of the inhibitor, whose level was above 1.5 mg-equivalent t-aminocyclohexane carboxylic acid per ml of the culture. A typical time course of *S. japonica* suspension culture showed that the concentration of the inhibitor increased with cell growth for 9 days. After that, it was accumulated continuously while the level of cell mass was decreased gradually (Figure 15). A semicontinuous culture was carried out with a 3-l bubble-column fermentor containing 2 l of the medium at 25 to 27°C and an aeration of 0.5 vvm. The cell yield for 18 days was 46.1 g, and the growth rate in dry cells was 1.29 g/l/day.

The level of the plasmin inhibitor in the cultured cells was compared with that in the intact plant. It was recognized that the activity was higher in the cultured cells and their producing rate was much faster than that of the intact *S. japonica*. This is another example in which a plant cell-suspension culture is superior to extraction from the natural plant for production of a metabolite.

The inhibitor purified with ion-exchange resins and trypsin-bound Sepharose® 4 B affinity chromatography was shown to have at least five components which were polypeptides of 3257 to 6050 mol wt. These molecular weights were much smaller than those of other proteinase inhibitors isolated from higher plants and of a bovine pancreatic trypsin inhibitor, Trasylol®.

As summarized in Table 6, these inhibitors of *S. japonica* cells showed stronger

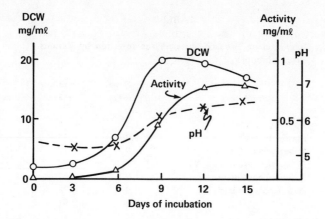

FIGURE 15.   Time course of cell growth and production of proteinase inhibitor by *Scopolia japonica* suspension culture. DCW;
dried cell weight activity was determined as plasmin-inhibitory activity. (Data from Misawa, M., Tanaka, H., Chiyo, O., and Mukai, N., *Biotechnol. Bioeng.*, 17, 305, 1975. With permission.)

TABLE 6

Inhibitory Activities of *Scopolia japonica* Inhibitors on Various Proteinases

	ID_{50} (μg/mℓ)					
Enzymes	I.1	I.3	I.4	I.5	Trasy-lol®[a]	*t*-AMCHA
Trypsin	1.05	0.61	2.00	1.50	1.90	>200[b]
α-Chymotrypsin	5.60	1.60	70.0	9.50	22.0	>2,500[c]
Plasmin[d]	1.02	0.78	12.5	19.5	7.10	—
[e]	0.44	0.27	0.56	0.33	6.15	>500
Kallikrein	1.22	1.05	1.95	7.70	2.21	>10,000
Pepsin	17.7	6.61	1.77	6.22	>1,000	—
Papain	>150	>150	>150	>150	>1,750	>200[f]

[a] 1 KIU = 0.14 μg.
[b] α-*N*-Benzoyl-L-arginine amide HCl(BAA).
[c] Casein.
[d] BAPA.
[e] Casein.
[f] BAA.

Data from Sakato, K., Tanaka, H., and Misawa, M., *Eur. J. Biochem.*, 55,
211, 1975. With permission.

activities against various proteinases. Components I.3, particularly, had the most potent activity towards trypsin, α-chymotrypsin, plasmin, and kallikrein. Therefore, *Scopolia* inhibitors should be called "broad specificity proteinase inhibitors" rather than
"the plasmin inhibitor". In in vitro tests with rats and rabbits, the crude inhibitor
showed similar behavior with Trasylol® (Bayer Co., W. Germany).

E. L-DOPA

3,4-Dihydroxyphenylalanine (L-DOPA) has been used as a drug for treatment of
Parkinson's Disease. Brain recognized accumulation of L-DOPA in remarkable

amounts with *Mucuna pruriens* callus.[49] Although this work was not carried out in industry, it is very interesting for its applications of tissue cultures. A callus of *M. pruriens* was shown to accumulate more than 0.5% of L-DOPA in the dried cells and 0.4% of dry cell weight in the medium using Murashige-Skoog's agar medium containing 25 mg of 2,4-D per liter after 21 days of incubation at 25°C. As Brain described, its yields were surprisingly high, and it is interesting to note that maximum growth and L-DOPA accumulation occurred at 25 mg of 2,4-D per liter, a level toxic to many other cell lines.

F. Miscellaneous

A patent applied for by Nippon Shinyaku Co., Ltd.[50] in Japan described the preparation of crude antipeptic-ulcer substances by plant cell culture of *Isodon japonicus*. They administered the water extract of the cultured cells to rats and recognized that its antipeptic-ulcer activity was about the same level as the natural plant. The author also observed[51] that the infection of a protozoa (coccidium) in chickens was inhibited by the administration of more than 250 ppm of the dried cells of *Vinca rosea* in the feed. In neither case was the active principle isolated.

According to Staba's patent,[52] the allergens may be more economically produced by tissue-culture systems than by extraction from pollen. Their production is more desirable for patient hypersensitivity evaluation and assay of allergenic products. They isolated two allergenically active fractions from 2-week-old suspension and 4-week-old callus cultures of *Ambrosia elatior* L. by ammonium sulfate precipitation, DEAE-cellulose and Sephadex® G-100 chromatography. The specific activities of two fractions isolated were shown to be about 1/1000 of that from short-ragweed-pollen antigen E.

Accumulation of an insulin-like substance by *Momordica charantia* callus was also reported by Khanna et al.[53]

VII. CELL MASS

The mass culture of plant cells has been studied by many researchers. Since the studies by Nickell and Tulecke at Charles Pfizer Co. in the 1960s,[1] Staba,[54] Byrne[55] at the Quartermaster Food and Container Institute in the U.S., Tulecke[56] at the Boyce Thompson Institute with Air Force support, Martin[57] at the National Research Council of Canada, and others have provided much useful data for large-scale cultivation of plant cells. Mandels, Maguire and El-Bisi,[58] at the U.S. Army Natick Laboratories cultivated the cells of edible plants such as carrot, bean, lettuce, etc. in commercial laboratory fermentors in batch and in semicontinuous systems for periods of up to 61 days without contamination as seen in three examples in Table 7. Using lettuce cells, productivity in a fermentor was shown to be 2.3 g dry weight of cells per liter of culture per day. Their cell yield was up to 40% based on the weight of sucrose in the medium. In order to help prevent future world food shortage, the production of food by plant cell cultures appears to be attractive, in addition to the production of yeast from hydrocarbons or production of chlorella and spirulina. However, the higher plant cells produced in fermentors are still too expensive as foodstuffs. This is why their work was terminated.

Japan Tobacco and Salt Public Corporation[59] is working on production of tobacco cells as a raw material of cigarettes by suspension-culture techniques. From many experimental results on the improvement of cell growth, they found that an increase of phosphate concentration up to three times higher than that of the ordinary Murashige-Skoog's medium stimulated cell growth. Namely, the doubling time in the exponential-growth phase was decreased from 1.3 days to 0.9 day. With the medium containing three times the phosphate level, 3% sucrose, 1 ppm thiamine HCl, and 0.2 ppm 2,4-

TABLE 7

**Cell Mass Production by Semicontinuous Culture System
(Lettuce Cells)**

	Experiment number		
	1	2	3
Sucrose concentration (%)	3.0	3.0—2.0	2.0
Inoculum (g)	10.0	4.0	9.7
Days operated	14	61	44
Average culture volume (l)	4.9	7.1	6.1
Average feed rate (l/day)	0.97	1.04	1.57
Harvest total (l)	40.0	74.5	69.0
Average conc. grams (dry wt/l)	12.0	9.5	8.1
Dilution rate per day[a]	0.20	0.15	0.26
Yield (g/100 g sucrose)[b]	39	34	40
Productivity (g/l/day)[c]	2.3	1.6	2.1

Note: Cells were grown on Murashige medium with 0.10 mg/l naphthalene-acetic acid in a 15-l New Brunswick Continuous Fermenter, Model CF 500, inoculum 1 l suspension culture from shake flask, temp. 26 to 28°C, air 1 to 1.5 l/min, impeller 120 rpm. Experiment 1. Constant volume 1.5 to 2.5 l of culture harvested every 2 to 3 days and replaced with fresh nutrient. Experiments 2, 3. Constant Nutrient Feed 1 to 1.5 l/day. Intermittent harvest.

[a] $\dfrac{\text{Feed rate}}{\text{Av. volume}}$

[b] $\dfrac{\text{(Total harvest grams)} - \text{(inoculum)}}{\text{(Total } l\text{)} \times \text{(g sucrose/}l\text{)}}$

[c] $\dfrac{\text{(Total harvest grams)} - \text{(inoculum)}}{\text{(No. days)} \times \text{(av. culture volume)}}$

From Mandels, M., Maguire, A., and El-Bisi, H. M., Growth of Plant Culture, I., II., III. in U.S. Army Natick Laboratories Technical Rep., 68-6-F1, 69-22-FL, and 69-36-FL, Natick, Massachusetts, 1968—1969.

D, *Nicotiana tabacum* BY-2 cells were cultivated in a 20 kl tank at 28°C aerated at 0.3 vvm under the pressure of 0.5 kg/cm². The highest growth rate was obtained between 45 and 70 hr after the inoculation with a doubling time of about 15 hr, which corresponded to the specific growth rate, $\mu = 1.09$/day. Furthermore, they designed "two-stage two-stream culture" systems for harvesting the cells of low nitrogen contents continuously as shown in Figure 16, because a high nitrogen content in the cells is not desirable in the raw material of tobacco products. According to their explanation on this system, a medium with a 9/10 nitrogen source and three times the phosphate was continuously supplied to Tank I at a dilution rate of 0.54, and the inflow was balanced by the outflow of the corresponding volume of the culture which was transferred to Tank II. Another continuous inflow to Tank II consisted of standard medium with a one sixth nitrogen source and three times phosphate. These two inflows were

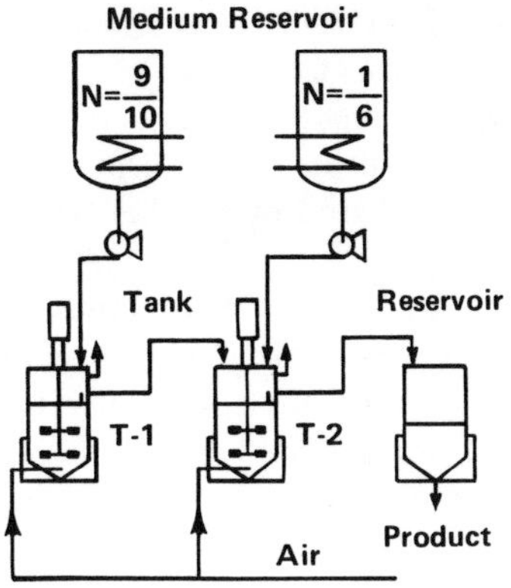

FIGURE 16. Two stage—two stream continuous culture system of tobacco cells. T - 1, Culture tank I (working culture volume 35 ℓ); T - 2, Culture tank II (working culture volume 35 ℓ). (From Noguchi, M., Matsumoto, T., Hirata, Y., Yamamoto, K., Katsuyama, A., Kato, A., Azechi, S., and Kato, K., in *Plant Tissue Culture and Its Bio-technological Applications,* Barz, W., Reinhard, E., and Zenk, M. H., Eds., Springer-Verlag, Berlin, 1977, 85. With permission.)

balanced by the outflow corresponding to the two inflows. The dilution rate with Tank II was 1.10. As a whole, the productivity of this culture system was, in dry weight, 6.9 g/ℓ/day, and the total nitrogen level of the cells was about 3.3%.

A mixture of the cells and adhesive agents such as carboxymethyl cellulose was dried and used as the raw materials. The differences in the production costs and in the qualities between the cultured cells and the intact plant leaves when used as raw materials for tobacco products were not clear. However, these studies seem to indicate one of the most realizable products for mass production. Hardy et al. at E. I. du Pont de Nemours Co.[60] claimed symbiotic fixation of atmospheric nitrogen in their patent. Undifferentiated plant cells derived from members of the Leguminosae and bacteria of the genus *Rhizobium* were incubated together in the liquid medium. The results showed that invasion of the plant cells by the bacteria occurred, and these cells had nitrogen-fixing activity. The final products containing plant cells and symbiotic bacteria may be valuable sources of usable nitrogen from the atmosphere, and they are expected to be used as feed for animals and for fertilizers.

VII. CONCLUSION

As mentioned in the Introduction, only a few recent studies on the production of biochemicals and cell mass carried out by, mainly, industrial and government laboratories were described in this chapter. These studies were selected on the basis of economic interest. Some of them seem to be applicable to industrial production. In addition, there are many other interesting reports and patents which had to be omitted because of space limitations. Furthermore, there must be many excellent unpublished research studies, particularly by industrial laboratories in the U.S. and in European countries. It is true that there are many difficulties, such as slow growth rate of the plant cells, low concentration of products, and unstable productivity, to be overcome before the application of plant tissue culture can be realized. However, several recently published reports gave satisfactory results as far as increasing the product levels. These will promote an advance of tissue culture for industrial applications, accompanied with progress of both basic and practical studies in other fields such as genetics and fermentation technology.

The most important matter for success in the industrial application of plant tissue culture is, of course, the decision as to what kind of compound should be produced. Because the production costs are still high, only useful and high-priced compounds are suitable as the tissue-culture products.

Although there are many difficulties in this field, the author believes that production of useful plant metabolites will soon be successful in industry.

REFERENCES

1. **Nickell, L. J.**, Submerged growth of plant cells, *Adv. Appl. Microbiol.*, 4, 213, 1962.
2. **Puhan, Z. and Martin, S. M.**, The industrial potentials of plant cell culture, *Prog. Ind. Microbiol.*, 9, 13, 1971.
3. **Johnson, I. S. and Border, G. B.**, Metabolites from animal and plant cell culture, *Adv. Appl. Microbiol.*, 15, 215, 1972.
4. **Misawa, M., Sakato, K., Tanaka, H., Hayashi, M., and Samejima, H.**, Production of physiologically active substances by plant cell suspension cultures, in *Tissue Culture and Plant Science 1974*, Street, H. E., Ed., Academic Press, London, 1975, 405.
5. **Tabata, M.**, Recent advances in the production of medicinal substances by plant cell cultures, in *Plant Tissue Culture and Its Bio-technological Application*, Barz, W., Reinhard, E., and Zenk, M. H., Eds., Springer-Verlag, Berlin, 1977, 3.
6. **Anon.**, Direct route to natural drugs, *Chem. Week*, p. 31, August 11, 1976.
7. **Zenk, M. H., El-Shagi, H., Arens, H., Stöckigt, J., Weiler, E. W., and Deus, B.**, Formation of the indole alkaloids serpentine and ajmalicine in cell suspension cultures of *Catharanthus roseus*, in *Plant Tissue Culture and Its Bio-technological Application*, Barz, W., Reinhard, E., and Zenk, M. H., Eds., Springer-Verlag, Berlin, 1977, 27.
8. **Tabata, M. and Hiraoka, N.**, Variation of alkaloid production in *Nicotiana rustica* callus cultures, *Physiol. Plant.*, 38, 19, 1976.
9. **Robinson, T.**, in *The Biochemistry of Alkaloids*, Springer-Verlag, Berlin, 1968, 1.
10. **Johnson, I. S.**, Historical background of Vinca alkaloid research and areas of future interest, *Cancer Chemother. Rep.*, 52, 455, 1968.
11. **Carew, D. P. and Krueger, R. J.**, Metabolism of vindoline, catharanthine HCl and vincaleukoblastine sulfate by suspension cultures of *Catharanthus roseus*, *Phytochemistry*, 16, 1461, 1977.
12. **Petiard, V. and Guinebault, P. R.**, Alkaloid Production by In Vitro Culturing of *Vinca minor* L. Cells, *German Patent* 2,603,588, 1976.
13. **Weiler, E. W.**, Radioimmuno screening methods for secondary plant products, in *Plant Tissue Culture and Its Bio-Technological Application*, Barz, W., Reinhard, E., and Zenk, M. H., Eds., Springer-Verlag, Berlin, 1977, 266.
14. **Wagner, F. and Vogelmann, H.**, Cultivation of plant tissue cultures in bioreactors and formation of secondary metabolites, in *Plant Tissue Culture and Its Bio-technological Application*, Barz, W., Reinhard, E., and Zenk, M. H., Eds., Springer-Verlag, Berlin, 1977, 245.
15. **Furuya, T. and Ishii, T.**, Production of Berberine, Japan Patent (open), 72-30897, 1972.
16. **Kuroda, H. and Ikekawa, T.**, Production of Berberine and Palmatine, Japan Patent (open), 75-13519, 1975.
17. **McCormick, J. R. D.**, Production of Plant Metabolites, Japan Patent (open), 48-4679, 1973.
18. **Sakato, K., Tanaka, H., Mukai, N., and Misawa, M.**, Isolation of camptothecin from cells of *Camptotheca acuminata* suspension cultures, *Agric. Biol. Chem.*, 38, 217, 1974.
19. **Wall, M. E., Wani, M. C., Cook, C. E., Palmer, K. H., McPhail, A. T., and Sim, G. A.**, Plant anti-tumor agents. I. The isolation and structure of camptothecin, a nobel alkaloidal leukemia and tumor inhibitor from *Camptotheca acuminata*, *J. Am. Chem. Soc.*, 88, 3888, 1966.

20. Delfel, N. E. and Rothfus, J. A., Antitumor alkaloids in callus cultures of *Cephalotaxus harringtonia*, *Phytochemistry*, 16, 1595, 1977.
21. Hartwell, J. L., Types of anticancer agents isolated from plants, *Cancer Treat. Rep.*, 60, 1031, 1976.
22. Misawa, M., Hayashi, M., Nagano, Y., and Kawamoto, T., Production of a plant pigment, Japan Patent (open), 73-6153, 1973.
23. Komatsu, K., Nozaki, W., Takemura, M., Umemori, S., and Nakaminami, M, Production of a Pigment by Plant Tissue Culture, Japan Patent (open), 75-24494, 1975.
24. Steck, W. and Constabel, F., Biotransformations in plant cell cultures, *Lloydia*, 37, 185, 1974.
25. Veliky, I., Synthesis of carboline alkaloids by plant cell cultures, *Phytochemistry*, 11, 1405, 1972.
26. Reinhard, E., Biotransformation by plant tissue cultures, in *Tissue Culture and Plant Science 1974*, Street, H. E., Ed., Academic Press, London, 1975, 433.
27. Alfermann, A. W., Boy, H. M., Döller, P. C., Hagedorn, W., Heins, M., Wahl, J., and Reinhard, E., Biotransformation of cardiac glycosides by plant cell cultures, in *Plant Tissue Culture and Its Bio-technological Application*, Barz, W., Reinhard, E., and Zenk, M. H., Eds., Springer-Verlag, Berlin, 1977, 125.
28. Staba, E. J. and Kaul, B., Production of Diosgenin by Plant Tissue-Culture Technique, U.S. Patent, 3,628,287, 1971.
29. Shibata, S., Saponins with biological and pharmacological activity, in *New Natural Products and Plant Drugs with Pharmacological, Biological or Therapeutical Activity*, Wagner, H. and Wolff, P., Eds., Springer-Verlag, Berlin, 1977, 177.
30. Furuya, T. and Ishii, T., Production of Ginseng Radix, Japan Patent (open), 73-31917, 1973.
31. Furuya, T. Kojoma, H., Syono, K., and Ishii, T., Isolation of panaxatriol from *Panax ginseng* callus., *Chem. Pharm. Bull.*, 18, 2371, 1970.
32. Yasuda, S., Satoh, K., Ishii, T., and Furuya, T., Studies on the cultural conditions of plant cell suspension culture, in *Fermentation Technology Today*, Terui, G., Ed., Society Fermentation Technology, Osaka, Japan, 1972, 697.
33. Staba, E. J., personal communication.
34. Tomita, Y. and Uomori, A., Production of Bupleuri Radix, Japan Patent (open), 76-12988, 1975.
35. Ikeda, T., Matsumoto, T., and Noguchi, M., Formation of ubiquinone by tobacco plant cells in suspension culture, *Phytochemistry*, 15, 568, 1976.
36. Mizukami, H., Konoshima, M., and Tabata, M., Effect of nutritional factors on shikonin derivative formation in *Lithospermum* callus cultures, *Phytochemistry*, 16, 1183, 1977.
37. Zenk, M. H., El-Shagi, H., and Schulte, U., Anthraquinone production by cell suspension cultures of *Morinda citrifolia*, *Planta Med.*, Suppl., 79, 1975.
38. Lin, A. and Mathes, M. C., The *in vitro* selection of growth regulators by isolated callus tissues, *Am. J. Bot.*, 60, 34, 1973.
39. Veliky, I. A. and Latta, R. K., Antimicrobial activity of cultured plant cells and tissues, *Lloydia*, 37, 611, 1974.
40. Misawa, M., Sakato, K., Tanaka, H., Hayashi, M., and Samejima, H., Production of physiologically active substances by plant cell suspension cultures, in *Tissue Culture and Plant Science 1974*, Street, H. E., Ed., Academic Press, London, 1975, 405.
41. Hartwell, J. L., Types of anticancer agents isolated from plants, *Cancer Treat. Rep.*, 60, 1031, 1976.
42. Kupchan, S., Novel plant-derived tumor inhibitors and their mechanisms of action, *Cancer Treat. Rep.*, 60, 1115, 1976.
43. Matthews, R. E. F., *Plant Virology*, Academic Press, New York, 1970, 447.
44. Misawa, M., Hayashi, M., Tanaka, H., Ko, K., and Misato, T., Production of a plant virus inhibitor by suspension culture of *Phytolacca americana*, *Biotechnol. Bioeng.*, 17, 1335, 1975.
45. Takayama, S., Misawa, M., Ko, K., and Misato, T., Effect of cultural conditions on the growth of *Agrostemma githago* cells in suspension culture and the concomitant production of an anti-plant virus substance, *Physiol. Plant*, 41, 313, 1977.
46. Wyatt, S. P. and Shepherd, R. J., Isolation and characterization of a virus inhibitor from *Phytolacca american*, *Phytopathology*, 59, 1787, 1969.
47. Misawa, M., Tanaka, H., Chiyo, O., and Mukai, N., Production of a plasmin inhibitory substance by *Scopolia japonica* suspension cultures, *Biotechnol. Bioeng.*, 17, 305, 1975.
48. Sakato, K., Tanaka, H., and Misawa, M., Broad-specificity proteinase inhibitors in *Scopolia japonica* (Solanaceae) cultured cells, *Eur. J. Biochem.*, 55, 211, 1975.
49. Brain, K. R., Accumulation of L-DOPA in Cultures from *Mucuna pruriens*, *Plant Sci. Lett.*, 7, 157, 1976.
50. Nishi, T. and Mitsuoka, S., Production of an Anti-Peptic Ulcer Substance by Plant Tissue Culture of Isodon, Japan Patent (open), 75-12288, 1975.
51. Misawa, M., Hayashi, M., Shimada, K., and Omotani, Y., Preservation and Therapy of Coccidiosis, Japan Patent (open), 75-101510, 1975.

52. **Staba, E. J.,** Production of Allergens by Plant Tissue Culture Technique, U.S. Patent 3,846,937, 1974.
53. **Khanna, P., Nag, T. N., Jain, S. C., and Mohan, S.,** Extraction of insulin from plant cultures in vitro, in *Abstr. 3rd Int. Congr. Plant Tissue and Cell Culture,* University of Leicester, England, 1974, 256.
54. **Staba, E. J.,** The biosynthetic potential of plant tissue and cultures, *Dev. Ind. Microbiol.,* 4, 193, 1963.
55. **Byrne, A. and Koch, R.,** Food production by submerged culture of plant tissue culture, *Science,* 135, 215, 1962.
56. **Tulecke, W.,** Growth of tissues of higher plants in continuous liquid culture and their use in a nutritional experiment, in Air Force Rep., AMRL-TR-65-101, Boyce Thompson Institute for Plant Science, Yonkers, 37, 1965.
57. **Martin, S. M.,** Mass culture systems for plant cell suspensions, in *Plant Tissue Cultures as a Source of Biochemicals,* Staba, J., Ed., CRC Press, Boca Raton, Fla., 1980.
58. **Mandels, M., Maguire, A., and El-Bisi, H. M.,** Growth of plant cell culture. I., II., III. in U.S. Army Natick Laboratories Technical Rep., 68-6-F1, 69-22-FL, and 69-36-FL, Natick, Massachusetts, 1968—1969.
59. **Noguchi, M., Matsumoto, T., Hirata, Y., Yamamoto, K., Katsuyama, A., Kato, A., Azechi, S., and Kato, K.,** Improvement of growth rates of plant cell cultures, in *Plant Tissue Culture and Its Bio-technological Application,* Barz, W., Reinhard, E., and Zenk, M. H., Eds., Springer-Verlag, Berlin, 1977, 85.
60. **Hardy, R. W. F. and Holsten R. D.,** Symbiotic Fixation of Atmospheric Nitrogen, U.S. Patent 3,704,546, 1972.

Chapter 9

PRODUCT COST ANALYSIS

Walter E. Goldstein
Linda L. Lasure
Morton B. Ingle

TABLE OF CONTENTS

I. INTRODUCTION

The future of plant cell culture will depend on its evolvement as a practical commercial entity, thereby resulting in a state of technology that is comparable or superior to that of industrial microbial fermentations. Successful solicitation of support for translation of this area into production scale requires convincing argument that a reasonable continuing profit will result.

A proper technical and economic data base does not presently exist to pose such an argument. However, based on principles and background of biochemical engineering and economics related to microbial fermentations, it is possible to propose a hypothetical framework suitable for development of a cost analysis for products from plant cell culture. This chapter is intended to provide cost information and relate such analyses to technological events required for commercial success.

A process description is proposed as a starting point where pertinent mass and flow balances and process constraints or information needs are defined. A specification of fermentor design is introduced where energy relationships appropriate to this aspect of the plant and other parts of the facility are examined. The cost analysis is then developed based on selected cases of improved technology that are proposed to lead to reduced costs. Capital and manufacturing cost analyses are presented, followed by a preliminary analysis of projected profitability and discussion of pertinent assumptions in this paper.

II. PROCESS DESCRIPTION

The basic steps required for obtaining product by plant cell culture might be as indicated in Figure 1, i.e., fermentation of the biomass, concurrent or subsequent induction of product formation in the biomass, separation of the product from the biomass, and, finally, purification. This task can be accomplished at laboratory scale basically in the manner described. However, when one considers translation of this into large scale producton, the process necessarily becomes more complex in order to promote economies in the facility, a matter possibly not of main concern at bench scale.

A framework representative of extension of the scheme in Figure 1 into a production facility is depicted in the schematic, Figure 2. The process diagram is intended to illustrate many of the features necessary for a plant. As indicated, substrate media for the fermentation is prepared in feed tankage with suitable residence time (i.e., tank volume/flow rate) selected to insure availability of sufficient fluid for demands downstream in the process. In batch preparation, feed tank volume is increased to accomodate increased exiting flow rate to a possibly time-varying continuous process.* At some point, based on economics and plant capacity, the feed stream may be prepared continuously by flow out of several reservoirs, each containing the individual ingredients to be used in the fermentor media. In either case, this media is then passed through continuous sterilization, passing then to fermentor feed tanks. Each fermentor feed tank is intended to supply one fermentor, where the feed tanks may also receive biomass that is to be reused.

From this point, fluid and possibly recycled biomass is passed to the fermentors designated to produce the biomass required for production of secondary product.**

---

* Process tankage of proper residence time serves the function of providing surge capacity to dampen out effects of process fluctuations and provide additional assurance of continuity in operations.

** Separate fermentors are allowed for biomass and product formation, since optimal conditions for growth of biomass and synthesis of product within the biomass may differ. The fermentors may be operated in batch or continuous mode, the choice based on economic, kinetic, as well as technological considerations.

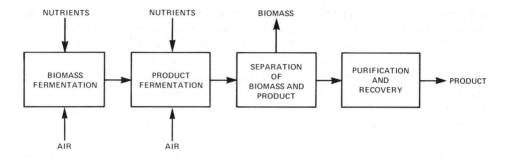

FIGURE 1.   Basic steps for plant cell culture.

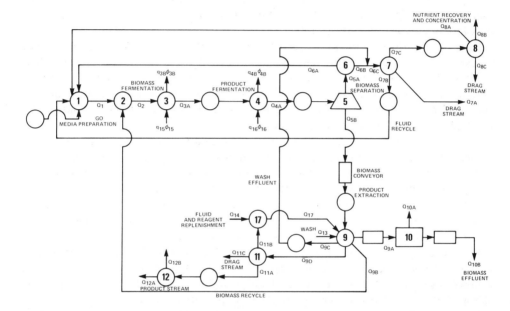

FIGURE 2.   Model process schematic for product from plant cell culture.

Several fermentors would be used, e.g., in continuous operation, replication of fermentors reduces risk of loss in production, while replication is necessary if batch operations are employed to promote continuity of operation in processes downstream of fermentors.

When biomass has reached the necessary concentration, effluent is passed to intermediate drop tanks where adjustments can be made preparatory to passage of the biomass slurry to the product fermentors (comments in regard to batch as opposed to continuous operation of these units also apply here).

Product is accumulated in the biomass in the secondary bank of fermentors, or else the product may be formed in the biomass and secreted extracellularly into the medium. The nature of product accumulation and release and the separation of the biomass from the product will influence the design of the product recovery section of the process. For example, if the product is extracellular, then the liquid resulting from primary separation of the biomass from the fluid (e.g., by filtration or centrifugation) would be treated to obtain pure product, and the biomass would then be subsequently treated by washing, etc. to recover additional product. In turn, intracellular product would require physical and/or chemical treatment to effect release of product from the biomass. However, a preferred embodiment of such a case requires that this treatment be nondestructive in the sense that the biomass could be reused for economic reasons. The example chosen for the case depicted in Figure 2 assumes the latter; i.e., intracellular formation with partially reusable biomass assumed to result.

Therefore, following the primary biomass/liquid separation, the concentrated biomass slurry is conveyed to a feed tank where the slurry then enters the product extraction area. The case presented in Figure 2 assumes aqueous extraction with possibly inline partial maceration of the biomass to promote release of the product.* The extraction system is assumed to involve a recycle format as indicated. Features incorporated in this system included removal of residual glucose by washing, recycle of a portion of the biomass for reuse, removal of part of the biomass as a drag stream, and of course, highly efficient appearance of product in the extractant. Nonproduct streams exiting the plant (such as the aforementioned biomass stream) are included to minimize accumulation of impurities and contaminants that would increase with time and potentially impair performance of the process.

The product stream is then transferred to a concentration unit for removal of water by reverse osmosis, introducing the assumption that the product can be separated from water by this membrane technique. This step reduces energy requirements for further concentration of the product stream to desired levels. The product is then dried to final level by vacuum evaporation or spray drying where the effluent as indicated is assumed to be a liquid as the case in Figure 2.

The diluent extractant stream from the reverse osmosis unit is then mixed with additional fluid added to maintain a water balance and provide replenishment of reagents, etc. necessary for the extraction or else preservation of the product. As indicated, this stream is then recycled to the extraction battery again.

Glucose washed from the biomass in the extraction system is recycled to another point in the process and the biomass drag stream is dried and exits the plant as a by-product, possibly suitable for sale as supplemental animal feed.

The liquid removed at the primary solid/liquid separation following fermentation is separated into two streams. One stream is recycled to the media makeup system for assumed reuse of nutrients where this stream would be subjected to continuous sterilization again before passage to fermentors. The other stream is mixed with the glucose-containing wash stream from the extraction area and fed to another reverse osmosis system for concentration. This operation is intended to separate sugar or glucose from the liquid, permitting discharge of a portion of the diluent stream from the reverse osmosis unit as a low B.O.D. waste and drag stream, the drag stream again included as a means to minimize build-up of contamination in the system without introducing an unacceptable environmental pollutant. The glucose is then further concentrated by evaporation and can be considered as another plant by-product for possible sale (e.g., animal feed) or else partly as a recycle for reusable nutrients. As indicated, part of the diluent from this reverse osmosis unit is recycled to media preparation, upstream of sterilization, to again maintain water balances. The waste stream treatment noted above could be replaced by a suitable solvent extraction system, if such a tact were technologically feasible and economically justified.

The process description is intended to include and represent the features necessary in a modern production facility. The process incorporates waste treatment and purification and nutrient recovery, as necessary steps in preparation of such a product. This process then forms the basis for development of the economic analysis.

---

* The aqueous extraction system can be assumed to also represent a possible solvent extraction system for recovery of product, where necessary water removal, extraction release of product from the solvent, and cleansing of the product could be accomplished.

III. MASS AND FLOW BALANCES AND PROCESS CONSTRAINTS

Material balances appropriate to development of an economic analysis for the model process in Figure 2 are listed in Table 1.* Each pertinent point in the process is labeled as a "node" where flow balances for total fluid influent and effluent are presented, these being effectively equivalent to mass balances, since density variations are minor. Concentration (mass) of constituents can be viewed as being expressed in terms of quantity of liquid.

The numerical quantities to be used in the mass balances will depend on process factors assumed necessary to achieve a desired amount of product of proper quantity in the stream exiting the plant, i.e., the volumetric flow rate, Q_{12A}, in Table 1. Selection of a process factor at a particular node will affect other points in the process because of the fluid recycles indicated in Figure 2. For example, concentrated glucose solution recycle to media preparation (Q_{8A}) is influenced by degree of water removal at node 8 (Q_{8B}) and the proportion removed from the facility in the drag stream (Q_{8C}). In turn, the amount of replenishment process nutrients such as glucose in stream G_0 is affected by glucose content in stream Q_{8A}, the magnitude of Q_{8A}, and the glucose metabolized to form biomass and product.

In general, then, the entries in Table 1 represent a set of simultaneous equations with specification of constraints (i.e., the process factors) required to reduce the number of unknowns to a quantity equaling the number of equations. The specification of constraints and assumptions for the mass balance in Table 1 is outlined in Table 2. Parameters and equations related to glucose can be assumed to represent those appropriate to other nutrients. As indicated in Table 2, establishment of process factors in a given sequence allows sequential specification of items in the material balance, with computations indicated much in the way they might be performed with a suitable computer program.

The first item requiring specification is the rate of product effluent from the facility, $Q_{12}P_{12A}$. In turn, this quantity is related to the yield of product per unit of biomass, assuming then that the quantity of biomass is important in relation to the amount of product formed. In certain cases, there may be an optimal concentration of biomass to yield secondary formation of product, and the quantity of biomass may be of secondary importance. The maximum biomass concentration that can be attained may be strongly governed by mass transfer and physical effects (e.g., mixing) in the fermentor. However, the combination of yield coefficient of product per unit of biomass and biomass concentration directly relates to amount of product formed, expressed in terms of quantity of fluid in the fermentor.

The fraction of biomass that can be recycled will directly relate to savings in nutrient addition and fermentor capacity. In addition, this fraction provides a measure of the degree of biomass reuse that is possible before the cell culture is no longer viable without introduction of fresh inoculum. Yield coefficients for nutrient use (e.g., glucose and oxygen) must be experimentally determined; however, they may be predicted to some extent through combination of possibly known stoichiometry and experiment.[2]

Inlet or initial concentrations for nutrients in the fermentor (e.g., glucose or oxygen) would be established based on experimentally determined mass transfer considerations and required concentration gradients needed for uptake of nutrient by the biomass. In addition, the concentrations would be limited by possible repression of growth and product formation determined in kinetic studies. Nutrient consumption in the product fermentor might be assumed to be governed by needs for biomass maintenance, this

---

* All tables appear at the end of the text. (See p.210)

factor possibly being large with respect to specific nutrient consumption for product formation, since the amount of product formed per unit of biomass is expected to be small. Therefore, for this study, the factors α_G and α_0 in Table 2 are introduced to allot nutrient consumption in product fermentors as a percentage of the consumption in formation of biomass. Specific determination of cell maintenance and stoichiometric needs for formation of product would allow nutrient consumption in product units to be expressed in a different manner.

Liquid removal efficiency at the biomass separator will be based on equipment design and the quantity of fluid that must remain with the biomass for ease of processing and to protect the viability of the biomass. Extractant requirements for processing a given quantity of biomass to release and separate product should really be based on mass transfer/diffusional considerations as well as equilibrium limitations related to solubility of the product in the extractant once the particular system is specified. The extraction system is represented as consisting of an aqueous fluid, although the system can be assumed to embody use of a solvent. As indicated, the extractant must absorb the product, release the product, be subject to necessary purification, and be reintroduced as indicated by the recycle system in Figure 2.

It is assumed that residual nutrient would be eliminated from the biomass in the extraction process for recycle and reuse or partially discharged as a nonpolluting waste stream following treatment. Therefore, the volumetric quantity of fluid required to efficiently effect such a wash (item 10) must be specified.

The degree of drying necessary for spent biomass would be based on ease of handling of this plant effluent, disposal hopefully based on sale as a by-product. Primary concentration of the product stream, Q_{11A}, in Figure 2 would be nonenergy intensive (e.g., reverse osmosis) or release from the solvent in the case of a solvent extraction system. Process development studies would be necessary to establish feasibility of product isolation and concentration by these techniques. In this case, the work should lead to specification of the degree of primary concentration possible.

The extraction recycle system must be cleansed due to expected periodic build-up of impurities. This aspect is represented in Figure 2 and by comments in Table 2 (item 13) by specification of a drag stream fraction (Q_{11C}/Q_{11B}) that is to be discharged from the process to hold impurity levels in the extractant to a maximal accepted level. In the case of a solvent extraction system, the solvent would be treated to remove such impurities, but again, in effect, producing a drag stream from the process of a nonpolluting nature. As indicated in Table 2, mass balance considerations then require fluid replenishment (Q_{14} in Figure 2) to maintain fluid balances in the case of the aqueous system as well as a certain degree of fluid removal (Q_{12B}) to provide a product stream (Q_{12A}) of proper concentration.

The liquid from primary separation of the biomass, stream Q_{5A} in Figure 2, will either be recycled for reuse of nutrient or else treated for possible discharge as a nonpolluting waste stream, again to minimize accumulation of impurities in the process. Bench scale/pilot plant studies would be required for a real facility to determine the amount of drag stream necessary to maintain a viable process and, therefore, to allow specification of the ratio, Q_{6B}/Q_{5A}. It should be noted that recycle streams containing low concentrations of glucose invite undesirable introduction of contaminating organisms in the system. Therefore, judicious choice of operating temperatures for these streams and possibly additional sterilization at different points in the process (e.g., stream Q_{6A}) might be necessary. As indicated in Figure 2, all recycle streams directed to points ahead of the biomass fermentor are subjected to sterilization.

The nutrient stream Q_{6C}, consisting partially of fluid from primary separation at node 5 and partially of aqueous wash liquid from node 9, would be concentrated by nonenergy intensive membrane or solvent techniques, the degree of concentration to be specified by experimental study. The aqueous diluent from this step would either be discharged as an environmentally acceptable waste stream (Q_{7A}) or else recycled to the front end of the process (Q_{7B}) to maintain fluid balances. Further concentration by, for example, evaporation would be used to eliminate additional fluid from the nutrient concentrate, stream Q_{7C}. Part of this concentrated solution (primarily glucose or sucrose) would be recycled for reuse (Q_{8A}) and part discarded (Q_{8C}), possibly for by-product sale. Reuse of nutrient is desirable for economic reasons; however, the nutrient might require treatment to avoid introduction of inhibitory/poisoning influences to the fermentation. Transfer of concentrated streams in the process may assist in minimization of possibilities of growth of contaminating microorganisms. As indicated in Table 2, the replenishment of nutrient required is governed in part by the nature of handling of recycle streams and necessary inclusion of drag streams in the process for control of contaminant levels.

Definition of the material balance and associated process constraints provide a portion of the input required for the economic analysis. Stream flows and separation factors will allow estimation of capital/operating costs for much of the process. Surge and storage tankage volumes can be specified, as indicated previously, by assignment of reasonable residence times for satisfactory process operation and control. Additional considerations are, however, required to specify sizes and numbers of fermentors.

IV. SPECIFICATION OF FERMENTORS

Both the biomass and product fermentors must have sufficient residence time to produce a desired quantity of biomass/unit volume of fluid and to, in turn, allow the required amount of product to be formed in the biomass. The product is then either released into extracellular fluid as a natural course of events or else retained internally for forced release as part of the process. Fermentor design can result in a variety of geometric configurations. However, the kinetics of biomass and product formation indicate which of several idealized types is most appropriate. The three basic types are batch, plug flow, and continuously stirred tank reactors (CSTR).[3] Continuous feeding or semibatch operation is considered to be a special case of batch fermentation, which is really a process control technique to introduce nutrient in an optimal manner for reaction, avoiding inhibitory effects. In addition, both batch and plug flow are kinetically the same, where reaction time in the case of batch operation is the real time to complete the conversion required. In the case of the plug flow reactor, reaction time is the residence time, i.e., the reactor volume per flow rate. In general, however, volume requirements for batch fermentation will exceed that for plug flow due to time for emptying, filling, etc. The assumption of continuous sterilization as opposed to batch sterilization allows for savings in processing time in both cases.

Therefore, continuous plug flow operation would be preferred over batch fermentation, assuming that such continuous operation is technically feasible, i.e., that frequent contamination and undesired mutation of the growth does not occur and that residence times are not too large so as to preclude operation in the continuous mode from a practical engineering standpoint. This latter point also applies to consideration of use of the CSTR.

Table 3 presents expressions for time requirements for growth of biomass and formation of product for different reactor types. In the case of the biomass reactor, idealized autocatalytic growth based on cell mitosis is assumed. In this case, the CSTR is preferred, since the residence time (volume required per given flow rate) will be less than in the other cases, with residence times or volume requirements for CSTR and plug flow reactors being almost equivalent only in the case of nearly complete recycle or reuse of biomass. For example, use of a 5% inoculum (or reuse of only 5% of the biomass) would require that the volume of the plug flow fermentor be 3.16 times that of the CSTR fermentor. The equations also point out that the volume requirements or residence time are inversely proportional to the specific growth rate, μ_B, μ_B being equal to 0.693 per doubling time. Therefore, determination of doubling time or specific growth rate is important since this quantity directly affects fermentor volume requirements.

In Table 3, product formation is assumed to be directly proportional to biomass content and occurs at a specific rate, μ_p, a factor also requiring experimental determination. This imposes a zero order fermentation, thereby resulting in equivalent residence times for either the plug flow or CSTR mode of operation.

In reality, the specific growth rate, μ_B, and specific rate of product formation, μ_p will not be constant and may vary in accord with conditions in the fermentation. Certainly, to maintain stable process control, these factors will be related to supply of nutrient and, in particular, to supply of the nutrient most limiting in the fermentation. If the specific growth rates and/or yield coefficients degrade with time, stable plant operation will require periodic reinoculation, (possibly continuously) with plant output then appearing as cyclic. The variance in this cycle can be minimized by specification of sufficient fermentors in parallel. Certainly, in the case of batch operation, fermentor operation would be staggered and sufficient fermentors provided to minimize time variations in plant productivity.

The expressions of Table 3 combined with the mass balances in Tables 1 and 2 permit computation of fermentor volume requirements necessary for computation of costs.

V. ENERGY REQUIREMENTS

A. Electrical

Electrical energy requirements for the facility can be determined for pumps, general tankage, and separation factors based on the material balance and some knowledge of engineering aspects such as general pressure drops to be overcome, etc. Determination of electrical energy input for fermentation is based in this paper on determination of a minimum operating cost based on depreciation from investment in mechanical agitators, depreciation from investment in the compressor or turboblower for supply of aeration, and operating costs in power for mechanical agitation and delivery of air. The method presented in this paper for determination of this minimum is presented in Table 4.

As indicated in Table 4, a fermentor height per diameter ratio of 2 is assumed as acceptable for the reasons stated. However, other geometric ratios can be assumed and factored into the analysis. Similarly, the equation in item 2 in Table 4 points out that practical plant design should minimize pressure losses in delivery of air to fermentors. Choice of the impeller diameter as two thirds tank diameter deviates from normal practice (where one third is usually the case).[4] However, such a design will reduce rotational speeds and effect reduced shear for a given required input of mechanical power.* New agitator designs appropriate to this situation and plant cell culture may be desirable. The designs should effect gentle mixing throughout the radius of the fermentor vessel.

In all cases, the analysis assumes that rheological characteristics will be Newtonian and that turbulent conditions will prevail. Since apparent viscosity will affect mechanical power requirements, experimental determination of this parameter for the real

---

* This is evident if one considers that mechanical power input for agitation of a Newtonian fluid is proportional to N^3D_i,[5] while shear is proportional to ND_i.[5]

situation is desirable. Certainly, a high volume ratio of cells to fermentor fluid will result in apparent viscosities that differ from the fluid alone on the basis of theory.[12] However, the exact manner in which this translates to power requirements is presently unknown, except for certain few cases in the literature.[12]

The assumption of maintenance of 10% gas hold-up and the correlation of Richards[7] as measures of proper power input and aeration merely provide a reasonable basis to carry out the assignment of this paper. Similar comments apply in regard to use of the correlation of Ohyama[8] to determine the ratio of gassed and ungassed power requirements. In any case, the equations of Table 4 provide a means to determine an estimate of economic power input for plant cell culture. In particular, the operating cost due to depreciation of agitator and turboblower and input of electrical energy for this equipment is given by the sum of items 2, 7, 8, and 9 in Table 4. This sum plus the first derivative of the sum with respect to aeration rate is presented in Table 5.* Therefore, given other factors in the equation (number of fermentors, fermentor volume, and cost of electricity), the economic optimum aeration rate to minimize costs of depreciation and electrical energy for fermentation can be calculated. It should be noted at this point that the analysis could be expanded to consider fermentor volume, electrical cost, fermentor height per diameter, and number of fermentors, etc. as additional variables, transforming the problem to multivariate determination of a minimal cost. However, such an approach would be inappropriate to this paper in view of the paucity of design information available.

In use of equations in Table 5, the number of fermentors, N_F, is established based on practical size and number for reduced risk in operation. This then establishes the volume required per fermentor. For all cases studied in this paper, the value of the second derivative of the function in Table 5 is positive when evaluated at the optimum cost conditions determined through use of the expression for the first derivative, this being necessary to show that the optimum is a minimum cost.

Following determination of the optimum aeration condition, mechanical horsepower requirements, superficial velocity, and VVM (volume of air per volume of liquid per minute), can be calculated. In turn, through use of the equation in Table 4 derived from Ohyama's data, the rotational speed can be implicitly determined.

B. Steam

1. Sterilization

In this cost estimate, continuous sterilization is assumed for media prior to entry to the biomass fermentor. As indicated in Aiba and Humphrey,[13] the media are passed through a preheater, steam injected, and the steam passes through a holding loop of sufficient duration. The steam then passes back through the preheater for reclaiming of heat and finally through a cooling heat exchanger for entry to the fermentor. An optimum sterilizer tubing diameter[14] is calculated, and the sterilized fluid is assumed to pass through the sterilizer in a plug flow where contaminant level is assumed to be reduced by a factor of 10^6. Further, provision for complete sterilization of the facility nine times per year, based on estimates of metal to be heated up and correcting for ambient loss, is included in determination of steam requirements. This frequency of nine times per year assumes a 1-day doubling time for contaminating microorganisms and growth from 10^{-9} organisms per milliliter to 10^3 organisms per milliliter in 40 days.

2. Evaporation and Drying

Steam is provided for the waste glucose evaporator, the biomass dryer, and the prod-

---

* The terms of delivery of air and mechanical power in Table 5 include conversion of hp to kW and multiplication by 8640 hr/year.

uct evaporator. Requirements for steam are based on the process mass balances, except provision for steam economy is introduced through use of multieffect evaporators where appropriate.

3. Heating of Building and Structures

Cost of buildings is estimated at 50% of the cost of purchased equipment. The floor area is computed based on $80/ft² with ceiling height approximated at 30 ft. Following computation of the surface area of the building structure (building length assumed to be twice the width), the heat loss is computed, assuming a 25°C temperature difference and an overall heat transfer coefficient from inside the structure to the outside of 0.05 kcal/m²min°C. In this case, then, steam required for this purpose is 1278 kg/year/m² of exposed building surface.

C. Cooling Water

Cooling water needs relate primarily to the cooler needed in sterilization of media and for possible heat removal in the biomass and product fermentors. The latter items can be depicted in terms of the heat balances presented in Tables 6 and 7. As indicated, for batch and plug flow types, cooling requirements vary with fermentation time or equivalently for plug flow, the residence time. For this estimate, cooling requirements are calculated at the final product condition (worst case), since heat exchangers or heat transfer surface must be adequate to control temperature in this situation. In effect, then, heat transfer calculations are based on the CSTR case if the temperature in the fermentor is to be maintained equivalent to the feed temperature to the fermentor.

Examination of equations in Tables 6 and 7 indicates that concentrations of biomass and product as well as specific rates of growth or formation, respectively, affect heat generation. In addition, as expected, fermentor volume increases result in increased cooling load. Determination of the heat of formation of biomass and product would be needed for specific design. Finally, variation of specific rates of growth and product formation with temperature has been ignored, although such dependencies could be important in real situations for maximization of productivity.[16]

VI. COST ANALYSIS

A. Selected Cases

Material previously described establishes the design basis for computation of projected capital and operating costs in this paper. Table 8 presents the cases to be considered for evaluation. Case A is intended to represent a base state of technology. Case B assumes that technology can be developed to allow reuse of 90% of the biomass, and product formation rates can increase tenfold. In addition, case C also assumes that fermentation technology can allow production of 500 g of biomass per liter of fluid (this is 100 g of dry cell mass per liter of fluid, assuming that hydrated cells are 80% water). Finally, case D assumes a tenfold increase in the amount of product that can be formed in a given amount of biomass. As indicated by the references in Table 8, values for yield coefficients and heat generation for formation of biomass are assumed to match those in the literature for microbial cells in absence of similar data for plant cell cultures. Example material balances appropriate to 10⁴ kg/year are presented in Tables 9 and 10 for cases A and B, respectively.

B. Capital Cost

Capital cost relationships or sources are listed in Table 11. All prices are modified to include inflationary factors for 1978 as given by the Marschall and Stevens cost indexes.[10] The extraction system was assumed to consist of tankage plus a separations device, cost for the latter based on the estimated cost of a centrifuge as the separations device.

Table 12 presents a sample calculation of a capital cost summary for case A (10^4 kg/year), while Table 13 indicates the reduction in purchased capital cost achieved ($1,717,673 from $5,402,246) through reuse of 90% of the biomass (case B) rather than reuse of 50% (case A), plus a tenfold increase in the rate of the product formation (to 6.93 days^{-1} from 0.693 days^{-1}). As indicated, fermentor associated cooling requirements and aeration needs dramatically decrease for case B as compared to case A. For case B, the small fermentor volumes and, in particular, the reduced residence time in the product fermentor indicate that success for continuous fermentation (CSTR) is more probable. Increased costs for reverse osmosis (sugar concentration) reflect a higher concentration level of glucose in the system for case B (less glucose is used in the biomass fermentor, while the inlet glucose concentration to this fermentor might still be near 0.05 kg/ℓ for mass transfer considerations).

Expansion of case B from 10^4 to 10^6 kg/year to effect economies of scale is depicted in the capital cost summary presented as Table 14. The results of this are apparent as a 100-fold increase in production capacity results in only an approximately tenfold increase in capital cost. However, the resulting installed capital cost at this larger capacity is very high. Therefore, even without reviewing the manufacturing costs presented later in this paper, ways of reducing such cost are relevant, the reason for exploration of cases C and D, further technological improvement, as defined in Table 8. Therefore, capital costs for cases A, B, C, and D are presented in Table 15, illustrating the combined effect of technological development and operation at larger scale. Figure 3 then presents graphs of total capital investment (installed cost plus building) per unit kg/year production as a function of production level for the four different cases considered. The effects of the technological improvements noted in this paper and of scale of operation are evident.

C. Manufacturing Costs

Parameters related to specification of fermentor design for this analysis were already discussed. Results of sample computations for the information needed in projection of manufacturing costs are presented in Table 16. For the range of cases in this study, at minimal operating cost, mechanical horsepower input per volume of ungassed liquid ranges from 0.8 to 1.0 hp/m^3 for 200 down to 4 m^3 of liquid volume. Horsepower input to provide aeration ranges from 1.1 to 1.3 hp/m^3 for (4 m^3 up to 200 m^3), where approximately 40% of this latter horsepower is provided to overcome liquid head in the fermentor. Assuming the horsepower used to overcome liquid head is converted to mixing, then the sum of this figure and the power from mechanical agitation results in a horsepower input for mixing of 1.3 to 1.5 hp/m^3 of ungassed fluid at the economic optimum prescribed by the method in the fermentor specification section.* From Table 16, it should be noted that rotational speeds are between 20 and 60 rpm and superficial air velocities between 100 and 140 m/hr.

Table 17 presents the manufacturing cost summary for case A at 10^4 kg of DS product per year, while Table 18 presents additional data used to obtain figures in Table 17. Major items contributing to manufacturing cost are raw materials, labor, and depreciation (reflecting capital investment). Raw material cost can be reduced by reuse of biomass to a greater extent and through possible economies of purchase at larger scale operation. Labor cost per unit of product will also substantially decrease with

---

* All coefficients for oxygen transfer (kla) are near 10 min^{-1} for aeration of water by the bisulfite method using $K_L a = 0.45$ (pg/V)$^{0.95}$ $(V_s)^{0.67}$ min$^{-1.24}$ The economic optimum occurs at conditions where aeration reduces requirements for mechanical agitation by approximately 30%.

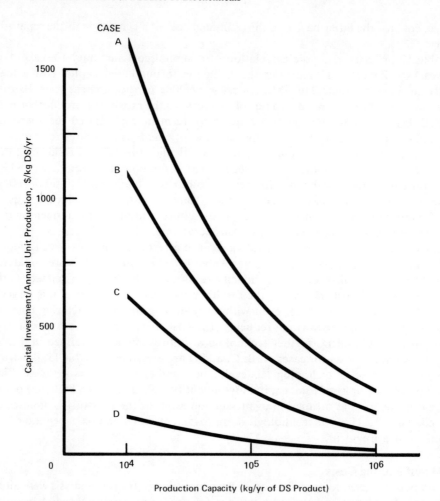

FIGURE 3.   Capital investment required per unit annual production as a function of production capacity.

increased production for such highly continuous processes.* Depreciation is reduced through technical innovation. Therefore, for case B (Table 19), reduction in manufacturing cost is effected ($551/kg to $324/kg) through reuse of 90% of the biomass and a 10 times increased rate of product accumulation. Then increasing production to 10^6 kg/year for case B brings the manufacturing cost down to $61.46/kg (Table 20).

Further reduction in manufacturing cost results through technological innovation again (cases C and D, previously described). Therefore, Figure 4 and Table 21 summarize the proposed dependence of manufacturing cost on production level for the different proposed technological achievements. Results indicate that case D at 10^6 kg/year yields a manufacturing cost of $17.52/kg of product, a dramatic improvement over case A at 10^4 kg/year.

VII. PROFITABILITY

If a 5-year payout on capital is required, if a tax rate of 50% is assumed, and if overhead/administrative costs are assumed equal to the manufacturing cost, then the

---

*   In this paper, labor cost is assumed to be proportional to $(capacity)^{0.25}$.[25]

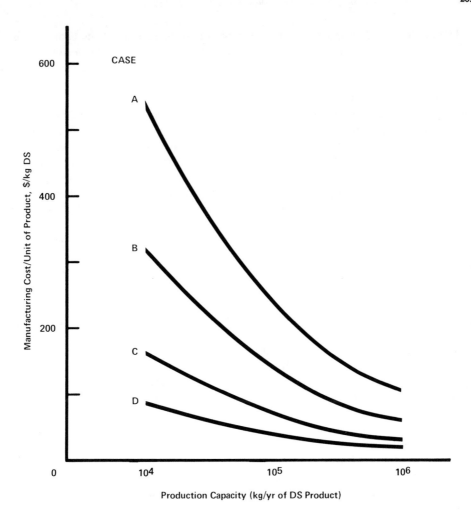

FIGURE 4. Manufacturing cost for product from plant cell culture as a function of production capacity.

projected selling price can be calculated. In this analysis, part of the depreciation is returned as a cash flow. Then

$$\frac{\text{Selling Price}}{\text{kg}} = 2\ \frac{\text{Manufacturing Cost}}{\text{kg}} + \frac{0.4\ (\text{total invested capital})}{\text{kg}}$$

$$- \text{Depreciation/kg}$$

Using the above formula, Table 22 presents results for selling price per kilogram and net profit as a percentage of sales to satisfy the 5-year payout criterion. The results indicate that $43/kg selling price would be necessary for case D at 10^6 kg/year.

VIII. DISCUSSION

Comparison of the results of this cost analysis with others in the literature is not possible, since comparative analyses for plant cell culture are not, to the authors' knowledge, available. However, other points, particularly in relation to the fermentation portion of the process, can be discussed in relation to the literature.

The method used to specify fermentor design and operation for the economic analysis in this paper results in shear-related values of rotational speed (N) times impeller diameter (Di) of 50 to 80 m/min. As a crude assumption, if this dissipates linearly over the tank radius for a water-like Newtonian fluid, the velocity gradient is approximately 60 min^{-1}. Wagner and Vogelmann's rheological studies of *Morinda citrifolia* culture for production of anthraquinones in a draft tube fermentor indicate satisfactory results at a shear rate of 360 min^{-1} (Newtonian fluid assumed).[26] Results with mechanical agitation and aeration were less positive with mechanical agitation (10 min^{-1}). However, Kato et al. were able to obtain growth of *Nicotiana tabacum* L. Bright Yellow-2 at values of ND$_i$ near 10 min^{-1}.[27] Kato and co-workers noted large increases in both viscosity and non-Newtonian behavior in study of tobacco cells induced from the above, a finding that would, of course, influence specification of mechanical power input/aeration factors and mass transfer considerations.[28] Therefore, the broth rheology and shear characteristics for particular systems may dictate particular fermentor designs, but should not significantly change the overall conclusions of this cost analysis. The important point is that engineering rheological data must be obtained to permit specification of fermentor design for particular plant cell culture systems.

Consideration of new fermentor designs can be represented by the note of Minami et al.[29] These workers report K$_L$a values (sulfite method) of 30 to 50/min, higher even than the calculated value resulting at the economic optimums in this estimate (10/min). The design couples aeration and mechanical agitation in a modified draft tube design. The draft tube has been used by many workers in investigations of plant cell culture at small scale. As noted by Hattori and Imada, the draft tube fermentor can reduce requirements for mechanical agitation power and aeration, one measure being gas hold-up, the basis for calculations in this analysis for plant cell culture.[30] The effect might be viewed as increasing superficial velocity of gas, thus improving entrainment of gas in the liquid. However, effective use of such a device may require concomitant use of mechanical agitation to effect proper mixing throughout the vessel.[29] In any case, the economic analysis of this paper does, in principle, implicitly account for the possibility of use of a draft tube design.

Consideration of the literature (e.g., Fowler[31]) indicates that the specific growth rate of biomass assumed in this analysis (0.693/day) is not unattainable, although attainment of 500 g hydrated biomass per liter will require technological advance. The maximum product formation rate assumed in this analysis (case D, 500 g hydrated biomass per liter, 0.005 kg of product per kilogram of hydrated biomass, formation rate of 6.93/day) corresponds to 17.5 product per liter per day. This rate is well in excess of current technology, e.g., Vogelmann et al. indicated 2 g/ℓ/day of anthraquinones.[32] The main factor of difference in this case would appear to be the formation rate of product. However, the cost analysis indicates that increased concentration of product in the biomass can compensate for reduced rate of product formation; that is, beneficial effects on the manufacturing cost and capital investment need per unit of product produced can be attained even if the reaction proceeds more slowly if the product accumulation per unit of biomass is increased in accord with the equations in Table 3. This result would then allow shorter residence times, or, equivalently, reduced product fermentor volume.

IX. SUMMARY

In order to develop an economic analysis, a process description is proposed as generally representative of fermentation and recovery of product from plant cell culture at commercial scale. The process separates biomass and product fermentations to emphasize that optimal conditions for each may differ and to allow possibilities for continuous culture in such a situation.[1] Extracellular product is preferred since intracellular product requires special measures to release same from the biomass, making economically desirable reuse of the biomass a more difficult proposition. The process scheme embodies aqueous extraction with nonenergy intensive membrane techniques such as reverse osmosis for necessary concentration. However, the product extraction/recovery area can also be used to symbolically represent nonaqueous extraction for recovery of product or concentration of solutions when such an alternative is economically and/or technically more attractive. Recovery of raw materials, important economically, is included in the hypothetical process, as are drag streams, suitably treated for elimination as nonpolluting effluent, but serving the purpose of minimization of contaminants and impurities in the process, a potentially important step for successful continuous operation at large scale, avoiding complete replacement of media.

Pertinent process constraints are listed as being relevant for complete specification of the plant mass balances. These include achievable biomass concentrations, assumed to be 40 g (dry) per liter or 200 g hydrated biomass per liter (80% water) and then 100 g (dry) per liter or 500 g hydrated biomass per liter. Product content per gram hydrated biomass is allowed to vary from 0.05% in one case to 0.5% in another case (hydrated basis). Doubling times for product accumulation are varied from one per day to ten times per day in separate cases, whereas a 1-day doubling time for biomass is assumed. Biomass is assumed to be reused in ratios of 50% and then 90%. Various assumptions were made in regard to volumes of liquid required at different points in the process as well as separation efficiencies. For example, a volume of extractant ten times the volume of biomass slurry to be treated was assumed to be required for removal of product.

Comments in relation to fermentor design note that the CSTR reactor will be optimal (minimal volume required) for ideal (autocatalytic) biomass growth. Product formation that is in proportion to time and biomass content will be linear (zero order), and therefore kinetic considerations in this case do not favor any particular reactor design for product formation. However, actual growth and product formation curves would have to be assessed in order to properly select a fermentation design format in practice. Continuous operation may be technically difficult at large scale if very large residence times are required, both in terms of engineering considerations as well as onset of contamination and undesirable mutation. As noted in this paper, an example fermentor design scheme is proposed based on existing engineering correlations in the literature, and the relative power input from mechanical agitation/aeration is determined through calculation of an economic optimum. The analysis assumes that 10% hold-up of air in the fluid is a desirable state and then proceeds from that point. In all cases, the economic optimum resulted in a mass transfer coefficient for oxygen (air-water-sulfite method) of approximately 10 min^{-1} and a power input from agitation/aeration of 1.3 to 1.5 hp/m^3. It is evident that mechanical agitation is being suggested in combination with aeration for economic benefit. However, as noted further in this paper, special agitator design could be necessary to prevent harmful shearing effects. Use of an air-lift fermentor, common in plant cell culture, need not be the only route.

Calculations and costs for continuous sterilization of media and periodic sterilization of facilities assume a 1-day doubling time for contaminating microorganisms, resulting in growth from 10^{-9} to 10^3 organisms per milliliter in 40 days. In regard to energy balances, literature values for heat evolution information for microorganisms are assumed in absence of such data for plant cell culture.

Analysis of costs for a base case (A) indicates approximately $551/kg product manufacturing cost and total capital investment of $1625/kg of product at a production level of 10^4 kg/year. These costs are reduced to a manufacturing cost of approximately

$17/kg and a capital cost of approximately $25/kg at a production level of 10^6 kg/ year, assuming 90% reuse of biomass, product content in the hydrated biomass of 0.5%, a specific rate of formation of product of 6.93 days^{-1}, a specific growth rate for biomass of 0.693 days^{-1}, attainable biomass concentrations of 100 g (dry) per liter of fluid, and significant recycle and reuse of liquid media. Approximately 67% of the cost of the liquid media is due to the carbon source, e.g., the extent of recycle, etc. will depend on glucose concentration levels required in biomass and product fermentors.

The analysis indicates that a 5-year payout on invested capital can be attained at a selling price of $43/kg, corresponding to 10^6 kg/year dry basis product production and the $17/kg manufacturing cost. Therefore, with sufficient technical innovation, plant cell culture can be economically competitive for production of specialty, more sparingly used items. However, this work possibly shows that the item need not be restricted to a rare pharmaceutical drug, if one considers as an example a product such as food-coloring agent, produced in other ways and selling at $20 to $40/kg. In conclusion, the authors believe that plant cell culture can have a viable commercial future, and the institution/organization developing the necessary technology to achieve production of, for example, near 10^6 kg/year, selling a product at $43/kg, should be able to apply such fermentation processing skills to other areas of interest.

NOMENCLATURE

A	=	heat surface for cooling or heating, area.
A_v	=	heat transfer surface per unit length of exchanger, area.
B_2	=	biomass content in the feed to the biomass fermentor, mass/vol.
B_{3A}	=	biomass content in the effluent from the biomass fermentor, mass/vol.
B_{4A}	=	biomass content in the effluent from the product fermentors, mass/vol.
B_{5B}	=	biomass content in slurry from biomass separation, mass/vol.
B_{9A}	=	biomass content in biomass effluent slurry, mass/vol.
B_{9B}	=	biomass content in biomass recycle slurry, mass/vol.
B_{10B}	=	biomass content in the biomass effluent, mass/vol.
C_c	=	heat capacity of the cooling water, energy/mass-temperature.
C_E	=	cost of electricity, $/kWh.
C_P	=	heat capacity of the fermentor media, energy/mass-temperature.
D	=	fermentor diameter.
D_i	=	impeller diameter.
D_P	=	depreciation period, time.
F	=	multiplication factor on capital cost of fermentors as subjective assessment of effects of technical difficulty.
G_o	=	glucose (representative of nutrient) makeup to media preparation, mass/ time.
G_1	=	glucose content in stream supply to biomass fermentor feed tanks, mass/vol.
G_2	=	glucose content in stream supply to biomass fermentors, mass/vol.
G_{3A}	=	remaining glucose content in stream effluent from biomass fermentors, mass/vol.
G_{4A}	=	remaining glucose content in stream effluent from product fermentors, mass/vol.
G_{5A}	=	content of glucose in liquid effluent from biomass separation, mass/vol.
G_{5B}	=	content of glucose in concentrated biomass slurry from biomass separation, mass/vol.

G_{6B} = glucose content in stream from biomass separation intended for concentration/treatment, mass/vol.

G_{6C} = glucose content in combined fluid fractions to be treated and concentrated, mass/vol.

G_{7A} = glucose content in the diluent drag stream from primary concentration, mass/vol.

G_{7B} = glucose content in the diluent stream from primary concentration intended for recycle to media preparation, mass/vol.

G_{7C} = glucose content in influent concentrate to secondary concentration, mass/vol.

G_{8A} = glucose content in recycle stream to media preparation from final concentration, mass/vol.

G_{8C} = glucose content in waste drag stream from final concentration, mass/vol.

G_{9C} = glucose content in stream effluent from biomass wash, mass/vol.

HP = agitator motor size, h.p.

$HP_{aeration}$ = turboblower power requirements, hp.

L = liquid depth in the fermentor, distance.

N = rotation speed, 1/time.

N_a = aeration number, Q/ND_i^3.

N_F = number of fermentors.

P = mechanical power input under turbulent conditions in absence of aeration, hp.

P_{4A} = product content in terms of volume of effluent from the product fermentor, mass/vol.

P_{5B} = product content in terms of fluid volume in biomass slurry from primary separation, mass/vol.

P_{9D} = product content in stream to primary concentration, mass/vol.

P_{11A} = product content in stream to final concentration, mass/vol.

P_{12A} = product content in product stream effluent after final concentration, mass/vol.

P_g = power input from mechanical agitation under conditions of simultaneous aeration, hp.

q_{15}, q_{3B} = supply and exhaust gas flow from biomass fermentors, vol/time.

q_{16}, q_{4B} = supply and exhaust gas flow from product fermentors, vol/time.

Q = flow rate of air, vol/time.

Q_1 = flow to biomass fermentor feed tanks, vol/time.

Q_2 = flow to biomass fermentors, vol/time.

Q_{3A} = effluent from biomass fermentors, vol/time.

Q_{4A} = effluent from product fermentors, vol/time.

Q_{5A} = liquid from primary biomass separation, vol/time.

Q_{5B} = biomass slurry from primary biomass separation, vol/time.

Q_{6A} = fluid recycle to media preparation, vol/time.

Q_{6B} = fluid portion from biomass separation to be treated and concentrated, vol/time.

Q_{6C} = combined fluid fractions from biomass separation and effluent from biomass waste to be treated and concentrated, vol/time.

Q_{7A} = drag stream of diluent following primary concentration of stream Q_{6C} vol/time.

Q_{7B} = portion of diluent follwing primary concentration of stream Q_{6C} to be recycled to media preparation, vol/time.

Q_{7C}	=	concentrate of stream Q_{6C} as influent to secondary concentration, vol/time.
Q_{8A}	=	fraction of final concentrate to be recycled to media preparation, vol/time.
Q_{8B}	=	water removed in the secondary concentration of nutrient, vol/time.
Q_{8C}	=	bottoms or drag stream following secondary concentration of nutrient vol/time.
Q_{9A}	=	portion of concentrated wet biomass to be dired as eventual effluent from the process, vol/time.
Q_{9B}	=	portion of concentrated wet biomass to be recycled to biomass fermentation.
Q_{9C}	=	effluent from biomass wash to be treated and concentrated, vol/time.
Q_{9D}	=	extract to be treated and concentrated for product recovery, vol/time.
Q_{10A}	=	water removal in drying of biomass effluent, vol/time.
Q_{10B}	=	biomass waste effluent, vol/time.
Q_{11A}	=	product liquid stream after primary concentration, vol/time.
Q_{11B}	=	recycled extraction diluent following primary concentration of the product stream, vol/time.
Q_{11C}	=	diluent drag stream from the extraction recycle, vol/time.
Q_{12A}	=	product stream after final concentration, vol/time.
Q_{12B}	=	water removal from final concentration of the product stream, vol/time.
Q_{13}	=	fluid for washing of the biomass, vol/time.
Q_{14}	=	fluid and reagent replenishment to extraction recycle, vol/time.
Q_{17}	=	influent of extractant to extraction, vol/time.
R_{B2}	=	biomass formed in the biomass fermentor, mass/vol.
R_{G3A}	=	glucose content depleted in the biomass fermentor, mass/vol.
R_{G4A}	=	glucose content depleted in the product fermentor, mass/vol.
$R_{\bullet 3A}$	=	oxygen (expressed in terms of liquid volume) depleted in the biomass fermentor, mass/vol.
$R_{\bullet 4A}$	=	oxygen (expressed in terms of liquid volume) depleted in the product fermentor, mass/vol.
R_{P4A}	=	product formed in the product fermentors, mass/vol.
t	=	batch fermentation time, time.
T_3, T_4	=	temperature of the biomass and product fermentors.
T_c	=	mean cooling water temperature.
T_0	=	reference temperature.
U	=	overall heat transfer coefficient, energy/area-time-temperature.
V	=	volume of ungassed liquid in the fermentor, vol.
V_3	=	volume of liquid content in the biomass fermentor, vol.
V_4	=	volume of liquid content in the product fermentor, vol.
V_s	=	superficial velocity of the air in the fermentor, distance/time.
W_c	=	flow rate of cooling water, mass/time.
α_G	=	proportion of glucose required in the product fermentor in terms of glucose utilization in the biomass fermentor, mass/mass.
α_O	=	proportion of oxygen required in the product fermentor in terms of oxygen utilization in the biomass fermentor, mass/mass.
$\gamma_{G/B}$	=	yield coefficient, glucose required per unit of biomass produced, mass/mass.
$\gamma_{O/B}$	=	yield coefficient, oxygen required per unit of biomass produced, mass/mass.
γ_P	=	yield coefficient, product from biomass, mass/mass.
ΔH_B	=	heat generated in formation of wet cells, energy/mass.

ΔH_p = heat generated due to residence of active biomass in the product fermentor and formation of product, energy/mass.

Δt_c = temperature rise in the cooling water.

θ = residence time, volume/flow.

μ_B = specific growth rate of the biomass, 1/time.

μ_P = specific growth rate of the product, 1/time.

ϱ = density of the fermentor media and cells, mass/vol.

ψ = fraction of total batch fermentation time for filling and emptying, time.

ϕ_{3B} = oxygen content in gas effluent from biomass fermentor, mass/vol.

ϕ_{4B} = oxygen content in gas effluent from product fermentors, mass/vol.

ϕ_{15} = oxygen content in gas influent to the biomass fermentors, mass/vol.

ϕ_{16} = oxygen content in gas influent to the product fermentors, mass/vol.

ACKNOWLEDGMENT

The authors express their gratitude to Ms. Mary Kay Quier for typing this manuscript.

TABLE 1

Material Balances — Process for Product from Plant Cell Culture

Node 1
Media preparation
vessel

$$Q_{7B} + Q_{8A} + Q_{6A} = Q_1$$

Overall

$$G_0 + G_{8A}Q_{8A} + G_{6A}Q_{6A} = Q_1 G_1$$

Glucose

Node 2
Biomass fermentor
feed vessel

$$Q_1 + Q_{9C} = Q_2$$

Overall

$$Q_1 G_1 = Q_2 G_2$$

Glucose

$$Q_{9c} B_{9C} = Q_2 B_2$$

Biomass

Node 3
Biomass fermentor

$$Q_2 = Q_{3A}$$

Overall

$$Q_2 G_2 = Q_{3A}G_{3A} + Q_{3A}R_{G3A}$$

Glucose

$$q_{15}\phi_{15} = q_{3B}\phi_{3B} + Q_{3A}R_{\phi 3A}$$

Oxygen

$$Q_2 R_{B2} + Q_2 B_2 = Q_{3A} B_{3A}$$

Biomass

(R_i represents depletion/appearance due to biomass formation)

Node 4
Product fermentor

$$Q_{3A} = Q_{4A}$$

Overall

$$Q_{3A}G_{3A} = Q_{4A}G_{4A} + Q_{4A}R_{G4A}$$

Glucose

$$q_{16}\phi_{16} = q_{4B}\phi_{4B} + Q_{4A}R_{\phi 4A}$$

Oxygen

$$Q_{3A}B_{3A} = Q_{4A}B_{4A}$$

Biomass

$$Q_{4A}P_{4A} = Q_{4A}R_{P4A}$$

Product

(R_i represents depletion/appearance due to product formation)

Node 5
Biomass separation

$$Q_{4A} = Q_{5A} + Q_{5B}$$

Overall

$$Q_{4A}G_{4A} = Q_{5A}G_{5A} + Q_{5B}G_{5B}$$

Glucose

$$Q_{4A}B_{4A} = Q_{5B}B_{5B}$$

Biomass

$$Q_{4A}P_{4A} = Q_{5B}P_{5B}$$

Product

Node 6
Liquid receiver from
biomass separation,
stream splitting

$$Q_{5A} = Q_{6A} + Q_{6B}$$

Node 6—7
Mix Point, feed
stream to primary
nutrient concentration

$$Q_{6B} + Q_{9C} = Q_{6C}$$

$$Q_{6B}G_{6B} + Q_{9C}G_{9C} = Q_{6C}G_{6C}$$

Glucose

Node 7
Primary nutrient
concentration

$$Q_{6C} = Q_{7A} + Q_{7B} + Q_{7C}$$

$$Q_{6C}G_{6C} = Q_{7C}G_{7C}$$

Glucose

TABLE 1 (continued)

Material Balances — Process for Product from Plant Cell Culture

Node 8
  Final concentration
    of nutrient stream

$$Q_{7C} = Q_{8A} + Q_{8B} + Q_{8C}$$

$$Q_{7C}G_{7C} = Q_{8C}G_{8C} + Q_{8A}G_{8A}$$

Glucose

Node 9
  Product extraction
  biomass separation
  nutrient removal

$$Q_{5B} + Q_{13} + Q_{17} = Q_{9A} + Q_{9B} + Q_{9C} + Q_{9D}$$

$$Q_{5B}G_{5B} = Q_{9C}G_{9C}$$

Glucose

$$Q_{5B}B_{5B} = Q_{9A}B_{9A} + Q_{9B}B_{9B}$$

Biomass

$$Q_{5B}P_{5B} = Q_{9D}P_{9D}$$

Product

Node 10
  Drying of biomass
  effluent

$$Q_{9A} = Q_{10A} + Q_{10B}$$

Biomass

$$Q_{9A}B_{9A} = Q_{10B}B_{10B}$$

Node 11
  Primary product concen-
  tration and drag stream
  from extraction cycle

$$Q_{9D} = Q_{11A} + Q_{11B} + Q_{11C}$$

$$Q_{9D}P_{9D} = Q_{11A}P_{11A}$$

Product

Node 12
  Final product concentration

$$Q_{11A} = Q_{12A} + Q_{12B}$$

$$Q_{11A}P_{11A} = Q_{12A}P_{12A}$$

Product

Node 17

  Fluid replenishiment
  to extraction cycle

$$Q_{11B} + Q_{14} = Q_{17}$$

TABLE 2

Specification of Process Parameters and Constraints

1. Rate of product effluent from the plant, $Q_{12}P_{12A}$
2. Yield of product per unit of biomass, γ_P
3. Maximum biomass concentration in the fermentor, B_{3A}

$$B_{4A} = B_{3A}$$

$$P_{4A} = \gamma_p B_{4A}$$

$$Q_{4A} = Q_{12}P_{12A}/P_{4A}$$

$$Q_{4A} = Q_{3A} = Q_2$$

4. Fraction of biomass that is recycled (B_{2A}/B_{3A})

$$B_{2A} = (B_{2A}/B_{3A}) \cdot B_{3A}$$

$$B_{4A} = B_{3A}$$

5. Yield coefficients for glucose and oxygen per unit biomass, $\gamma_{G/B}, \gamma_{O/B}$
6. Inlet or initial concentration of glucose and oxygen in the biomass fermentor, G_2, ϕ_{15}

$$G_{3A} = G_2 - \gamma_{G/B} (B_{3A} - B_{2A})$$

$$q_{15}\phi_{15} = q_{3B}\phi_{3B} - \gamma_{O/B} (B_{3A} - B_{2A})$$

7. Glucose and oxygen consumption factors in the product fermentor, α_G, α_o

$$G_{3A} - G_{4A} = \alpha_G (G_2 - G_{3A})$$

$$q_{16}\phi_{16} - q_{4B}\phi_{4B} = \alpha_o \gamma_{O/B} (B_{2A} - B_{3A})$$

8. Liquid removal efficiency at the biomass separator, Q_{5A}/Q_{4A}

$$Q_{5A} = (Q_{5A}/Q_{4A}) Q_{4A}$$

$$Q_{5B} = Q_{4A} - Q_{5A}$$

$$B_{5B} = Q_{4A}B_{4A}/Q_{5B}$$

$$P_{5B} = Q_{4A}P_{4A}/Q_{5B}$$

$$G_{5B} = G_{4A} = G_{5A}$$

$$G_{5B} = Q_{4A}G_{4A}/Q_{5B}$$

TABLE 2 (continued)

Specification of Process Parameters and Constraints

9. Volume rate of extractant required per volume rate of biomass slurry, Q_{17}/Q_{5B}

$$Q_{17} = (Q_{17}/Q_{5B})\, Q_{5B}$$

10. Volume rate of wash for removal of residual glucose per volume rate of biomass slurry, Q_{13}/Q_{5B}

$$Q_{13} = (Q_{13}/Q_{5B})\, Q_{5B}$$

With complete removal of glucose by use of the wash,

$$G_{9C}Q_{9C} = G_{5B}Q_{5B}$$

With complete recycle of the wash liquid,

$$Q_{9C} = Q_{13}$$

$$G_{9C} = \frac{G_{5B}Q_{5B}}{Q_{9C}}$$

With complete removal of the biomass after extraction of product and removal of residual glucose

$$Q_{9B}B_{9B} + Q_{9A}B_{9A} = Q_{5B}B_{5B}$$

if $B_{9B} = B_{9A} = B_{5B}$

$$Q_{9B} + Q_{9A} = Q_{5B}$$

Biomass to be recycled is specified before as B_{2A}/B_{3A}

$$\frac{Q_{9B}}{Q_{5B}} = B_{2A}/B_{3A}$$

$$Q_{9B} = (B_{2A}/B_{3A})\, (Q_{5B})$$

$$Q_{9A} = Q_{5B} - Q_{9B}$$

11. Degree of drying of spent biomass, Q_{10B}/Q_{9A}

$$Q_{10B} = (Q_{10B}/Q_{9A})\, Q_{9A}$$

$$Q_{10A} = Q_{9A} - Q_{10B}$$

$$B_{10B} = \frac{Q_{9A}B_{9A}}{Q_{10B}}$$

TABLE 2 (continued)

Specification of Process Parameters and Constraints

12. Degree of primary concentration for the product stream, Q_{11A}/Q_{9D}

$$Q_{11A} = [Q_{11A}/Q_{9D}]\ Q_{9D}$$

$$P_{11A} = \frac{Q_{9D}P_{9D}}{Q_{11A}}$$

13. Fraction of diluent from primary concentration of the product stream to be discharged from the process as a drag stream, Q_{11C}/Q_{11B}

$$Q_{11C} + Q_{11B} = Q_{9D} - Q_{11A}$$

$$\frac{Q_{11C}}{Q_{11B}} + 1 = \frac{Q_{9D} - Q_{11A}}{Q_{11B}}$$

$$Q_{11B} = \frac{Q_{9D} - Q_{11A}}{1 + \dfrac{Q_{11C}}{Q_{11B}}}$$

$$Q_{11C} = Q_{9D} - Q_{11A} - Q_{11B}$$

Then fluid replenishment to the extraction cycle must be

$$Q_{14} = Q_{17} - Q_{11B}$$

Fluid removal in final drying of the product stream must be

$$Q_{12B} = Q_{11A} - Q_{12A}$$

14. Volume rate of liquid from primary separation to be treated for possible discharge as a drag stream, Q_{6B}/Q_{5A}

$$Q_{6B} = (Q_{6B}/Q_{5A})\ Q_{5A}$$

$$Q_{6A} = Q_{5A} - Q_{6B}$$

$$G_{6A} = G_{5A} = G_{5B}$$

$$Q_{6C} = Q_{9C} + Q_{6B}$$

$$G_{6C} = \frac{Q_{9C}G_{9C} + Q_{6B}G_{6B}}{Q_{6C}}$$

15. Degree of primary concentration for stream Q_{6C}, Q_{7C}/Q_{6C}

$$Q_{7C} = (Q_7/Q_{6C})\ Q_{6C}$$

$$G_{7C} = Q_{6C}G_{6C}/Q_{7C}$$

TABLE 2 (continued)

Specification of Process Parameters and Constraints

$$Q_{7A} = \left[\frac{Q_{7A}}{(Q_{6C} - Q_{7V})} \right] (Q_{6C} - Q_{7C})$$

$$Q_{7B} = Q_{6C} - Q_{7A} - Q_{7C}$$

$$Q_{8B} = (Q_{8B}/Q_{7C})\, Q_{7C}$$

18. Fraction of final concentrate to be discarded as a drag stream, $Q_{8C}/(Q_{7C} - Q_{8B})$

$$Q_{8C} = \left[\frac{Q_{8C}}{(Q_{7C} - Q_{8B})} \right] (Q_{7C} - Q_{8B})$$

$$Q_{8A} = Q_{7C} - Q_{8B} - Q_{8C}$$

$$G_{8A} = G_{8C} = \frac{Q_{7C}\, G_{7C}}{[Q_{8A} + Q_{8C}]}$$

Then at Node 2,

$$Q_1 = Q_2 + Q_{9B}$$

$$B_2 = \frac{Q_{9B}\, B_{9B}}{Q_2}$$

At Node 1,

$$G_1 = \frac{Q_2 G_2}{Q_1}$$

$$G_o = Q_1 G_1 - Q_{8A} G_{8A} - Q_{6A} G_{6A}$$

TABLE 3

Expressions for Fermentation Time for Different Reactor Types

Biomass Formation — idealized autocatalytic growth, $dB/dt = \mu_B B$

$$\text{CSTR} \qquad \frac{V_3}{Q_2} = \frac{1 - B_2/B_{3A}}{\mu_B}$$

$$\text{Plug Flow} \quad \frac{V_3}{Q_2} = \frac{\ln B_{3A}/B_2}{\mu_B}$$

$$\text{Batch} \qquad t_3 = (1 + \psi) \frac{\ln\left(\dfrac{B_{3A}}{B_2}\right)}{\mu_B}$$

Product formation — zero order growth in proportion to biomass present, $dP/dt = \gamma_p B_{3A} \mu_p$

$$\begin{matrix}\text{CSTR or} \\ \text{plug flow}\end{matrix} \qquad \frac{V_4}{Q_{3A}} = \frac{P}{\gamma_p B_{3A} \mu_p}$$

$$\text{Batch} \qquad t_4 = \frac{P}{\gamma_p B_{3A} \mu_p} (1 + \psi)$$

Note: ψ = filling, emptying time fraction.
μ_B = specific growth rate of biomass.
μ_p = specific rate of formation of product in the biomass.

TABLE 4

Determination of Electrical Energy Requirements for Fermentation

1. Assume fermentor height/diameter is 2 to minimize capital investment in tankage and avoid excessive energy to pass air through fluid in the fermentor. In this case, then,

$$D = \left(\frac{2V}{\pi}\right)^{1/3} \quad \text{Fermentor diameter}$$

$$L = \left(\frac{16V}{\pi}\right)^{1/3} \quad \text{Liquid depth in fermentor}$$

$$V = \text{Volume of liquid in the fermentor}$$

2. Assume power required to pass necessary air through the fermentor is based on adiabatic decompression, where overall pressure drop to be overcome is three times the liquid height in the fermentor to account for losses through sterile filters, piping, control valves, and spargers. In the case where fluid density is nearly that of water and an 80% efficiency for conversion of electrical energy to compression is assumed,

TABLE 4 (continued)

Determination of Electrical Energy Requirements for Fermentation

$$HP_{aeration} = 0.172\, N_F Q\, [(0.4984\, V^{1/3} + 1)^{0.274} - 1]^9$$

Q = air flow in m^3/hr

V = fermentor liquid volume in m^3

N_F = number of fermentors

3. Assume impeller diameter for mechanical agitators to be 2/3 the tank diameter, resulting in less shear (product of rotational speed and impeller diameter) for given input of mechanical power. Then,

$$D_1 = \left[\frac{16V}{27\pi}\right]^{1/3} \quad \text{impeller diameter}$$

4. Assume that a desirable combination of aeration, mechanical agitation maintains a gas/liquid hold-up percentage of 10. Then from the correlation of Richards,[7]

$$10 = (Pg/V)^{0.4}\, (Vs)^{.5}$$

Pg/V = power input from mechanical agitation/volume of ungassed
    fluid under conditions of simultaneous aeration

Vs = superficial velocity of the air, Q/A

A = cross section of the fermentor for aeration

5. Mechanical power input under conditions of aeration is obtained from the data of Ohyama and Endoh.[8]

$$\frac{Pg}{P} = 0.3 + 0.7\, e^{-10.5\, Na}$$

P = mechanical power input under turbulent conditions in absence
    of aeration, $\dfrac{6N^3 D^5}{g}$ for turbine impellers

Na = aeration number $\left(\dfrac{Q}{ND_i^3}\right)$, dimensionless

Q = volume of air/unit time, m^3/hr

N = rotational speed

6. Solving the equation in 4 above for Pg, expressing V_s in terms of volumetric air flow Q, and fermentor volume V, and assuming 80% efficiency in conversion of electrical energy to mechanical agitation, the gassed power for one fermentor is given by

$$\frac{200.5\, V^{1.833}}{Q^{1.25}}$$

TABLE 4 (continued)

Determination of Electrical Energy Requirements for Fermentation

and N_F times this value for N_F fermentors.

7. The expense due to depreciation of purchased mechanical agitators is assumed given by

$$\frac{1806 \, N_F \, [HP]^{0.56}}{Dp}$$

N_F = No. of fermentors

HP = motor size, h.p.

Dp = depreciation period

This equation is based on literature cost data,[9] modified for inflationary effects using the Marschall and Stevens cost index.[10]

8. The expense due to depreciation of purchased turboblowers for aeration is given by

$$\frac{1360 \, [N_F Q]^{0.488}}{Dp}$$

the equation based on literature cost data modified again for inflation.[11]

9. The expression in item 6 can replace the HP term in item 7, yielding

$$\frac{3514.8 \, N_F V^{1.026}}{Q^{0.7}}$$

as the contribution to cost for depreciation of N_F agitator units.

TABLE 5

Preliminary Analysis for Minimal Cost Due to Aeration/Agitation

$$\text{Annual Cost} = \frac{3514.8 \, N_F \, V^{1.026}}{Q^{0.7}} + 136 \, (N_F Q)^{0.488} + 1108.2 \, C_E N_F Q$$

$$[(0.4984 \, V^{1/3} + 1)^{0.274} - 1] + \frac{1{,}291{,}812 \, C_E \, N_F V^{1.833}}{Q^{2.25}}$$

$$\frac{d \, [\text{Annual Cost}]}{d \, Q} = 0 = \frac{-2460.36 \, N_F V^{1.026}}{Q^{1.7}} + \frac{66.368 \, N_F^{0.488}}{Q^{.512}} + 1108.2 \, C_E N_F$$

$$[(0.4984 \, V^{1/3} + 1)^{0.274} - 1] - \frac{1614765 \, C_E N_F \, V^{1.833}}{Q^{2.25}}$$

TABLE 6

Heat Balances to Establish Cooling Requirements for Biomass Fermentors

Batch

$$-UA\,(T_3 - T_c) + VB_2\,\Delta H_B \mu_B e^{\mu_B t} = \rho C_p \frac{V_3\,dT_3}{dt}$$

t	=	fermentation time
W_c	=	cooling water flow rate
T_c	=	mean cooling water temperature
C_c	=	heat capacity of the cooling water
ϱ	=	density of fermentor media
C_p	=	heat capacity of fermentor media
T_3	=	fermentor temperature
V_3	=	fermentor volume
ΔH_B	=	heat generated in formation of a gram of wet cells
U	=	heat transfer coefficient for cooling
A	=	total heat transfer surface for cooling

CSTR

$$-UA\,(T_3 - T_c) + \mu_B B_2\,\Delta H_B V_3 = Q\rho C_p\,(T_3 - To)$$

To = inlet reference temperature

Plug Flow

$$-UA_v\,(T_3 - T_c) + B_4\,\Delta H \mu_B e^{\mu_B \Theta} = \rho\, C_p \frac{dT_3}{d\Theta}$$

θ	=	V/Q residence time
A_v	=	heat transfer surface/unit length of exchanger

If heat removal requirements are calculated at the final value of the biomass and the temperature is maintained at a precise value, then in all cases

$$-UA\,(T_3 - T_c) + B_4\,\Delta H \mu_B e^{\mu_B \Theta} V_3 = 0$$

and cooling water requirements are computed from

$$W_c C_c T_c = UA(T_3 - T_c) = B_2\,\Delta H_B \mu_B e^{\mu_B \theta} V_3$$

ΔT_c = temperature rise in the cooling water

TABLE 7

Heat Balances to Establish Cooling Requirements for Product Fermentors

Batch

$$\rho C_p V_4 \frac{dT4}{dt} = V_4 B_4 \gamma_p \mu_p \Delta H_p - UA\,(T_4 - T_c)$$

T_4 = temperature of the fermentor
ΔH_p = heat generation/g product formed
V_4 = volume of the biomass fermentor

CSTR

$$Q\rho C_p\,(T_4 - To) = V_4 B_2 \gamma_p \mu_p \Delta H_p + UA\,(T_4 - T_c)$$

Plug Flow

$$\rho C_p \frac{dT_4}{d\Theta} = V_4 B_4 \gamma_p \mu_B e^{\mu_B \Theta} - UA_V\,(T_4 - T_c)$$

With similar assumptions as in Table 6,

$$W_c C_c\,\Delta T_c = V_4 B_4 \gamma_p \mu_p\,\Delta H_p$$

TABLE 8

Cases for Cost Analysis (To be Evaluated at Levels of Product/Annum of 10^4, 10^5, and 10^6 kg/year)

	Case A
γ_p =	0.0005 g product/g hydrated biomass
B_{3A} =	200 g hydrated biomass/liter of fluid, final biomass concentration
B_{2A}/B_{3A} =	0.5 recycled biomass
$\gamma G/B$ =	0.4 g/g wet biomass, glucose yield coefficient[17]
α_G =	0.2, glucose consumption in the product fermentor is 20% of that in the biomass fermentor
Q_{5A}/Q_{4A} =	0.9, liquid removal at the biomass separator
Q_{17}/Q_{5B} =	10, volume of extractant/volume of biomass slurry
Q_{13}/Q_{5B} =	2, wash volume/volume of biomass slurry
Q_{10B}/Q_{9A} =	0.044, degree of dryness for spent biomass
Q_{11A}/Q_{9D} =	0.2, degree of primary concentration, product stream
Q_{11C}/Q_{11B} =	0.1, drag stream fraction from extraction cycle
Q_{6B}/Q_{5A} =	0.478, liquid fraction from primary separation to be treated for possible discharge from process
Q_{7C}/Q_{6C} =	0.0085, degree of primary concentration, nutrient stream
$Q_{7A}/Q_{6C} - Q_{7C}$ =	0.23, fraction of low B.O.D. fluid to be discarded as a drag stream
Q_{8B}/Q_{7C} =	0.8, fraction additional fluid removal from nutrient concentrate
$Q_{8C}/Q_{7C} - Q_{8B}$ =	1.0, fraction of final concentrate to be eliminated as a drag stream
μ_B =	0.693 days^{-1}, one day doubling time for biomass
μ_p =	0.693 days^{-1}, one day doubling time for product formation
ΔH_B =	0.5 kcal/g hydrated biomass[17]
ΔH_p =	0.1 kcal/g hydrated biomass

TABLE 8 (continued)

Cases for Cost Analysis (To be Evaluated at Levels of Product/Annum of 10^4, 10^5, and 10^6 kg/year)

Case B

B_{2A}/B_{3A}	=	0.9, increase biomass reuse
$Q_{8C}/Q_{7C}-Q_{8B}$	=	0.9, recycle most of glucose concentrate
Q_{13}/Q_{5B}	=	6, increased wash volume due to increased glucose present
Q_{7C}/Q_{6C}	=	0.21, reduce to reach 0.2 g/cc concentration
$Q_{7A}/Q_{6C}-Q_{7C}$	=	0.38, increase due to higher levels of nutrient concentration and relatively greater fluid addition to process
Q_{8B}/Q_{7C}	=	0.8, to maintain fluid balances
μ_p	=	6.93 days,$^{-1}$ tenfold increase in rate of product formation

Case C

As Case B except

B_{3A}	=	500 g/l of fluid, increase biomass concentration possible in fermentor

Case D

As Case C except

γ_p	=	0.005 g product/g hydrated biomass, tenfold increase

TABLE 9

Material Balance — 10,000 kg/year of Product Case A

Stream	Flow rate (m^3/hr)	Biomass (kg/l)	Glucose (kg/l)	Product (kg/l)
Q_{7B}	5.55	—	—	—
Q_{6A}	5.42	—	0.002	—
Q_{8A}	—	—	—	—
Glucose + nutrients	—	—	566.7 kg/hr glucose	—
Q_1	10.97	—	0.05	—
Q_{9B}	0.58	2.0	—	—
Q_2	11.55	0.1	0.05	—
Q_{3A}	11.55	0.2	0.01	—
Q_{4A}	11.55	0.2	0.002	0.0001
Q_{5B}	1.155	2.0	0.002	0.001
Q_{5A}	10.395	—	0.002	—
Q_{6B}	4.97	—	0.002	—
Q_{6C}	7.28	—	0.0017	—
Q_{7A}	1.67	—	—	—
Q_{7C}	0.062	—	0.2	—
Q_{8B}	0.049	—	—	—
Q_{8C}	0.0124	—	0.99	—
Q_{9A}	0.58	2.0	—	—
Q_{10A}	1.48	—	—	—
Q_{10B}	0.025	254.1 kg/hr (10%-H$_2$O)	—	—
Q_{13}	2.31	—	—	—
Q_{9C}	2.31	—	0.001	—
Q_{9D}	11.55	—	—	0.0001
Q_{11A}	2.31	—	—	0.0005
Q_{11B}	9.24	—	—	—
Q_{12A}	0.58	—	—	0.002
Q_{12B}	1.73	—	—	—
Q_{11C}	0.92	—	—	—
Q_{14}	3.23	—	—	—
Q_{17}	11.55	—	—	—

TABLE 9 (continued)

Material Balance — 10,000 kg/year of Product Case A

Stream	Flow rate (m³/hr)	Biomass (kg/ℓ)	Glucose (kg/ℓ)	Product (kg/ℓ)
Q_{11B}	9.24	—	—	—
Q_{12A}	0.58	—	—	0.002
Q_{12B}	1.73	—	—	—
Q_{11C}	0.92	—	—	—
Q_{14}	3.23	—	—	—
Q_{17}	11.55	—	—	—

TABLE 10

Material Balance — 10,000 kg/year of Product Case B

Stream	Flow rate (m³/hr)	Biomass (kg/ℓ)	Glucose (kg/ℓ)	Product (kg/ℓ)
Q_{7B}	4.87	—	—	—
Q_{6A}	5.42	—	0.0404	—
Q_{8A}	0.23	—	1.0	—
Glucose + nutrients	—	—	135.64 kg/hr glucose	—
Q_1	10.51	—	0.055	—
Q_{9B}	1.04	2.0	—	—
Q_2	11.55	0.18	0.05	—
Q_{3A}	11.55	0.2	0.042	—
Q_{4A}	11.55	0.2	0.0404	0.0001
Q_{5B}	1.155	2.0	0.0404	0.001
Q_{5A}	10.395	—	0.0404	—
Q_{6B}	4.97	—	0.0404	—
Q_{6C}	11.90	—	0.02	—
Q_{7A}	4.56	—	—	—
Q_{7C}	2.48	—	0.2	—
Q_{8B}	2.23	—	—	—
Q_{8C}	0.025	—	1.0	—
Q_{9A}	0.12	2	—	—
Q_{10A}	0.3	—	—	—
Q_{10B}	0.005	56.4 kg/hr (10%-H_2O)	—	—
Q_{13}	6.93	—	—	—
Q_{9C}	6.93	—	0.0067	—
Q_{9D}	11.55	—	—	0.0001
Q_{11A}	2.31	—	—	0.0005
Q_{11B}	9.24	—	—	—
Q_{12A}	0.58	—	—	0.002
Q_{12B}	1.73	—	—	—
Q_{11C}	0.92	—	—	—
Q_{14}	3.23	—	—	—
Q_{17}	11.55	—	—	—

TABLE 11

Relationships or Sources for Determination of Capital Costs

Item	Purchased cost equation or source	Units	Ref.
Agitated tanks	$247 (V)^{0.5}$	ℓ	18
Pumps (centrifugal)	Chart × 4.25		19
Fermentors (agitated/-aerated)	$247 F (V)^{0.5}$ F = factor for subjective assessment of technical difficulty in design (1, 2, 3, or 4)	ℓ	18
Biomass centrifuge	$8500 [Q_{4A}]^{0.5}$	ℓ/min[20]	
Conveyor (biomass or other)	$871 [W]^{0.4}$	kg/hr	21
Reverse osmosis system	$16316 [Q_{6C} \text{ or } Q_{9D}]^{0.6}$	ℓ/min	
Spray dryer	$5806 [W]^{0.25}$	kg/hr water	22
Evaporator (multi-effect)	$9550 [A]^{0.65}$	m^2	23
Turboblower	$1360 [Q]^{0.488}$	m^3/hr	11
Mechanical agitator	$1806 [HP]^{0.56}$	HP	9

TABLE 12

Capital Cost Summary
(Case A, 10,000 kg/year — Table 8)

Agitated Tanks

Fermentor Preparation Area

Item	Volume (m³)/ each	Quantity	$ Cost/each	Total cost ($)
Media makeup	50	1	55,231	55,231
Fermentor feed	55	1	57,927	57,927
Fermentation Area				
Fermentors (biomass)				
(1F) CSTR	20	10	(F = 4) 139,364	1,393,640
(1F) Batch	45	10	(F = 2) 104,793	1,047,930
(1F) Plug flow	35	10	(F = 4) 184,836	1,848,360
Intermediate tanks	1.5	10	9,566	95,660
Fermentors (product)				
(1F) Plug flow or CSTR	45	10	(F = 4) 209,586	2,095,860
(1F) Batch	55	10	(F = 2) 115,885	1,158,850
Drop tanks	1.5	10	9,566	95,660
Product Recovery Area				
Extraction feed tank	30	1	42,782	42,782
Extraction unit	30	1	42,782	42,782
Extraction product tank	30	1	42,782	42,782
Product dryer feed	3	1	13,529	13,529
Recovery tank — reverse osmosis	30	1	42,782	42,782
Sugar evap. feed	0.15	1	3,025	3,025
Primary separation liquid receiver	12	1	27,057	27,057

TABLE 12 (continued)

Capital Cost Summary
(Case A, 10,000 kg/year — Table 8)

Liquid receiver — glucose conc.	15	1	30,251	30,251
Wash receiver	8	1	22,092	22,092

Subtotal — agitated tanks (assuming batch fermentors)

$2,778,340

Pumps

Fermentor Preparation Area

Item	Flow (ℓ/min)/each	Quantity	$ Cost/each	Total cost ($)
Media discharge	192.5	1	4,250	4,250
Fermentor feed (biomass)	19.25	10	2,975	29,750
Fermentor Area				
Fermentor feed (product)	19.25	10	2,975	29,750
Fermentor discharge (biomass) tank	19.25	10	2,975	29,750
To drop tank	19.25	10	2,975	29,750
To primary separation	19.25	10	2,975	29,750
Biomass cooling	1083	2	7,990	15,980
Product cooling	265	2	4,505	9,010
Product Recovery Area				
Pump to product RO unit	192.5	1	28,475	28,475
Pump to product dryer	38.5	1	4,250	4,250
Pump — extraction recycle	208	1	4,250	4,250
Pump to glucose RO unit	121	1	13,200	13,200
Pump to sugar evap.	1.7	1	500	500
Recycle pump — to media tank from glucose RO receiver	100	1	4,250	4,250
To extraction	100	10	4,250	42,500

Subtotal — pumps $275,415

Heat Exchangers

Fermentor Preparation Area

Item	Surface area (m²/each)	Quantity	$ Cost/each	Total cost ($)
Media preheater	9.2	1	7,093	7,093
Post steril. cooler media sterilizer	9.2	1	7,093	7,093
Media sterilizer		1	10,000	10,000
Fermentor Area				
Biomass cooling	27.1	10	56,884	568,844
Product cooling	6.6	10	23,020	230,200

Subtotal — heat exchangers $823,230

225

TABLE 12 (continued)

Capital Cost Summary
(Case A, 10,000 kg/year — Table 8)

Agitated Tanks

Fermentor Preparation Area

Item	Volume (m³)/ each	Quantity	$ Cost/each	Total cost ($)

Miscellaneous

Fermentor Area

Item	Parameter/ each	Quantity	$ Cost/each	Total cost ($)
Turboblower biomass ferms.	8,530 m³/hr	1	112,698	112,698
Turboblower product ferms.	10,620 m³/hr	1	125,397	125,397

Product Recovery Area

Item	Parameter/ each	Quantity	$ Cost/each	Total cost ($)
Centrifuges — primary separation	192.5 ℓ/min	2	117,933	235,866
Biomass conveyor	2310 kg/hr	1	19,296	19,296
Centrifuge — extraction	211.8 ℓ/min	1	123,689	123,689
Solids conveyor to biomass dryer	1155 kg/hr	1	14,623	14,623
Biomass dryer	3210 kg/hr H₂O	1	30,000	30,000
Product weighing/handling system	—	1	10,000	10,000
Product conc. — reverse osmosis	192.5 ℓ/min	1	383,065	383,065
Product dryer	693 ℓ/min H₂O	1	127,500	127,500
Product handling	577.5 ℓ/hr	1	11,082	11,082
Glucose conc. — reverse osmosis	121.4 ℓ/min	1	290,470	290,470
Glucose evaporator		1	40,000	40,000
Biomass recycle conveyor		1	11,575	11,575

Subtotal — miscellaneous $1,535,261

Note: Purchased equipment total = $5,412,246; Installation factor (2.5) installed cost = $13,530,615; Building cost at 50% of purchased equipment = $2,706,123.

TABLE 13

Comparison of Capital Costs for Cases A and B at 10000 kg/year

Item	Case A	Case B
General tankage	$2,778,340	$2,802,612
Biomass fermentors	1,047,030 (batch) 10 at 45 m³ each F = 2ᵃ	523,907 (CSTR) 10 at 5 m³ each F = 3

TABLE 13 (continued)

Comparison of Capital Costs for Cases A and B at 10000 kg/year

Item	Case A	Case B
Product fermentors	1,158,853	497,080
	(batch)	(CSTR)
	10 at 55 m³ each	10 at 4.5 m³ each
	F = 2	F = 3
Turboblower — biomass	112,698	53,104
Turboblower — product	125,397	52,161
Conveyor	26,198	19,842
Sugar concentration — reverse osmosis	290,470	390,057
High pressure pump	13,200	28,475
Sugar evaporator	40,000	130,716
Fermentor heat exchangers for cooling	798,640	181,970

Note: Net difference Case A — Case B = $1,717,673; Purchased capital for Case B = $3,684,573; Installed cost (Case B) = $9,211,432; Building cost = $1,842,286.

ᵃ   F = factor of technical difficulty used in computing the capital cost (see Table 11).

TABLE 14

Capital Cost Summary
(Case B, 1,000,000 kg/year — Table 8)

Agitated Tanks

Fermentor Preparation Area

Item	Volume (m³)/ each	Quantity	$ Cost/each	Total cost ($)
Glucose bin	136	1	90,968	90,968
Media makeup	120	10	85,563	855,630
Fermentor feed	130	10	89,006	890,060
Fermentor Area				
Fermentors (biomass), CSTR	250	20	(F = 1) 123,500	2,470,000
Intermediate tanks	65	20	62,973	1,259,460
Fermentors (product), CSTR	250	20	(F = 1) 123,500	2,470,000
Drop tanks	65	20	62,973	1,259,460
Product Recovery Area				
Extraction feed tanks	55	5	57,927	289,635
Extraction tanks	300	10	135,287	1,352,870
Extraction receiver — product RO feed	400	4	156,216	624,864
Concentrate receiver — product RO and product dryer feed	130	4	89,057	356,228
Diluent receiver — product RO	700	4	206,655	826,620
Wash tanks	200	4	110,462	441,848

TABLE 14 (continued)

Capital Cost Summary
(Case B, 1,000,000 kg/year — Table 8)

Agitated Tanks

Fermentor Preparation Area

Item	Volume (m³)/ each	Quantity	$ Cost/each	Total cost ($)
Glucose conc. receiver — RO and evap. feed	70	4	65,350	261,400
Liquid receivers — primary sep.	300	4	135,287	541,148
Recycle fluid from RO	550	1	183,180	183,180

Subtotal — agitated tanks $14,173,371

Pumps

Fermentor Preparation Area

Item	Flow (m³/min)/each	Quantity	$ Cost/each	Total cost ($)
Media discharge	1.75	10	5,610	56,100
Fermentor feed	1.925	10	5,610	56,100
Fermentor Area				
Fermentor discharge (biomass)	0.96	20	5,015	100,300
Fermentor feed (product ferm.)	0.96	20	5,015	100,300
To drop tank	0.96	20	5,015	100,300
To primary separation	1.925	10	5,610	56,100
Biomass cooling	6.02	20	1,836	36,720
Product cooling	1.20	20	1,003	20,060
Product Recovery Area				
Feed to extraction	0.38	5	4,250	21,250
HP pumps to product RO unit	4.81	4	340,000	1,360,000
Product dryer feed	0.24	4	5,015	20,060
Pumps RO diluent (extraction recycle)	5.2	4	7,990	31,960
From biomass wash receiver	2.89	4	6,562	26,250
HP pumps to glucose RO unit	4.96	4	340,000	1,360,000
Pump to sugar evap.	4.13	1	7,990	7,990
From receiver — primary sep.	2.17	8	5,610	44,880
Diluent recycle — glucose RO area	8.11	1	9,180	9,180

Subtotal — pumps $3,407,550

Heat Exchangers

Fermentor Preparation Area

Item	Surface area (m²)/each	Quantity	$ Cost/each	Total cost ($)
Media preheater	87.6	10	30,118	301,180
Post steril. cooler	87.6	10	30,118	301,180
Media sterilizer	142.6	10	20,000	200,000

TABLE 14 (continued)

Capital Cost Summary
(Case B, 1,000,000 kg/year — Table 8)

Agitated Tanks

Fermentor Preparation Area

Item	Volume (m³)/ each	Quantity	$ Cost/each	Total cost ($)
Fermentor Area				
Biomass cooling	150.4	20	170,226	3,404,520
Product cooling	30.1	20	60,769	1,215,380
			Subtotal — heat exchangers	$5,422,260

Miscellaneous

Fermentor Preparation Area

Item	Parameter/ each	Quantity	$ Cost/each	Total cost ($)
Nutrient conveyor (glucose)	1.36 mt/hr	1	320,783	320,783
Fermentor Area				
Turboblower (biomass ferm.)	59,000 m³/hr	1	289,544	289,544
Turboblower (product ferm.)	59,000 m³/hr	1	289,544	289,544
Product Recovery Area				
Centrifuges (primary separation)	1.92 m³/min	10	372,936	3,729,360
Biomass conveyor	46.2 mt/hr	5	63,955	319,775
Centrifuges (extraction)	2.12 m³/min	10	391,139	3,911,390
Product RO units		4		10,570,514
Product evaporator (multieffect)				2,225,752
Product handling system	57.8 mt/hr	1	69,926	69,926
Biomass conveyor to dryer	34.6 mt/hr	1	57,003	57,003
Biomass dryer	29.5 mt/hr H_2O	1	76,104	76,104
Dry biomass handling	51.3 kg/hr	1	4,208	4,208
Glucose conc. RO units		4	2,642,628	10,570,512
Glucose conc. evap. (multieffect)	222.8 mt/hr H_2O	1	2,621,478	2,621,478
Biomass conveyor recycle	311.8 mt/hr		21,757	21,757

Subtotal — miscellaneous $ 35,073,442
Purchased equipment total 58,076,623
Installation factor (2.5)
Installed cost 145,191,560
Building cost at 50% of purchased equipment 29,038,312

TABLE 15

Variations in Capital Cost as a Function of Technological Advance and Scale of Production

Production Capacity (kg/year DS of Product)

Case	Purchased equipment	10,000 installed cost	Building	Purchased equipment	100,000 installed cost	Building	Purchased equipment	1,000,000 installed cost	Building
A	5,416,859	13,542,148	2,708,430	21,554,800	53,912,000	10,782,400	85,851,016	214,627,540	42,925,508
B	3,699,186	9,247,965	1,849,593	14,726,800	36,817,000	7,363,400	58,081,100	145,202,700	29,040,550
C	2,118,633	5,296,583	1,059,317	8,432,161	21,080,402	4,216,080	33,560,000	83,900,000	16,780,000
D	530,290	1,325,724	265,145	2,110,553	5,276,382	1,055,276	8,400,000	21,000,000	4,200,000

TABLE 16

Fermentor Parameters for Minimal Cost

10,000 (kg/year DS Product)

Case	Fermentor	Mechanical horsepower input (hp)	Agitator diameter (m)	Rotational speed (rpm)	Aeration quantity (m³/hr)	Power input aeration	Power input to overcome liquid head	Superficial velocity (m/hr)	Volume air/-vol. liquid/-min (VVM)	tank diam. (m)	Liquid volume (m³)
A	Biomass (batch)	32.5	1.91	37	853	45.1	18.8	133	0.38	2.86	37
	Product (batch)	43.0	2.11	34	1062	60.4	25.5	135	0.35	3.17	50
B	Biomass (CSTR)	4.2	0.98	57	183	5.5	2.1	108	0.72	1.47	4.2
	Product (CSTR)	4.0	0.95	59	176	5.2	2.0	111	0.73	1.42	4
	1,000,000 kg/year DS Product										
B	Biomass (CSTR)	167.5	3.41	24	2950	233	105	143	0.23	5.12	211
	Product (CSTR)	167.5	3.41	24	2950	233	105	143	0.23	5.12	211

TABLE 17

Manufacturing Cost Summary Case A, 10⁴ kg of DS Product/ Year

		$ Cost/kg product
Raw materials at $0.022/$\ell$		$215.55
Operating labor and supervision		104.33
Utilities		
Electricity	14.21	
Steam	6.56	
Cooling water	7.88	
Process water	0.25	
Sewage	0.12	
Utilities subtotal		29.02
Depreciation		
Equipment (10 year)	135.13	
Building (30 year)	9.03	
Depreciation subtotal		144.16
Maintenance (3% of installed equipment cost)		40.54
Taxes and insurance (3% of installed equipment cost)		40.54
Total before credit		573.84
Credit for sale of biomass by-product		(21.45)
Credit for sale of nutrient by-product		(1.06)
Net manufacturing cost		$551.33/kg

TABLE 18

Support Data for Manufacturing Cost Summary Case A, 10⁴ kg/year

Operating labor and supervision	
Fermentation area	2/shift
Product recovery/extraction area	2/shift
Recycle handling	1/shift
Laboratory	1/shift
Utility operator	1/shift
Total	7/shift

(7/shift) [8 hr/Individual] (3 shifts/day) (360 days/ year) =	60,480 man hours/year
Supervision and clerk at 15% =	9,072 man hours/year
	69,552 man hours/year
69,552 × $15/hr (with benefits) =	$1,043,280
or	$104.33/kg

Electrical summary	
Pumps	96 hp
Conveyor	8
Fermentor mechanical agitation	755
Compressed air	1055
General tank agitation at 0.5 hp/m³	132
Centrifuges	160
	2206 hp

(2206 hp) (kW/1.341 hp) (8640 hr/year) ($0.01/kWh) = $142,112 or $14.21/kg product

TABLE 18 (continued)

Support Data for Manufacturing Cost Summary Case A, 10^4 kg/year

	Steam
Sterilization of equipment	3.75×10^6 kg/year
Media sterilization	2.81×10^6 kg/year
Evaporation and drying	19.28×10^6 kg/year
Heating of building	3.97×10^6 kg/year
Total	29.81×10^6 kg/year
at \$2.2/1,000 kg →	\$65,587
or	\$6.56/kg product
Cooling water	

1.49×10^9 kg/year $\times$ \$0.0528/1,000 kg = \$78,772 or \$7.88/kg product

TABLE 19

Manufacturing Cost Summary Case B, 10^4 kg/year

		\$ Cost/kg product
Raw materials at \$0.0052/l		\$ 51.56
Operating labor and supervision		104.33
Utilities		
Electricity	3.90	
Steam	9.82	
Cooling water	1.26	
Process water	0.46	
Sewage	0.25	
Utilities subtotal		15.69
Depreciation		
Equipment (10 year)	92.48	
Building (30 year)	6.17	
Depreciation subtotal		98.65
Maintenance		27.74
Taxes and insurance		27.74
Total before credit		\$325.71
Credit for sale of biomass by-product		(0.04)
Credit for sale of glucose by-product		(2.14)
Net manufacturing cost		\$323.53/kg

TABLE 20

Manufacturing Cost Sunmary Case B, 10^6 kg/year

		$ Cost/kg product
Raw materials at $0.0028/$ℓ		$25.78
Operating labor and supervision		3.30
Utilities		
Electricity	3.24	
Steam	5.13	
Cooling water	1.27	
Process water	0.46	
Sewage	0.25	
Utilities subtotal		10.35
Depreciation		
Equipment (10 year)	14.52	
Building (30 year)	0.97	
Depreciation subtotal		15.49
Maintenance		4.36
Tafes and insurance		4.36
Total before credit		$63.64
Credit for sale of biomass by-product		(0.04)
Credit for sale of glucose by-product		(2.14)
Net manufacturing cost		$61.46/kg

TABLE 21

Manufacturing Cost Summary Cases A, B,
C, and D at 10^4, 10^5, 10^6 kg/year

	Production level kg/year		
Cases	10^4	10^5	10^6
A	$551.33/kg	241	106
B	323.53	142	61.46
C	165.31	72.16	31.50
D	91.96	40.14	17.52

TABLE 22

Profitability of Plant Cell Culture Production Level kg DS/year

	10^4		10^5		10^6	
Case	Selling price (kg)	% Profit (Sales)	Selling price (kg)	% Profit (Sales)	Selling price (kg)	% Profit (Sales)
A	1608	15.7	683	14.7	290	13.8
B	992	17.4	421	16.3	177	15.3
C	528	18.7	223	17.6	94	16.6
D	233	10.6	100	9.8	43	9.1

REFERENCES

1. Mandels, M., The culture of plant cells, *Adv. Biochem. Eng.*, 2, 201, 1972.
2. Cooney, C. L., Wang, H. Y., and Wang, D. I. C., Computer-aided material balancing for prediction of fermentation parameters, *Biotechnol. Bioeng.*, 19, 55, 1977.
3. Carberry, J., *Chemical and Catalytic Reaction Engineering*, 1st ed., McGraw-Hill, New York, 1976.
4. McCabe, W. L. and Smith, J. C., *Unit Operations of Chemical Engineering*, 1st ed., McGraw-Hill, New York, 1956.
5. Perry, R. H. and Chilton, C. H., *Chemical Engineers' Handbook*, 5th ed., McGraw-Hill, New York, 1973.
6. Peters, M. S. and Timmerhaus, K. D., *Plant Design and Economics for Chemical Engineers*, 2nd ed., McGraw-Hill, New York, 1968.
7. Richards, J. W., Studies in aeration and agitation, *Prog. Ind. Microbiol.*, 3, 143, 1961.
8. Ohyama, Y. and Endoh, K., Power characteristics of gas-liquid contacting mixers, *Kagaku Kogaku*, 19, 2, 1955.
9. Peters, M. S. and Timmerhaus, K. D., *Plant Design and Economics for Chemical Engineers*, 2nd ed., McGraw-Hill, New York, 1968, 478.
10. *Chemical Engineering*, McGraw-Hill, New York, any issue.
11. Peters, M. S. and Timmerhaus, K. D., *Plant Design and Economics for Chemical Engineers*, 2nd ed., McGraw-Hill, New York, 1968, 470.
12. Bailey, J. C. and Ollis, D. F., *Biochemical Engineering Fundamentals*, 1st ed., McGraw-Hill, N. Y., 1977, 456.
13. Aiba, S., Humphrey, A. E., and Millis, N. F., *Biochemical Engineering*, 2nd ed., Academic Press, New York, 1973, 257.
14. Peters, M. S. and Timmerhaus, K. D., *Plant Design and Economics for Chemical Engineers*, 2nd ed., McGraw-Hill, New York, 1968, 306.
15. Peters, M. S. and Timmerhaus, K. D., *Plant Design and Economics for Chemical Engineers*, 2nd ed., McGraw-Hill, New York, 1968, 112.
16. Kato, A., Hashimoto, Y., and Soh, Y., Effect of temperature on the growth of tobacco cells, *J. Ferment. Technol.*, 54, 10, 754, 1961.
17. Bailey, J. C. and Ollis, D. F., *Biochemical Engineering Fundamentals*, 1st ed., McGraw-Hill, New York, 1977, 479.
18. Peters, M. S. and Timmerhaus, K. D., *Plant Design and Economics for Chemical Engineers*, 2nd ed., McGraw-Hill, New York, 1968, 477.
19. Peters, M. D. and Timmerhaus, K. D., *Plant Design and Economics for Chemical Engineers*, 2nd ed., McGraw-Hill, New York, 1968, 465.
20. Fermentation Equipment Catalog, New Brunswick Scientific Co., Inc., Edison, New Jersey, 1978.
21. Peters, M. S. and Timmerhaus, K. D., *Plant Design and Economics for Chemical Engineers*, 2nd ed., McGraw-Hill, New York, 1968, 507.
22. Peters, M. S. and Timmerhaus, K. D., *Plant Design and Economics for Chemical Engineers*, 2nd ed., McGraw-Hill, New York, 1968, 660.
23. Peters, M. S. and Timmerhaus, K. D., *Plant Design and Economics for Chemical Engineers*, 2nd ed., McGraw-Hill, New York, 1968, 572.
24. Aiba, S., Humphrey, A. E., and Millis, N. F., *Biochemical Engineering*, 2nd ed., Academic Press, New York, 1973, 183, 189.
25. Peters, M. S. and Timmerhaus, K. D., *Plant Design and Economics for Chemical Engineers*, 2nd ed., McGraw-Hill, New York, 1968, 130.
26. Wagner, F. and Vogelmann, H., Cultivation of plant tissue cultures in bioreactors and formation of secondary metabolities, in *Plant Tissue Culture and Its Bio-technological Application*, Barz, W., Reinhard, E., and Zenk, M. H., Eds., Springer-Verlag, Berlin, 1977, 245.
27. Kato, A., Shimizo, Y., and Nagai, S., Effect of initial K_la on the growth of tobacco cells in batch culture, *J. Ferment. Technol.*, 53, No. 10, 744, 1975.
28. Kato, A., Kawazoe, S., and Soh, Y., Viscosity of the broth of tobacco cells in suspension culture, *J. Ferment. Technol.*, 56, No. 3, 224, 1978.
29. Minami, K., Yamamura, M., Shimizu, S., Ogawa, K., and Sekine, N., A new fermentor with a high oxygen transfer capacity, *J. Ferment. Technol.*, 56, No. 1, 64, 1978.
30. Hattori, K., Shuji, Y., and Imada, O., Performance of draft tube fermentor for hydro carbon fermentation, *J. Ferment. Technol.*, 52, No. 8, 583, 1974.
31. Fowler, M. W., Growth of cell cultures under chemostat conditions, in *Plant Tissue Culture and Its Bio-technological Application*, Barz. W., Reinhard, E., and Zenk, M. H., Eds., Springer-Verlag, Berlin, 1977, 253.
32. Vogelmann, H., Zenk, M., and Wagner, F., Secondary metabolite formation by plant tissue culture in bioreactors, in *Abstr. 5th Int. Fermentation Symp.*, Berlin, 1976.

Chapter 10

PRODUCTS

Louis G. Nickell

TABLE OF CONTENTS

I. INTRODUCTION

Theoretically, it should be possible to produce in culture any compound that is produced in nature by the plant from which the culture was obtained. Practically, the true situation is not quite that simple — in certain cases. When the desired product is made in specialized cells which do not grow or grow well in culture, or when the product is related to the maturation of the cell, rather than growth, there are a few more technical hurdles to clear.

There are three obvious possibilities, (1) production of the same materials in culture that are produced by the plant in natural habitat from which the culture was derived, at the same or different concentrations, (2) no production under cultural conditions, and (3) production of compounds in culture not produced in nature by the plant from which the culture originated. There have already been reported several instances of production of compounds in vitro, but not in vivo. Several were even new compounds. Gamborg and his colleagues[96] reported the presence of rutacultin in cultures of *Ruta graveolens*, but its absence in the plant from which the culture originated. Allison et al.[3] found three new sesquiterpene lactones in tissue cultures of *Andrographis paniculata* that were not found in the original plant in nature. Heble and his co-workers[116] found 24-methylenecholesterol in tissue cultures of *Holarrhena antidysenterica*, but not in the original plants. In his study of anthraquinone production by cell-suspension cultures of *Morinda citrifolia*, Leistner[189] found lucidin, not hitherto reported to be a constituent of the plant, in the cell cultures as well as minor amounts in the root of the intact plant.

The list of types of compounds already shown to be produced in static or submerged culture is quite impressive (Table 1). However, the possibility of commercial use of this approach is still limited to high-cost items such as certain medicinals or to products under specific conditions, such as in space. Much progress has been made since the first patent was issued to Routien and Nickell in 1956[251] covering a group of substances produced by plant cell and tissue cultures. Until that time, most of the investigative effort was concerned with the isolation of tissues from different plants, from different groups of plants, and from different parts of plants. This thrust has been so successful that we can now say that, with rare exceptions, any tissue from any plant can be isolated and established as a culture.

This isolation stage was followed by a stage emphasizing the use of cultures to investigate problems in various disciplines: pathology, physiology, biochemistry, etc.[248] The next stage was the use of cultures in genetic studies, possible only after the establishment of submerged cell culture,[214] the proof of the totipotency of plant cells,[29] and the development of techniques for the production of protoplasts leading to the differentiation of entire plants from single cells. It should be noted that our knowledge of the factors controlling differentiation is very sparse and is preventing what could be spectacular advances in plant genetics.

Now we have come full circle and, once again, are investigating the synthetic capabilities of plant cell and tissue cultures — this time with a vastly superior background of experience and information. Also, the organizations supporting the research this time around have a better understanding of the potential of this usage and are, thus, able to better evaluate the probable return on their investment.

TABLE 1

List of Substances Reported Produced by Plant Cell and Tissue Cultures In Vitro

Alkaloids	Immunochemicals
Allergens	Insecticides
Amino acids	Insulin-like compounds
Anthraquinones	Latex
Antileukemic agents	Lipids
Antimicrobial agents	Medicinals, miscellaneous
Antitumor agents	Naphthoquinones
Benzoic acid derivatives	Nucleic acids and derivatives
Benzopyrones	Oils, commercial
Benzoquinones	Oils, volatile
Biotransformations	Opiates
Carbohydrates	Organic acids
Cardiac glycosides	Peptides
Chalcones	Perfumes
Condiments	Phenolics
Dianthrones	Pigments
Emulsifiers, food	Polysaccharides
Enzymes (isoenzymes)	Proteins
Enzyme inhibitors	Spices
Ethylene	Steroids, sterols, saponins, sapogenins
Flavanoids	Sugars
Flavors	Sweeteners
Food	Tannins
Fragrances	Terpenes, terpenoids
Furanochromones	Virus inhibitors, plant
Furanocoumarins	Vitamins
Growth regulators, plant	
Hormones	

II. PRODUCTS AND POTENTIAL PRODUCTS

It is interesting that alkaloids represent one of the first classes of useful products to be investigated and also represent one of the largest bodies of work in this area of investigation. Probably the first work showing alkaloid production in culture was that of West and Mika in 1957.[362] They demonstrated synthesis of atropine by belladonna root-callus cultures. Since that time, there have been many publications dealing with the production of a number of types of secondary products and enzymes, as well as the use of plant cell and tissue cultures for the biotransformation from starch of products ranging from steroids to sucrose. That a fantastic number of uses is possible is without doubt. What is questionable is how any could be economically worthwhile. The latter criterion, of course, changes with time and circumstances. With the upswing in interest in higher plant-derived compounds for antitumor activity, this and similar medicinal uses might well lead the way to a "second coming" of plant medicinals in medicine. After all, historically, medicine started with plants as the arsenal of the physician.

I would like to present a summary of the products already reported in the literature as having been produced by plant cell and tissue cultures. There are so many references and so many types of products that, for simplicity of presentation, the list will be given alphabetically, beginning with alkaloids.

A. Alkaloids

Several families of plants are well-known to be rich in alkaloids. Consequently, members of these families (Solanaceae, Apocynaceae, Amaryllidaceae, Leguminosae)

were the first to be studied in vitro to determine if the alkaloids produced in nature were produced in culture and, if so, at what level. A summary of this work is given in tabular form in Table 2.   x

The use of rye callus as host tissue for the inoculation with *Claviceps purpurea* for the production of clavine alkaloids has been investigated by Carew and his colleagues.[42,47]

Interest in the *Vinca (Catharanthus)* alkaloids for the treatment of cancer was discussed by Johnson et al. in 1963.[143] This announcement caused increased activity with *Catharanthus* isolates and the demonstration that many of the alkaloids can be produced in vitro.[328]

As a general rule, alkaloid production is considerably lower under cultural conditions than in nature. It is expected that an intense study of cultural conditions affecting alkaloid production will raise this level. In studying the levels of the alkaloids berberine and jatrorrhizine in *Coptis japonica* cultures, Ikuta et al.[132] found the levels to be low in callus, but the levels returned to normal levels upon regeneration of plantlets from the callus. In working with tissue cultures of *Hyoscyamus niger*, Dhoot and Henshaw[68] could find no clear-cut relationship between organization and alkaloid synthesis except, possibly, for hyoscyamine.

Interest in alkaloids has increased again recently because of the discovery that the giant scarlet poppy (*Papaver bracteatum*) contains significant quantities of thebaine.[8,52,80,81,268,372] Thebaine, through demethylation processes, is readily converted to codeine, the cough suppressant and pain killer that accounts for nearly 90% of the estimated 1500 metric tons of opium legally used in the world annually. Unlike the simple and efficient morphine-to-heroin conversion, the conversion of thebaine to heroin is extremely difficult. There is hope that thebaine from the giant scarlet poppy will offer a solution to the problem of codeine shortages brought on, in part, by the illegal conversion to heroin.

Recent investigations by Kamimura and his colleagues have shown the feasibility of establishing callus and cell cultures from *Papaver bracteatum*.[147] Subsequent work showed that, under standard conditions, the main alkaloids produced were stylopine and protopine, with the amount of thebaine being almost negligible.[148] These workers then showed that the production of thebaine is highly dependent on the appropriate cultural conditions,[149] the hormone level in the medium being of primary importance.

The multitude of problems when introducing a new plant to intensive agriculture, the shortage of codeine, the social and moral advantage of reducing the heroin supply, all suggest intensified study of tissue and cell culture of *Papaver bracteatum* as a method of thebaine production.

B. Allergens

A fertile, but little considered, field of study is that of plant allergen production in vitro. Staba and Shafiee[266,289] recently have started looking into this group of substances, starting with ragweed.

C. Amino Acids and Proteins

Although excellent use has been made of cell and tissue cultures for the study of amino acid biosynthesis by investigators such as Dougall[74-77] and Widholm[364-367], little wrk has been published concerned with the assaying of plant cultures for their amino acid contents or the effect of cultural conditions on the amino acid level.

Warwick and Hildebrandt[354] determined the free amino acids of grape cultures. Weinstein and his co-workers[360,361] studied *Agave toumeyana*, Paul's Scarlet Rose, and *Gingko biloba* cultures. Khanna and Nag[165] studied *Datura metel, D. tatula, Momardica charantia,* and *Trigonella foenum-graecum.* Wickremasinghe et al.[363] found in

TABLE 2

Alkaloid Production by Plant Cell and Tissue Cultures In Vitro

Alkaloid	Plant source	Ref.
Acetonyldihy-drosanguinarine	Papaver somniferum	101
Actinidine	Tecoma stans	70
Ajmalicine (cavincine)	Catharanthus roseus	73, 228, 250, 328, 378
Akuammicine	C. roseus	228, 328
Alstonine (serpentine)	C. roseus	228, 328
Amaryllidaceae alkaloids	Hippeastrum vittatum	313
Anabasine	Nicotiana tabacum	101
Anatabine	N. tabacum	101
Apoatropine	Scopolia parviflora	319
Atropine (DL-hyoscyamine)	Atropa belladonna	169, 362
	Duboisia myoporoides	63, 274
Berberine	Coptis japonica	101, 132
Boschniakine	Tecoma stans	70
Caffeine	Camellia sinensis	221, 222
	Coffea arabica	34, 159
Camptothecin	Camptotheca acuminata	254, 256
Candicine	Trichocereus spachianus	294
Capaurimine	Corydalis pallida	131
β-Carboline alkaloids	Peganum harmala	213
Cathalanceine	Catharanthus roseus	228, 328
Cathindine	C. roseus	328
Cavincidine	C. roseus	228, 328
Cavincine (ajmalicine)	C. roseus	228, 328
Cephalotaxine	Cephalotaxus harringtonia	66
Choline	Medicago sativa	265
Codeine	Papaver somniferum	161
Coptisine	Coptis japonica	101
Cuscohygrine	Hyocyamus niger	68
Desacetyl vindoline	Catharanthus roseus	25
Dihydrosanguin-arine	Papaver somniferum	101
Dihydrositsiri-kine	Catharanthus roseus	228, 328
Ephedrine	Ephedra foliata	238
	E. gerardiana	238
Glycoalkaloids	Solanum xanthocarpum	114
Haemanthamine	Narcissus pseudonarcissus	314

TABLE 2 (continued)

Alkaloid Production by Plant Cell and Tissue Cultures In Vitro

Alkaloid	Plant source	Ref.
Harman	*Phaseolus vulgaris*	346, 347
Harmine	*Peganum harmala*	213
Harringtonine	*Cephalotaxus harringtonia*	66
Homoharringtonine	*C. harringtonia*	66
Homodeoxyharringtonine	*C. harringtonia*	66
Hydroxy-3-methoxy-*N*-methyl-acridone	*Ruta graveolens*	259
Hydroxy-*N*-methylacridone	*R. graveolens*	259
Hyoscine (scopolamine)	*Datura stramonium*	46
	Duboisia myoporoides	63, 274
	Hyocyamus niger	68
Hyoscyamine	*Duboisia myoporoides*	63
	Hyocyamus niger	68
	Scopolia acutangula	379, 380
	S. parviflora	319
Indole alkaloids	*Catharanthus roseus*	63
Isoharringtonine	*Cephalotaxus harringtonia*	66
Jatrorrhizine	*Coptis japonica*	101, 132
Lanceine	*Catharanthus roseus*	228, 328
Lochneridine	*C. roseus*	228, 328
Magnoflorine	*Coptis japonica*	101
Mitraphylline	*Catharanthus roseus*	328
Morphine	*Papaver somniferum*	161
	P. rhoes	161
Narceine	*P. somniferum*	161
Narcotine	*P. somniferum*	161
	P. rhoes	161
Nicotine	*Nicotiana tabacum*	101, 269, 280
Norharman	*Phaseolus vulgaris*	346, 347
Norsanguinarine	*Corydalis pallida*	131
	Macleaya cordata	131
	Papaver somniferum	101, 131
Oxysanguinarine	*P. somniferum*	101
Palmatine	*Coptis japonica*	101
Papaver bracteatum alkaloids	*Papaver bracteatum*	63, 131
Papaverine	*P. somniferum*	161
Perivine (perosine)	*Catharanthus roseus*	328
Perosine (perivine)	*C. roseus*	228, 328

TABLE 2 (continued)

Alkaloid Production by Plant Cell and Tissue Cultures In Vitro

Alkaloid	Plant source	Ref.
Protopine	*Papaver bracteatum*	149
Reserpine	*Alstonia constricta*	41, 44
	Rauwolfia serpentina	207
Rutacridone	*Ruta graveolens*	259
Sanguinarine	*Papaver somniferum*	101, 131
Scopolamine	*Datura stramonium*	46
(hyoscine)	*Duboisia myoporoides*	63, 274
	Scopolia acutangula	379, 380
	S. parviflora	319
Serpentine	*Catharanthus roseus*	72, 73, 228, 250, 328, 378
(alstonine)		
Sitsirikine	*C. roseus*	228, 328
Skytanthine	*Tecoma stans*	70
Solamargine	*Solanum acculeatissimum*	146
Solasodine	*S. acculeatissimum*	146
Solasonine	*S. xanthocarpum*	114
Stachydrine	*Medicago sativa*	265
Stylopine	*Papaver bracteatum*	149
Tecomanine	*Tecoma stans*	70
Thebaine	*Papaver bracteatum*	61, 131, 149, 267
	P. somniferum	161
	P. rhoes	161
Tomatine	*Lycopersicon esculentum*	249
Trigonelline	*Trigonella foenum-graecum*	162
Tropane	*Datura inermis*	317
alkaloids	*D. innoxia*	46, 88, 124, 317
	D. metel	46, 88
	D. meteloides	60
	D. quercifolia	46, 80, 317
	D. stramonium	46, 80, 317
	D. tatula	46, 80, 317
	Scopolia japoniia	88, 317
	S. parviflora	317
Valtropine	*Duboisia myoporoides*	274
Vinca alkaloids	*Catharanthus roseus*	25
Vindoline	*C. roseus*	25
Vindolinine	*C. roseus*	25

cultures of *Acer pseudoplatanus* that free amino acids greatly increased in cultures grown with a limited air supply compared with tissues grown with free access to air. Tobacco and carrot cultures have been studied by Kanamaru et al.[150] and by Lacharme and Netien,[182] respectively. Uddin[338] studied the production of amino acids in suspension cultures of *Ephedra*, and Constabel and colleagues[57] did the same for *Juniperus communis.*

D. Antileukemic and Antitumor Agents

The change from emphasis on synthetic chemicals back to plant and animal extracts as starting points for pharmacologically active compounds has been hastened by the isolation of antileukemic principles from a number of plants. One of the earliest of these was *Camptotheca acuminata* from which the alkaloid camptothecin was isolated and identified.[261,352] Subsequent work by Misawa and his colleagues[204,254,256] demonstrated the production of camptothecin in cell cultures of *Camptotheca acuminata*. More recent work by Kupchan and his co-workers has demonstrated active antileukemic principles in *Croton tiglium*,[180] *Euphorbia esula*,[180] *Maytenus buchananii*,[178,179] and *Maytenus ovatus*.[179,181]

Work on antitumor agents from plants is almost identical to the work on antileukemic agents. Wall[352] found extracts (which later was found to be the alkaloid camptothecin) of *Camptotheca acuminata* to be active against Walker-256 rat carcinosarcoma. The production of camptothecin in cell culture was demonstrated by Misawa and his co-workers.[204,254,256] Kupchan et al. demonstrated activity in extracts of *Maytenus ovatus* against KB nasopharnyx carcinoma[181] and in extracts of *Euphorbia esula* against sarcoma 180, Walker carcinosarcoma, and Lewis lung carcinoma. This, plus previous work by this same group with thalicarpine from the purple meadow rue, elephantin and elephantopin from *Elephantopus elatus*, withaferin A from *Acnistus arborescens*, solamarine from *Solanum dulcamara*, and tetrandrine from *Stephania hernandifolia* and work by the Lilly group with vincaluekoblastine, leurosine, leurocristine, leurosidine, leurosivine, and rovidine from *Vinca (Catharanthus) rosea* and acronycin from the Australian scrub ash (*Acronychia baueri*), emphasize a fertile field for secondary products from plant cell and tissue culture. In fact, this area meets almost all of the requirements discussed in the introduction for successful commercial utilization of plant cultures: (1) important product, (2) scarce product, and (3) potentially expensive product. At least one example has already been produced in vitro, camptothecin.

Recent work by Delfel and Rothfus[66] showed cephalotaxine and its antitumor esters (harringtonine, isoharringtonine, and homoharringtonine) to be produced by callus cultures of *Cephalotaxus harringtonia*. As this tree is slow-growing and available supplies have been essentially exhausted, the potential value of production by tissue and/ or cell cultures is greatly increased. A new alkaloid, homodeoxyharringtonine, was detected in the medium.

E. Antimicrobial Agents

Although antimicrobial agents have been found throughout the plant kingdom,[216] little has been done in studying their occurrence in plant cell and tissue cultures. Mathes[199] tested several dozen selected plant tissue cultures for antimicrobial activity and found most of them to produce some detectable activity. The most active were *Populus grandidentata* and *Salix babylonica*. Both secreted the active material(s) into the medium. Heble et al.[119] showed the production of plumbagin by cultures of *Plumbago zeylanica*. Campbell et al.[40] demonstrated the production of antimicrobial principles which were secreted into the medium by cultures of both lettuce and cauliflower. More recently, Khanna and his co-workers have studied the production of antimicrobial agents from tissue cultures of a number of plants.[166-168] Veliky and Genest showed strong antimicrobial activity in extracts of suspension cultures of *Cannabis sativa*.[348]

F. Benzo-Compounds

1. Benzoic Acid Derivatives

Paupardin[229] found gentisic acid (2,5-dihydroxybenzoic acid), *p*-hydroxybenzoic

TABLE 3

Benzoquinone Production by Plant Cell and Tissue Cultures In Vitro

Compound	Plant source	Ref.
Benzoquinones	*Petunia hybrida*	190
(nonspecified)	*Pimpinella anisum*	190
Plastohydro-	*Hordeum vulgare*	190
quinone	*Nicotiana tabacum*	190
	Petunia hybrida	190
	Pimpinella anisum	190
Plasto-	*Hordeum vulgare*	190
quinone	*Nicotiana tabacum*	190
	Petunia hybrida	190
	Pimpinella anisum	190
Tocopherol	*Hordeum vulgare*	190
	Nicotiana tabacum	190
	Petunia hybrida	190
	Pimpinella anisum	190
Tocoquinone	*Hordeum vulgare*	190
	Nicotiana tabacum	190
	Petunia hybrida	190
	Pimpinella anisum	190
Ubiquinone	*Nicotiana tabacum*	129, 130
	Parthenocissus sp.	227
Vitamin K	*Hordeum vulgare*	190
	Nicotiana tabacum	190
	Petunia hybrida	190
	Pimpinella anisum	190

acid, and vanillic acid (4-hydroxy-3-methoxy benzoic acid) to be produced by tuber cultures of *Helianthus tuberosus*.

2. Benzopyrones

Routien and Nickell[251] showed that coumarin is produced by cultures of *Melilotus officinalis* under submerged conditions. Furuya and Ikuta[89] showed the production of maackiain and pterocappin in callus cultures of *Sophora angustifolia*.

3. Benzoquinones

Ubiquinone has been isolated from cultured cells of tobacco[130] and callus cultures of *Parthenocissus* sp.[227] The other investigation of benzoquinones occurring in a number of plant cultures (shown in Table 3) was carried out by Lichtenthaler and Straub.[190]

G. Carbohydrates

1. Simple Sugars

Strangely enough, there are few reports on sugars in plant cultures. Most of the reports have been concerned with the utilization of sugars as energy sources. Durzan et al.[79] reported on sugars in white-spruce cultures as did Weinstein and his colleagues for *Agave toumeyana*[360] and Paul's Scarlet Rose.[361]

2. Polysaccharides

A number of investigators have reported the production of extracellular polysaccharides by a number of plant cultures. These include English sycamore,[6,15] bush bean,[195] red kidney bean,[113] and tobacco.[152,153] Hanower[112] reported the formation of polyfructosans in *Helianthus annuus* cultures.

H. Cardiac Glycosides and Other Cardioactive Substances

The production of cardiac glycosides by tissue cultures of varies species of *Digitalis* has been reported by a number of investigators.[33,233,284,286,288,300] For example, Medora and his co-workers[201] reported the production of cardioactive substances by callus tissue derived from *Digitalis mertonensis.*

I. Enzymes and Inhibitors

Most of the work concerning the presence or absence of enzymes in plant cell and tissue cultures has been conducted for the study of biochemical pathways, control systems, biotransformations, and the like. The studies specifically aimed at determining the production of a given enzyme(s) and/or the amount of that production are presented in Table 4.

Misawa and his colleagues[204,255] demonstrated the production of "broad specificity" proteinase inhibitors by cultures of *Scopolia japonica.*

J. Ethylene

Gamborg and La Rue in 1968[105] showed the production of ethylene by tissue cultures of mung bean, soybean, rose, flax, wheat, rice, and several other plants. Their results suggested that ethylene formation depends not only on the kind of plant from which the cells originated, but also on the physiological state of the cells. Later, Gamborg and his colleagues[106] in working with cultures of rose and *Ruta graveolens* showed a 2,4-D stimulation of ethylene production by the *Ruta* culture, but not by the rose.

K. Foods, Flavors, and Sweeteners

Because of the low value of food products in general, relatively little work has been carried out with this objective in mind, except that supported by space research. Tulecke and Nickell in 1959[335,336] reported the first "large scale" (at that time) production of plant-cell material under submerged cultural conditions. Their work was with holly, rose, *Lolium*, and ginkgo tissues. Bryne and Koch in 1961[32] worked with a number of plant cultures including those from tomato, potato, rose, grape, and tobacco, but their large scale emphasis was on carrot cultures. Fukami and Hildebrandt in 1967[87] worked with carrot, endive, lettuce, parsley, and spinach tissues.

Freeman et al.[65,84] reported that undifferentiated callus cultures of onion contained only very small amounts of its flavor components. This was due to the absence of precursors, not the enzyme, alliinase. Tissues which had differentiated roots, on the other hand, produced flavor intensities approaching those of fresh onions. Two groups of investigators have demonstrated flavor production by cultures of licorice.[324,370]

The continually increasing interest in nonnutritive sweeteners[11] and the shift in preference away from synthetic chemicals to natural products has stimulated the search for new types of sweeteners from plants. Examples include (1) a series of intensely sweet-tasting dihydrochalcones developed by USDA investigators which can be derived from flavone glycosides that occur naturally in citrus peels,[125] (2) miraculin (miralin) from the fruits of *Synsepalum dulcificum* (*Richardella dulcifica*),[236,342] (3) stevioside from *Stevia rebaudiana*,[230] (4) thaumatin (monellin) from *Thaumatococcus daniellii*,[210,343] (5) 8,9-epoxyperillartine from *Perilla nankinensis*, and (6) the hydrofluorene diterpenoids from pine-tree rosin.[321,322] The occurrence of glycyrrhizin in licorice has already been discussed.[324]

Because of the scarcity of many of these plant species and the numerous problems of domesticating a "wild" species, the potential for the tissue- and cell-culture approach becomes apparent. Cultures of *Stevia rebandiana* have been established to study steviol biosynthesis.[111] Berlin and Barz reported the presence of trihydrochalcone in cell cultures of *Phaseolus aureus.*[24]

TABLE 4

Enzyme Production by Plant Cell and Tissue Cultures in Vitro

Enzyme	Plant source	Ref.
Alanine aminopeptidase	*Atropa belladonna*	273
Amylases	*Cupressus funebris*	308
	Nicotiana tabacum	138, 139, 150, 271
	Oryza sativa	253
	Phaseolus vulgaris	349
	Rosa multiflora	308
	Rumex acetosa	27, 28 218
	Saccharum spp.	196, 219
	Zea mays	308
Arginase	*Datura stramonium*	141
Ascorbic acid oxidase	*Lycopersicon esculentum*	281, 282, 283
Catalase	*Helianthus tuberosus*	104
	Parthenocissus tricuspidata	104
	Scorzonera hispanica	104
	Vitis vinifera	104
Catechol oxidase	*Pyrus malus*	351
Chlorogenic acid oxidase	*Lycopersicon esculentum*	283
Coumarate:CoA ligase	*Petroselinum hortense*	174
Esterase	*Datura stramonium*	141
Flavanone synthase	*Happlopappus gracilis*	257
Glucanase	*Capsicum frutescens*	194
	Daucus carota	194
	Lactuca sativa	194
Glucose phosphate cycloaldolase	*Acer pseudoplatanus*	193
Glucose phosphate dehydrogenase	*Nicotiana tabacum*	357
Glutamate dehydrogenase	*N. tabacum*	355
Glutamate; oxaloacetate transaminase	*Atropa belladonna*	273
Glutamate synthetase	*Nicotiana tabacum*	356
Glutamine synthetase	*N. tabacum*	356
Glyceraldehyde phosphate dehydrogenase	*N. tabacum*	358
Hexokinase	*N. tabacum*	358

TABLE 4 (continued)

Enzyme Production by Plant Cell and Tissue Cultures in Vitro

Enzyme	Plant source	Ref.
Indoleacetic acid oxidase	*Lycopersicon esculentum*	308
	Nicotiana tabacum	308
	Pelargonium sp.	308
	Zea mays	308
Invertase	*Cupressus funebris*	307
	Ephedra sp.	307
	Libocedrus decurrens	307
	Nicotiana tabacum	307
	Pyrus communis	307
	Rosa multiflora	307
	Zea mays	307
Isocitrate dehydrogenase	*Pinus elliotii*	62
Lysopine dehydrogenase	*Nicotiana tabacum*	224
Malic enzyme	*N. tabacum*	357
Myrosinase	*Armoracia lapathifolia*	170
	Eruca sativa	170
	Iberis sempervirens	170
	Nasturtium officinale	170
	Reseda luteola	170
	Sinapis alba	170
	Tropaeolum majus	170
Nitrite reductase	*Nicotiana tabacum*	355
Peroxidase	*Arachis hypogaea*	344, 350
	Atropa belladonna	273
	Lycopersicon esculentum	308
	Nicotiana tabacum	231, 257, 270, 308
	Phaseolus vulgaris	349
	Rosa multiflora	308
	Zea mays	308
Phenylalanine ammonia lyase	*Citrus paradici*	330
	Trigonella foenum-graecum	67
Phosphatase (acid)	*Atropa belladonna*	273
	Cupressus funebris	308
	Lycopersicon esculentum	308
	Nicotiana tabacum	308
	Pelargonium sp.	308
	Rosa multiflora	308
	Zea mays	308
Phosphodiesterase	*Nicotiana tabacum*	271
	Vinca rosea	204, 339
Phosphogluconate dehydrogenase	*Nicotiana tabacum*	337

TABLE 4 (continued)

Enzyme Production by Plant Cell and Tissue Cultures in Vitro

Enzyme	Plant source	Ref.
Polyphenoloxid-ase	*Picea glauca*	242
Proteolytic enzymes	*Nicotiana tabacum*	102, 103
Pyruvate kinase	*Pinus elliotii*	62
Ribonuclease	*Atropa belladonna*	273
RNA polymerase	*Nicotiana tabacum*	264
Transaminase	*Datura stramonium*	141
Trytophan synthetase	*Parthenocissus tricuspidatus*	173
Tyrosine ammonium lyase	*Arachis hypogaea* *Lycopersicon esculentum*	240 281

L. Fragrances and Perfumes

Jones[144] has shown that cultures of Lady Seton Rose were able to metabolize geraniol to geranial, neral, nerol, and citronellol.

M. Furano-Compounds

Visnagin was shown to be produced by cultures of *Ammi visnaga* by Staba and his co-workers.[50,154,155] Furanochromones are found only in the genus *Ammi* (Umbelliferae) and the genus *Eranthus* (Ranunculaceae) and are used medicinally for the treatment of coronary thrombosis and angina pectoris and to increase coronary blood flow. Visnagin is similar structurally and pharmacologically to khellin and khellol.

Gamborg et al.[106] found that cultures of *Ruta graveolens* produced psoralen, anthotoxin, bergapten, isopimpinellin, and rutamarin. These are furanocoumarins produced in nature by *Ruta graveolens*. They also found that the cultures produced rutacultin, but that the plant does not.

N. Growth Regulators, Plant

The only report of the production of plant growth regulators by tissue cultures is that of Lin and Mathes[191] working with *Lemna*. Not included in this consideration is the production of indoleacetic acid, nor of gibberellic acid-like materials which will be discussed under hormones below.

Nickell[215] demonstrated the production of gibberellin-like substances by cultures from a number of plants.

O. Immunochemicals

The immunochemical cross-reactivity of plant tissue-culture antigens was reported by Wu et al.[371] This seems to be the only report of research in this field.

P. Latex

One of the earliest studies concerned with the production of secondary products by plant tissue cultures was that of Arreguin and Bonner in 1950.[5] They showed that stem-callus cultures of guayule (*Parthenium argentatum*) would synthesize rubber when leaf extracts of guayule were added to the culture medium. Later work showed that acetate, acetone, and β-methylcrotonic acid could duplicate the effect of the leaf extracts.

Q. Lipids

Song and Tattrie[279] studied the lipid composition of morning-glory cell suspensions. Radwan et al.[237] conducted similar studies with callus and suspension cultures of *Brassica napus, Hydnocarpus anthelminthica, Artemisia absinthium,* and *Petroselinum hortense.* Other lipid studies with a variety of cultures have been reported by Staba et al.[290] and Tattrie and Veliky.[327]

R. Medicinals, Miscellaneous

Misawa and colleagues[204,205] demonstrated the production of a potent inhibitory agent against human plasmin by callus tissue of *Scopolia japonica.* Plasmin is a fibrinolytic proteinase and its overproduction causes a number of disorders.

The precise pharmacological effects of ginseng and its constituents are still not well defined, but there has been considerable traditional use of ginseng roots and extracts in the Orient for centuries. In more recent times, there has been considerable activity in the field of plant cell and tissue culture to establish cultures of the various ginseng species and to determine their production of active materials by investigators in Russia,[37,38,235,276-278] Japan,[90,91,99-101,171] Korea,[186] Germany,[203] and the U.S.[140]

S. Monofluorocarbon Compounds

Peters and Shorthouse[232] demonstrated that cell cultures of *Glycine max* can convert inorganic fluoride to fluoroacetate and fluorocitrate, a trait previously known to be an inherent property of the soybean plant.

T. Nucleic Acids and Derivatives

Other than the total RNA and DNA content of tissue and cell cultures as part of other investigations, little work has been done in studying the actual production of nucleic acids or their derivatives. Chen and Hall[49] studied the biosynthesis of N^6-(Δ^2-isopentenyl) adenosine in the transfer RNA of cultured tobacco-pith tissue. Keller et al.[159] reported on the synthesis of caffeine in tissue cultures of *Coffea arabica* (coffee). Ogutaga and Northcote reported on caffeine production in tissue cultures of *Camellia sinensis* (tea).[221,222]

The changing nucleotide pattern of *Acer pseudoplatanus* cells in suspension culture was studied by Brown and Short.[31]

U. Oils

1. Commercial

Jones,[144,145] in his discussion of the potential use of plant tissue and cell culture approaches for the commercial production of palm oil, gives a good summary of the situation as it currently exists. He believes that large-scale production of plant oils by cell culture is "not a practical proposition because of the limited output and high costs involved, and these are fundamental rather than technical problems. Major production of vegetable oils is, and will remain, an agricultural process."

2. Volatile

The production of volatile oils in tissue culture has been studied in *Mentha piperita* by Bricout and Paupardin,[30] in *Ruta graveolens* by Corduan and Reinhard,[61] in *Ocimum basilicum* by Lang and Horster,[185] and in *Matricaria chamomilla* by Reichling and Becker.[241]

V. Organic Acids

Organic-acid contents of the tissue and cell cultures of a number of plants have been determined. The results are given in Table 5.

TABLE 5

Organic Acid Production by Plant Cell and Tissue Cultures
in Vitro

Acid	Plant source	Ref.
Caffeic	*Helianthus tuberosus*	229
	Tecoma stans	71
Chlorogenic	*Crataegus monogyna*	260
	Helianthus tuberosus	229
	Tecoma stans	71
Cinnamic	*Coffea arabica*	34
	Crataegus monogyna	260
	Daucus carota	182, 310
Citric	*Agave toumeyana*	360
	Paul's Scarlet Rose	361
Coumaric	*Helianthus tuberosus*	229
	Tecoma stans	71
Ferulic	*Helianthus tuberosus*	229
	Tecoma stans	71
Fumaric	*Agave toumeyana*	360
	Paul's Scarlet Rose	361
Glyceric	*Paul's Scarlet Rose*	361
α-Ketoglutaric	*Paul's Scarlet Rose*	361
Malic	*Agave toumeyana*	360
	Paul's Scarlet Rose	361
Malonic	*Paul's Scarlet Rose*	361
Melilotic	*Melilotus officinalis*	251
Oxalic	*Rumex acetosa*	251
Quinic	*Paul's Scarlet Rose*	361
Shikimic	*Paul's Scarlet Rose*	361
Sinapic	*Tecoma stans*	71
Succinic	*Agave toumeyana*	360
	Paul's Scarlet Rose	361
Vanillic	*Tecoma stans*	71

W. Phenolics

Surprisingly little has been published concerning the phenolic content of plant cultures. Reports are available concerning *Perilla*,[127] *Nicotiana tabacum*,[23] cocoa,[137] and Paul's Scarlet Rose.[64] Forrest[83] studied the polyphenol metabolism of tissue cultures derived from the tea plant (*Camellia sinensis*) and found that it was not characteristic of the parent plant. Recently, Phillips and Henshaw,[234] working with cell cultures of *Acer pseudoplatanus*, showed that protein synthesis acts as the principal rate-limiting step in phenolics synthesis by means of a competition for common metabolites. Zenk and co-workers[377] found both sucrose concentration (7%) and the addition of the precursor L-phenylalanine increased the yield of rosmarinic acid in cell-suspension cultures of *Coleus blumei*. The highest concentration exceeded the concentration reached in the differentiated plant by a factor of five.

Suzuki et al.[316] reported the isolation of two polyphenols (hydrangenol and umbelliferone) from cultured cells of *Hydrangea macrophylla* leaves. The occurrence of phenolic compounds linked to putrescine has been studied in tobacco cultures by Mizusaki and his colleagues.[209] Recent work by Subbaiah and Mehta[309] with *Datura metel* callus cultures suggests that polyphenol synthesis can be controlled by the auxin concentration in the medium.

X. Pigments

Pigment production in plant cell and tissue cultures has been extensively studied, with the most emphasis on chlorophyll, carotenoids, and anthocyanins (Table 6).

TABLE 6

Pigment Production by Plant Cell and Tissue Cultures in Vitro

Compound	Plant source	Ref.
Acetylshikonin	*Lithospermum erythrorhizon*	208
Alizarin	*Galium mollugo*	11
Anthocyanins	*Crataegus monogyna*	260
(nonspecified)	*C. oxyacantha*	260
	Daucus carota	2, 128, 310
	Ginkgo biloba	260
	Haplopappus gracilis	4, 58, 86 106, 183 243
	Helianthus tuberosus	128
	Linum usitatissimum	128
	Parthenocissus tricuspidata	292
	Paul's Scarlet Rose	64
	Urginea maritima	272
	Vitis vinifera	275
	Zea mays	306
Apigenin	*Glycine max*	110
Aureoxanthin	*Paul's Scarlet Rose*	108
	Ruta graveolens	63
α-Carotene	*R. graveolens*	63
β-Carotene	*Daucus carota*	311
	Plumbago zeylanica	119
	Ruta graveolens	63
Carotenoids	*Hordeum vulgare*	190
(nonspecified)	*Nicotiana tabacum*	190
	Petunia hydrida	190
Chlorophyll	*Cichorum endivia*	87, 345
	Daucus carota	87, 345
	Hordeum vulgare	190
	Lactuca sativa	87, 345
	Lycopersicon esculentum	345
	Mentha arvensis	69
	Nicotiana tabacum	190
	Petroselinum hortense	87, 345
	Petunia hydrida	190
	Pimpinella anisum	190
	Rosa sp.	345
	Rumex acetosa	35, 220
	Ruta graveolens	63
	Spinacia oleracea	87
Cryptoxanthin	*Ruta graveolens*	61
Daidzein	*Phaseolus aureus*	24
Deoxyshikonin	*Lithospermum erythrorhizon*	208
Digitolutein	*Digitalis lanata*	92
Dimethylacryl-shikonin	*Lithospernum erythrorhizon*	208
Flavanoid	*Citrus limon*	88

TABLE 6 (continued)

Pigment Production by Plant Cell and Tissue Cultures in Vitro

Compound	Plant source	Ref.
(nonspecified)	Glycine max	88
	Prunus sp.	82
	Silybum marianum	13
Formononetin	Cicer arietinum	?
Hydroxydigitolu-tein	Digitalis lanata	92
Hydroxyisoral-erylshikonin	Lithospermum erythrorhizon	208
Hydroxy-4'-methoxy-isoflavone	Cicer arietinum	?
Leucoanthocyan-ins	Acer pseudoplatanus	107
	Cassia tora	320
(nonspecified)	Juniperus communis	55
	Lithospermum erythrozhizon	318
Lucidin	Galium mollugo	11
Lutein	Ruta graveolens	63
Luteoxanthin	R. graveolens	63
Lycopene	Daucus carota	311
Mollugin	Galium mollugo	11
Neoxanthin	Ruta graveolens	63
Purpurin	Galium mollugo	11
Purpurincar-boxylic acid	G. mollugo	11
Rutin	Stevia rebaudiana	315
Shikonin	Lithospermum erythrorhizon	208
Violaxanthin	Ruta graveolens	63
Zeaxanthin	R. graveolens	63

1. Anthraquinones

Other than the studies of *Cassia tora* by Tabata et al.[320] and *Cassia angustifolia* by Friedrich and Baier[10,85] showing the production of chrysophanol, emodin, and physcion, most of the work concerning anthraquinones in plant cultures has been with *Morinda citrifolia*. Zenk and his colleagues[376] found no anthraquinones to be present in the callus cultures when 2,4-D was used as the auxin in the medium, as opposed to their presence when NAA was the auxin used. Leistner[189] found lucidin, an anthraquinone previously not reported to occur in *Morinda citrifolia*, in the cell cultures, as well as minor amounts in the root of the intact plant. Other anthraquinones isolated and identified by Leistner were alizarin, moridone, nordamnacanthal, and rubiadin. droxy-4'-methoxy-isoflavone), and *Stevia rebaudiana* rutin).[315] Furuya and co-work-

2. Flavanoids and Chalcones

Flavanoid production by plant cultures has been shown in soybean, lemon,[88] and *Prunus*.[82] Production of specific flavanoids has been shown for soybean (apigenin),[110] *Phaseolus aureus* (the isoflavone diadzein),[24] *Cicer arietinum* (formononetin, 7-hydroxy-4'-methoxy-isoflavone), and *Stevia rebaudiana* (rutin).[315] Furuya and co-workers[97] isolated a new chalcone named echinatin from the tissue culture of *Glycerrhiza echinata*.

3. Tannins

Tannins have been reported in cultures of *Picea glauca*[45.79] and of *Juniperus communis.*[55.56]

Y. Steroids, Sterols, Saponins, Sapogenins

By far the greatest effort in the study of secondary products, their production, their metabolism, and their conversion has been devoted to the steroids, sterols, saponins, and sapogenins. The scope of these efforts is convincingly shown in Table 7.

Z. Terpenes and Terpenoids

Monoterpenes have been reported in cultures of *Perilla.*[312] Phytol, the diterpenoid alcohol component of chlorophyll, has been studied in cultures of *Kalanchoe crenata.*[295] Two diterpenoid alcohols, cafestol and kahweol, which are major components of coffee-bean-oil unsaponifiables, have been shown to be present in cell cultures of *Coffea arabica.*[341] Triterpenes have been reported in cultures of *Solanum xanthocarpum.*[117] The triterpene, aroundoin, has been reported in rice cultures.[373]

The occurrence of maslinic and 3-epimaslinic acids has been reported for cultures of *Isodon japonicus,*[331] while amyrine and ursolic and oleanolic acids have been found in cultures of *Tecoma stans.*[71]

Three new sesquiterpene lactones not found in the original plant have been reported in tissue cultures of *Andrographis paniculata.*[3.36] Terpenoids in Paul's Scarlet Rose cultures have been reported by Goodwin and Williams.[108.368] Similarly, terpenoids have been reported in cultures of pumpkin by Yanagawa et al.[374]

A'. Virus Inhibitors, Plant

Misawa and his colleagues[204.206] have reported the production of plant-virus inhibitors by suspension cultures of pokeweed (*Phytolacca americana*).

B'. Vitamins

Surprisingly, few reports on the production of vitamins by plant cell and tissue cultures are available. Routien and Nickell[251] reported ascorbic acid production by tobacco cultures, and Skoog and his co-workers have reported thiamin synthesis in the same tissue.[78]

III. SUMMARY

The field of plant cell and tissue culture has been developed sufficiently during the past 2 decades so that it is now ready to be utilized for its productive capabilities for synthesis of secondary products in vitro. Emphasis in recent years has been on its utilization for metabolic and genetic studies. Advances connected with these studies have been of considerable help in aiding our understanding of, and ability to overcome, previous impediments to exploitation of the potential productive capacity of plant materials in vitro.

Economics in most instances will dictate the first type(s) of materials to be produced for commercial purposes. These will most probably be medicinals of one kind or another. Among the most obvious are antileukemic and antitumor agents in particular, opiates, and alkaloids and steroids in general. Of nonmedical products, the most probable will be in the areas of nonnutritive sweeteners, perfumes, and flavors.

As new and important plant products are discovered in wild, rare, and/or difficult-to-grow plants, the tissue and cell culture approach will become increasingly important. The fact that little use of techniques common to the related field of "fermenta-

TABLE 7

Steroid, Sterol, Sapogenin, and Saponin Production by
Plant Cell and Tissue Cultures in Vitro

Compound	Plant source	Ref.
Amyrin	Corchorus olitorius	326
	Lindera strychnifolia	333
	Oryza sativa	373
	Paul's Scarlet Rose	368
	Tylophora indica	16
	Withania somnifera	375
Brassicasterol	Brassica napus	237
Campesterol	Artemisia absinthium	237
	Brassica napus	237
	Coffea arabica	341
	Digitalis lanata	122
	Dioscorea deltoidea	157, 198, 305
	D. tokora	334
	Hydnocarpus anthelminthica	237
	Ipomoea sp.	279
	Nicotiana tabacum	18, 20, 101
	Petroselinum hortense	237
	Yucca glauca	302
Cholesterol	Digitalis lanata	122
	Dioscorea deltoidea	157, 198
	D. tokoro	334
	Holarrhena antidysenterica	116, 120, 121
	Momordica charantia	164
	Nicotiana tabacum	101
	Sesamum indicum	135
	Yucca glauca	302
Citrostadienol	Nicotiana tabacum	20
Cycloartenol	Digitalis lanata	122
	Nicotiana tabacum	18, 19, 20, 101, 236
Cycloeucalenol	N. tabacum	17, 18
Diosgenin	Dioscorea composita	202, 287
	D. deltoidea	48, 156, 157, 197, 202, 304, 305
	D. floribunda	160, 202, 287
	D. spiculiflora	202, 287
	D. tokoro	334
	Momordica charantia	164
	Solanum aviculare	160
	S. elaeagnifolium	160
	S. laciniatum	340
	S. nigrum	160
	S. xanthocarpum	115, 118
	Trigonella occulta	136

TABLE 7 (continued)

Steroid, Sterol, Sapogenin, and Saponin Production by
Plant Cell and Tissue Cultures in Vitro

Compound	Plant source	Ref.
	D. tokoro	334
	Euphorbia cyparissias	188
	E. esula	188
	Holarrhena antidysenterica	116, 120
	Hydnocarpus anthelminthica	237
	Ipomoea sp.	279
	Lindera strychnifolia	333
	Momordica charantia	164
	Morus alba	177
	Nicotiana tabacum	18, 20
		101
	Oryza sativa	373
	Paul's Scarlet Rose	
	Petroselinum hortense	237
	Sesamum indicum	135
	Solanum xanthocarpum	115, 118
	Tecoma stans	71
	Trigonella occulta	136
	T. foenum-graecum	163
	Tylophora indica	16
	Withania somnifera	375
	Yucca glauca	302, 303
Solasodine	*Solanum acculeatissimum*	146
	S. aviculare	160
	S. melongena	134
	S. nigrum	160
Solasonine	*S. xanthocarpum*	114, 118
Spinasterol	*Cucurbita maxima*	374
Squalene	*Nicotiana tabacum*	21
Stigmasterol	*Artemisia absinthium*	237
	Brassica napus	237
	Coffea arabica	341
	Corchorus olitorius	326
	Digitalis lanata	122
	Dioscorea deltoidea	198, 305
	D. tokoro	334
	Holarrhena antidysenterica	116, 120
	Hydnocarpus anthelminthica	237
	Ipomoea sp.	279
	Lindera strychnifolia	333
	Momordia charantia	164
	Nicotiana tabacum	18, 20
		101
	Oryza sativa	373
	Paul's Scarlet Rose	108, 368
	Petroselinum hortense	237
	Sesamum indicum	135
	Trigonella foenum-graecum	163

TABLE 7 (continued)

Steroid, Sterol, Sapogenin, and Saponin Production by Plant Cell and Tissue Cultures in Vitro

Compound	Plant source	Ref.
	T. foenum-graecum	160, 163
Ergost-4-ene-3-one	*Glycine max*	359
	Stephania cepharantha	285
Ergost-4-ene-3,6-dione	*Glycine max*	359
	Stephania cepharantha	133
24-Ethylidene cholesterol	*Withania somnifera*	375
Gitogenin	*Trigonella occulta*	136
	T. foenum-graecum	163
	Yucca glauca	302, 303
28-Isofucosterol	*Digitalis lanata*	122
	Holarrhena antidysenterica	120
Lanesterol	*Dioscorea composita*	202
	Momordica charantia	164
	Paul's Scarlet Rose	108, 368
	Sesamum indicum	135
Manogenin	*Yucca glauca*	303
24-Methylcholesterol	*Holarrhena antidysenterica*	116, 120
	Withania somnifera	375
24-Methyl-cholest-7-en-3 β-ol	*Nicotiana tabacum*	18
24-Methylene-cycloartanol	*Digitalis lanata*	122
	Nicotiana tabacum	18, 19, 20, 101
24-Methyl-enelophenol	*N. tabacum*	18
28-Norcitrostandi-enol	*N. tabacum*	20
Oleanolic acid	*Isodon japonicus*	331
	Panax ginseng	100, 101
Obtusifoliol	*Nicotiana tabacum*	17, 18
Panaxadiol	*Panax ginseng*	101, 140
Panaxatriol	*P. ginseng*	90, 91, 100, 101
5 α-Pregnan-3β, ol-20-one	*Dioscorea deltoidea*	298
5 α-Pregnan-3β-20 β-diol	*D. deltoidea*	298
Protokoronin	*D. tokoro*	332
Sitosterol	*Apocynum cannabinum*	187
	Artemisia absinthium	279
	Brassica napus	237
	Coffea arabica	341
	Corchorus olitorius	326
	Digitalis lanata	122
	Dioscorea deltoidea	157, 198, 305

TABLE 7 (continued)

Steroid, Sterol, Sapogenin, and Saponin Production by
Plant Cell and Tissue Cultures in Vitro

Compound	Plant source	Ref.
	Tylophora indica	16
	Withania somnifera	375
	Yucca glauca	302, 303
Stigmasta-4,22-	*Glycine max*	359
diene-3-one	*Stephania cepharantha*	133
Stigmasta-4,22-	*Glycine max*	359
diene-3,6-dione	*Stephania cepharantha*	133
Stigmasta-7,22,25-triene-3 β ol	*Cucurbita maxima*	374
Stigmast-4-ene-3-	*Glycine max*	359
one	*Stephania cepharantha*	133
Stigmast-4-ene-	*Glycine max*	359
3,6-dione	*Stephania cepharantha*	133
Tigogenin	*Trigonella occulta*	136
	T. foenum-graecum	163
Tokorogenin	*Dioscorea tokoro*	334
Yonogenin	*D. tokoro*	334

tion'' for increased production of desirable products — mutation, strain selection, and process development to name a few — has been made reinforces the view for optimism concerning the potential for the future of plant cell and tissue culture for productive purposes.

REFERENCES

1. **Acton, E. M., Leaffer, M. A., and Stone, H.,** 8,9 Epoxy Perillartine Sweeteners, U. S. Patent 3,699,132, 1970.
2. **Alfermann, A. W., Merz, D., and Reinhard, E.,** Induktion der Anthocyanbiosynthese in Kalluskulturen von *Daucus carota, Planta Med.,* Suppl., 70, 1975.
3. **Allison, A. J., Butcher, D. N., Connolly, J. D., and Overton, K. H.,** Paniculides A, B and C, bisabolenoid lactones from tissue cultures of *Adrographis paniculatea, Chem. Commun.,* 23, 1493, 1968.
4. **Ardenne, R.,** Bestimmung der Natur der Anthocyane in Gewebekulturen von *Haplopappus gracilis, Z. Naturforsch.,* 20, 186, 1965.
5. **Arreguin, B. and Bonner, J.,** The biochemistry of rubber formation in guayule. II. Rubber formation aseptic tissue cultures, *Arch. Biochem.,* 26, 178, 1950.
6. **Aspinall, G. O., Molloy, J. A., and Craig, J. W. T.,** Extracellular polysaccharides from suspension-cultured sycamore cells, *Can. J. Biochem.,* 47, 1063, 1969.
7. **Austin, D. J. and Brown, S. A.,** Furanocoumarin biosynthesis in *Ruta graveolens* cell cultures, *Phytochemistry,* 12, 1657, 1973.
8. **Aynehchi, Y. and Jaffarian, S.,** Determination of thebaine in various parts of *Papaver bracteatum* Lindl, during the growing season, *Lloydia,* 36, 427, 1973.
9. **Babcock, P. A. and Carew, D. P.,** Tissue culture of the Apocynaceae. I. Culture requirements and alkaloid analysis, *Lloydia,* 25, 209, 1962.
10. **Baier, S. and Friedrich, H.,** Anthracen-Derivate in Kalluskulturen aus Senna, *Naturwissenschaften,* 56, 548, 1970.

11. **Bauch, H. J. and Leistner, E.**, Aromatic metabolites in cell suspension cultures of *Galium mollugo* L., *Planta Med.*, 33, 105, 1978.

12. **Beck, K. M.**, Sweeteners, non-nutritive, *Encyl. Chem. Technol.*, 19, 593, 1969.

13. **Becker, H. and Schrall, R.**, Callus — und Suspensions-kulturen von *Silybun marianum*. I. Mitteilung: Anlage und Wachstum der Callus — und Suspensionskulturen und Untersuchung auf flavonoide Inhaltsstoffe, *Planta Med.*, 31, 185, 1977.

14. **Becker, G. E., Hui, P. A., and Alberscheim, P.**, Synthesis of extracellular polysaccharide by suspensions of *Acer psuedoplatanus* cells, *Plant Physiol.*, 39, 913, 1964.

15. **Becker, H.**, Stoffproduktion in pflanzlichen Callus — und Organkulturen, *Mitt. Dtsch. Pharm. Ges.*, 39, 273, 1969.

16. **Benjamin, D. B. and Mulchandani, N. B.**, Biosynthesis of secondary constituents in tissue cultures of *Tylophora indica*, *Planta Med.*, 23, 394, 1973.

17. **Benveniste, P.**, La biosynthesis des sterols dans les tissus de tabac cultures *in vitro*. Mise en evidence du cycloeucalenol et de l'obtusifoliol, *Phytochemistry*, 7, 951, 1968.

18. **Benveniste, P., Hewlins, M. J. E., and Fritig, B.**, La biosynthese des sterols dan les tissus de tabac cultures *in vitro*. Cinetique de formation des sterols et de leurs precurseurs, *Eur. J. Biochem.*, 9, 526, 1969.

19. **Benveniste, P., Hirth, L., and Ourisson, G.**, La biosynthese des sterols dans les cultures de tissus de tabac. Identification du cycloartenol et du methylene-24 cycolartenol, *C. R. Acad. Sci.*, 259, 2284, 1964.

20. **Benveniste, P., Hirth, L., and Ourisson, G.**, La biosynthese des sterols dans les tissus de tabac cultives *in vitro*. I. Isolement de sterols et de triterpenes, *Phytochemistry*, 5, 31, 1966.

21. **Benveniste, P., Durr, A., Hirth, L., and Ourisson, G.**, La biosynthese des sterols dans les cultures de tissus de tabac. Mise en evidence de substances a marquage rapide et identification du squalene, *C. R. Acad. Sci.*, 259, 2005, 1964.

22. **Ben-Yehoshua, S. and Conn, E. E.**, Biosynthesis of prunasin, the cyanogenic glucoside of peach, *Plant Physiol.*, 39, 331, 1964.

23. **Bergmann, L., Thies, W., and Erdelsky, K.**, Das Vorkommen von Glucosaminestern der Hydroxyzimtsauren in Gewebekulturen von *Nicotiana tabacum*, *Z. Naturforsch.*, 20, 1297, 1965.

24. **Berlin, J. and Barz, W.**, Stoffwechsel von Isoflavonen und Cumöstanen in Zell-und Callussuspensionkulturen von *Phaseolus aureus* Roxb., *Planta*, 98, 300, 1971.

25. **Boder, G. B., Gorman, M., Johnson, I. S., and Simpson, P. J.**, Tissue culture studies of *Catharanthus roseus* crown gall, *Lloydia*, 328, 1964.

26. **Boulanger, D., Bailey, B. K., and Steck, W.**, Formation of edulinine and furoquinoline alkaloids from quinoline derivatives by cell suspension cultures of *Ruta graveolens*, *Phytochemistry*, 12, 2399, 2405, 1973.

27. **Brakke, M. K. and Nickell, L. G.**, Secretion of α-amylase by *Rumex* virus tumors *in vitro*. Properties and assay, *Arch. Biochem. Biophys.*, 32, 28, 1951.

28. **Brakke, M. K. and Nickell, L. G.**, Secretion of an enzyme from intact cells of a higher plant, *Ann. Biol.*, 31, 215, 1955.

29. **Braun, A. C.**, A demonstration of the recovery of the crowngall tumor cell with the use of complex tumors of single-cell origin, *Proc. Natl. Acad. Sci., U.S.A.*, 45, 932, 1959.

30. **Bricout, J. and Paupardin, C.**, The composition of the essential oil of *Mentha piperita* L. cultured *in vitro*: influence of several factors on its synthesis, *C. R. Acad. Sci. Ser.D*, 281, 383, 1975.

31. **Brown, E. G. and Short, K. C.**, The changing nucleotide pattern of sycamore cells during culture in suspension, *Phytomchemistry*, 8, 1365, 1969.

32. **Bryne, A. F. and Koch, R. B.**, Food production by submerged culture of plant tissue cells, *Science*, 135, 215, 1961.

33. **Büchner, S. A. and Staba, E. J.**, Preliminary examination of *Digitalis* tissue cultures for cardenolides, *J. Pharm. Pharmacol.*, 16, 733, 1964.

34. **Buckland, E. and Townsley, D. M.**, Coffee cell suspension culures. Caffeine and chlorogenic acid content, *J. Can. Inst. Food Sci. Technol.*, 8, 164, 1975

35. **Burkholder, P. R. and Nickell, L. G.**, Atypical growth of plants. I. Cultivation of virus tumors of *Rumex* on nutrient agar, *Bot. Gaz.*, 110, 426, 1949.

36. **Butcher, D. N. and Connolly, J. D.**, An investigation of factors which influence the production of abnormal terpenoids by callus cultures of *Andrographis paniculata* Nees., *J. Exp. Bot.*, 22, 314, 1971.

37. **Butenko, R. G.**, Tissue culture of medicinal plants and prospective of its usage in medicine, *Probl. Pharmacog.*, 21, 184, 1967.

38. **Butenko, R. G., Brushwitzky, I. V., and Slepyan, L. T.**, Organogenesis and somatic embryogenesis in the tissue culture of *Panax ginseng*, C. A. Meyer, *Bot. Zh. (Leningrad)*, 7, 906, 1968.

39. **Calam, D. H. and Callow, R. K.**, Crowngall and tomatine, *Science*, 147, 174, 1965.

40. **Campbell, G., Chan, E. C. S., and Blosker, W. G.,** Growth of lettuce and cauliflower tissues *in vitro* and their production of antimicrobial metabolities, *Can. J. Microbiol.,* 11, 785, 1965.
41. **Carew, D. P.,** Reserpine in a tissue culture of *Alstonia constricta* F. Muell, *Nature (London),* 207, 89, 1965.
42. **Carew, D. P. and Schwarting, A. E.,** Production of rye embryo callus, *Bot. Gaz.,* 119, 237, 1958.
43. **Carew, D. P. and Staba, E. J.,** Plant tissue culture: its fundamentals, application and relationship to medicinal plant studies, *Lloydia,* 28, 1, 1965.
44. **Carew, D. P., Nylund, H. B., and Harris, A. L.,** Tissue culture studies of certain members of the Apocynaceae, *Lloydia,* 27, 322, 1964.
45. **Chafe, S. C. and Durzan, D. J.,** Tannin inclusions in cell suspension cultures of white spruce, *Planta,* 113, 251, 1973.
46. **Chan, W. N. and Staba, E. J.,** Alkaloid production by *Datura* callus and suspension tissue cultures, *Lloydia,* 28, 55, 1965.
47. **Chang, C. K. and Carew, D. P.,** Clavine alkaloid production with rye callus tissue, *Lloydia,* 31, 38, 1968.
48. **Chaturvedi, H. C. and Srivastava, S. N.,** Diosgenin biosynthesis by tuber-callus tissue cultures of *Dioscorea deltoidea, Lloydia,* 39, 82, 1976.
49. **Chen, C. M. and Hall, R. H.,** Biosynthesis of N^6-(Δ^2-isopentenyl) adenosine in the transfer ribonucleic acid of cultured tobacco pith tissue, *Phytochemistry,* 8, 1687, 1969.
50. **Chen, S., Stohs, S. J., and Staba, E. J.,** The biosynthesis of visnagin from 2-14C-acetate by *Ammi visnaga* suspension cultures and the metabolism of 14C visagin and 14C khellin by *A. visaga* and *A. majus, Lloydia,* 32, 339, 1969.
51. **Chen, P. R. and Venketeswara, S.,** Acid phosphatase activity of normal and tumor tissue of tobacco grown *in vitro* and *in vivo, Plant Physiol.,* 41, 842, 1966.
52. **Cheng, P. C.,** Cultivation and analysis of *Papaver bracteatum* Lindley, M.S. thesis, University of Mississippi, London, 1972.
53. **Constabel, F.,** Zur Amylasesekretion pflanzlicher Gewebekulturen, *Naturwissenschaften,* 47, 17, 1960.
54. **Constabel, F.,** Quantitative Untersuchungen über die extracellulare Hydrolyse von Kohlenhydraten durch *Juniperus communis*—Gewebekulturn, *Planta,* 59, 330, 1963.
55. **Constabel, F.,** Über die Gerbstoffe in Gewebekulturn von *Juniperus communis* L., *Planta Med.,* 11, 417, 1963.
56. **Constabel, F.,** Gerbstoffproduktion der Calluskulturen von *Juniperus communis* L., *Planta,* 79, 58, 1968.
57. **Constabel, F., Kirsten, G., and Steiner, M.,** Die freien Aminosaüren in Gemekekulteren von *Juniperus communis* L. *Ber. Dtsch. Bot. Ges.,* 78, 348, 1966.
58. **Constabel, F., Shyluk, J. P., and Gamborg, O. L.,** The effect of hormones on anthocyanin accumulation in cell cultures of *Haplopappus gracilis, Planta,* 96, 306, 1971.
59. **Constabel, R., Gamborg, O. L., Kurz, W. F. W., and Steck, W.,** Production of secondary metabolites in plant cell cultures, *Planta Med.,* 25, 158, 1974.
60. **Corduan, G.,** Produktion von Tropanalkaloiden in Gewebekulturen, *Planta Med.* Suppl., 22, 1975.
61. **Corduan, G. and Reinhard, E.,** Synthesis of volatile oils in tissue cultures of *Ruta graveolens, Phytochemistry,* 11, 917, 1972.
62. **Cowles, J. R., Fowler, J. A., and Walkinshaw, C. H.,** Comparison of isocitrate dehydrogenase activity, pyruvate kinase activity, and polyphenol content in physiologically different pine callus tissue, *Physio. Plant.,* 33, 177, 1975.
63. **Czygan, F. C.,** Moglichkeiten zur Production von Arneistoffen durch pflanzliche Gewebekulturen, *Planta Med.,* Suppl., 169, 1975.
64. **Davies, M. E.,** Polyphenol synthesis in cell suspension cultures of Paul's Scarlet rose, *Planta,* 104, 50, 1972.
65. **Davey, M. R., MacKenzie, I. A., Freeman, G. G., and Short, K. C.,** Studies on some aspects of the growth, fine structure and flavour production of onion tissue grown *in vitro, Plant Sci. Lett.,* 3, 113, 1974.
66. **Delfel, N. E. and Rothfus, J. A.,** Antitumor alkaloids in callus cultures of *Cephalotaxus harringtonia, Phytochemistry,* 16, 1595, 1977.
67. **Dhandapani, M., Antony, A., and Subba Rao, P. V.,** Purification and properties of phenylalanine ammonium lyase from fenugreek callus cultures in *All India Symp. 3rd Conf. Plant Tissue Culture,* The Maharaja Sajajirao University of Baroda, Baroda, 1978, 28.
68. **Dhoot, G. K. and Henshaw, G. G.,** Organization and alkaloid production in tissue cultures of *Hyoscyamus niger, Ann. Bot.,* 41, 943, 1977.
69. **Dobberstein, R. H. and Staba, E. J.,** Chlorophyll production in Japanese mint suspension cultures, *Lloydia,* 29, 50, 1966.

70. **Dohnal, B.,** Investigations on some metabolites of *Tecoma stans* Juss. callus tissue. II. Chromatographical analysis of alkaloid and quinone compounds, *Acta. Soc. Bot. Pol.,* 45, 369, 1976.

71. **Dohnal, B.,** Investigations on some metabolities of *Tecoma stans* Juss. callus tissue, III. Chromatographical search for iridoids, phenolic acids, terpenoids and sugars, *Acta Soc. Bot. Pol.,* 46, 187, 1977.

72. **Döller, G.,** Influence of the medium on the production of serpentine by suspension cultures of *Catharanthus roseus* (L.) G. Don, in *Production of Natural Compounds by Cell Culture Methods,* Alfermann, A. W., and Reinhard, E., Eds., Proc. Int. Symp. Plant Cell Culture: BPT — Report 1/78, Gesellschaft für Strahlen und Umweltforschung mbH, Munich, 109, 1978.

73. **Döller, G., Alfermann, A. W., and Reinhard, E.,** Produktion von Indolalkaloiden in Calluskulturen von *Catharanthus roseus, Planta Med.,* 30, 14, 1976.

74. **Dougall, D. K.,** The biosynthesis of protein amino acids in plant tissue cultures. I. Isotope competition experiments using glucose-U-^{14}C and the protein amino acids, *Plant Physiol.,* 40, 891, 1965.

75. **Dougall, D. K.,** Biosynthesis of protein amino acids in plant tissue cultures. II. Further isotope competition experiments using protein amino acids, *Plant Physiol.,* 41, 1411, 1966.

76. **Dougall, D. K.,** Biosynthesis of protein amino acids in plant tissue culture. III. Studies on the biosynthesis of arginine, *Plant Physiol.,* 42, 387, 1967.

77. **Dougall, D. K.,** Biosynthesis of protein amino acids in plant tissue culture. IV. Isotope competition experiments using glucose-U-^{14}C and potential intermediates, *Plant Physiol.,* 42, 941, 1967.

78. **Dravnieks, D. E., Skoog, F., and Harris, R. H.,** Cytokinin activation of de novo thiamine biosynthesis in tobacco callus cultures, *Plant Physiol.,* 44, 866, 1969.

79. **Durzan, D. J., Chafe, S. C., and Lopushanski, S. M.,** Effects of environmental changes on sugars, tannins, and organized growth in cell suspension cultures of white spruce, *Planta,* 113, 241, 1973.

80. **Fairbairn, J. W.,** New plant sources of opiates, *Planta Med.,* 29, 26, 1976.

81. **Fairbairn, J. W. and Hakim, F.,** *Papaver bracteatum* Lindl. — a new plant source of opiates, *J. Pharm. Pharmacol.,* 25, 353, 1973.

82. **Feucht, W.,** Flavonoide in *Prunus* callus, *Planta. Med.,* Suppl., 112, 1975.

83. **Forrest, G. I.,** Studies on the polyphenol metabolism of tissue cultures derived from the tea plant (*Camellia sinensis* L.), *Biochem. J.,* 113, 765, 1969.

84. **Freeman, G. G., Whenham, R. J., MacKenzie, I. A., and Davey, M. R.,** Flavour components in tissue cultures of onion (*allium cepa,* L.), *Plant Sci. Lett.,* 3, 121, 1974.

85. **Friedrich, H. and Baier, S.,** Anthracene derivatives in callus cultures from *Cassia angustifolia, Phytochemistry,* 12, 1459, 1973.

86. **Fritsch, H. and Grisebach, H.,** Biosynthesis of cyanidin in cell cultures of *Haplopappus gracilis, Phytochemistry,* 14, 2437, 1975.

87. **Fukami, T. and Hildebrandt, A. C.,** Growth and chlorophyll formation in edible green plant callus tissues *in vitro* on media with limited sugar supplements, *Bot. Mag.,* 80, 199, 1967.

88. **Furuya, T.,** Metabolic products and their chemical regulations in plant tissue cultures, *Kitasato Arch. Exp. Med.,* 41, 47, 1968.

88. **Furuya, T.,** Metabolic products and their chemical regulations in plant tissue cultures, *Kitasato Arch. Exp. Med.,* 41, 47, 1968.

89. **Furuya, T. and Ikuta, A.,** The presence of *l*-maackian and pterocarpin in callus tissue of *Sophora angustifolia, Chem. Pharm. Bull.,* 16, 771, 1968.

90. **Furuya, T. and Ishii, T.,** Verfahren zur Herstellung eines Saponine enthaltenden Ginseng-Medikamentes, German Patent, 2143936, 1972.

91. **Furuya, T. and Ishii, T.,** The manufacturing of *Panax* plant tissue culture containing crude sapogenins and crude sapogenins which are identical with those of natural *Panax* roots, *Japanese Patent, 4831917, 1973.*

92. **Furuya, T. and Kojima, H.,** 4-hydroxy digitolutein, a new anthraquinone from callus tissue of *Digitalis lanata, Phytochemistry,* 10, 1607, 1971.

93. **Furyua, T., Hirotani, M., and Kawaguchi, K.,** Biotransformation of progesterone and pregnenolone by plant suspension cultures, *Phytochemistry,* 11, 1013, 1971.

94. **Furuya, T., Hirotani, M., and Shinohara, T.,** Biotransformation of digitoxin by suspension callus culture of *Digitalis purpurea, Chem. Pharm. Bull.,* 18, 1081, 1970.

95. **Furuya, T., Ikuta, A., and Syōno, K.,** Alkaloids from callus tissue of *Papaver somniferum, Phytochem,* 11, 3041, 1972.

96. **Furuya, T., Kojima, H., and Katsuta, T.,** 3-methylpurpurin and other anthraquinones from callus tissue of *Digitalis lanata, Phytochem.,* 11, 1073, 1972.

97. **Furuya, T., Matsumoto, K., and Hikichi, M.,** Echinatin, a new chalcone from tissue culture of *Glycyrrhiza echinata, Tetrahedron Lett.,* 27, 2567, 1971.

98. **Furuya, T., Syōno, K., and Ikuta, A.,** Isolation of berberine from callus tissue of *Coptis japonica, Phytochemistry,* 11, 175, 1972.

99. **Furuya, T., Kojima, H., Syōno, K., and Ishii, T.,** Isolation of panatriol from *Panax ginseng* callus, *Chem. Pharm. Bull.,* 18, 2371, 1970.

100. **Furuya, T., Kojima, H., Syōno, K., Ishii, T., Votani, K., and Nishio, M.,** Plant tissue cultures. XVII. Isolation of saponins and sapogenins for callus tissue of *Panax ginseng, Chem. Pharm. Bull.,* 21, 98, 1973.

101. **Furuya, T., Syōno, K., Kojima, H., Hirotani, M., Ikuta, A., Hikichi, M., Kawaguchi, K., and Matsumoto, K.,** Chemical constituents and transformation capacity of medicinal plant callus tissues, in *Proc. 4th Int. Ferm. Symp.,* Society of Fermentation Technology, Japan, Osaka, 705, 1972.

102. **Gainor, C. and Crisley, F. D.,** Proteolytic activity of crude stem extracts from normal and tumor tissues of plants, *Nature (London),* 190, 1031, 1961.

103. **Gainor, C. and Crisley, F. D.,** Factors affecting proteolytic activity of extracts from normal and tumor tissues of tobacco, *Nature (London),* 193, 1076, 1962.

104. **Galston, A. W.,** Sur la relation entre la croissance des cultures de tissus vegetaux et leur teneur en catalase, *C. R. Acad. Sci.,* 232, 1505, 1951.

105. **Gamborg, O. L. and La Rue, T. A. G.,** Ethylene produced by plant cells in suspension cultures, *Nature (London),* 220, 604, 1968.

106. **Gamborg, O. L., Constabel, F., La Rue, T. A. G., Miller, R. A., and Steck, W.,** The influence of hormones on secondary metabolite formation in plant cell cultures, *Colloq. Int. C.N.R.S.,* 193, 335, 1971.

107. **Goldstein, J. L., Swain, T., and Tjhio, K. H.,** Factors affecting the production of leucoanthocyanins in sycamore cambial cell cultures, *Arch. Biochem. Biophys.,* 98, 176, 1962.

108. **Goodwin, T. W. and Williams, B. L.,** Preliminary observations on terpenoids in plant tissue cultures, *Biochem. J.,* 85(2), 12P, 1962.

109. **Graves, J. M. H. and Smith, W. K.,** Transformation of pregnenolone and progesterone by cultured plant cells, *Nature (London),* 214, 1248, 1967.

110. **Hahlbrock, K.,** Isolation of apigenin from illuminated cell suspension cultures of soybeans, *Glycine max, Phytochemistry,* 11, 165, 1972.

111. **Handro, W., Hell, K. G., and Kerbauy, G. B.,** Tissue culture of *Stevia rebaudiana,* a sweetening plant, *Planta Med.,* 32, 115, 1977.

112. **Hanower, P.,** Formation des polyfructosanes dans les tissue des tubercules de topinambour cultives *in vitro, C. R. Acad. Sci.,* 258, 3081, 1964.

113. **Hawes, G. B. and Adams, G. A.,** Extracellular arabinogalactan from suspension-cultured red kidney bean root cells, *Phytochemistry,* 11, 1461, 1972.

114. **Heble, M. R., Narayanaswami, S., and Chadha, M. S.,** Solasonine in tissue cultures of *Solanum xanthocarpum. Naturwissenschaften,* 55, 350, 1968.

115. **Heble, M. R., Narayanaswami, S., and Chadha, M. S.,** Diosgenin and β-sitosterol: isolation from *Solanum xanthocarpum* tissue cultures, *Science,* 161, 1145, 1968.

116. **Heble, M. R., Narayanaswami, S., and Chadha, M. S.,** 24-Methylene-cholesterol in tissue cultures of *Holarrhena antidysenterica, Z. Naturforsch.,* 26, 12, 1971.

117. **Heble, M. R., Narayanaswami, S., and Chadha, M. S.,** Lupeol in tissue cultures of *Solanum xanthocarpum, Phytochemistry,* 10, 910, 1971.

118. **Heble, M. R., Narayanaswami, S., and Chadha, M. S.,** Hormonal control of steroid synthesis in *Solanum xanthocarpum* tissue cultures, *Phytochemistry,* 10, 2393, 1971.

119. **Heble, M. R., Narayanaswami, S., and Chadha, M. S.,** Tissue differentiation and plumbagin synthesis in variant cell strains of *Plumbago zeylanica* L. *in vitro, Plant Sci. Lett.,* 2, 405, 1974.

120. **Heble, M. R., Narayanaswami, S., and Chadha, M. S.,** Studies on growth and steroid formation in tissue cultures of *Holarrhena antidysenterica, Phytochemistry,* 15, 681, 1976.

121. **Heble, M. R., Narayanaswami, S., and Chadha, M. S.,** Metabolism of cholesterol by callus culture of *Holarrhena antidysenterica, Phytochemistry,* 15, 1911, 1976.

122. **Helmbold, H., Voelter, W., and Reinhard, E.,** Sterols in cell cultures of *Digitalis lanata, Planta Med.,* 33, 185, 1978.

123. **Hildebrandt, A. C., Wilmar, J. D., Johns, H., and Riker, A. J.,** Growth of edible chlorophyllous plant tissues *in vitro, Am. J. Bot.,* 50, 248, 1963.

124. **Hiraoka, N. and Tabata, M.,** Alkaloid production by plants regenerated from cultured cells of *Datura innoxia, Phytochemestry,* 13, 1671, 1974.

125. **Horowitz, R. M. and Gentili, B.,** Dihydrochalcone Derivatives and Their Use as Sweetening Agents, U.S. Patent 3,087,821, 1963.

126. **Howard, J., Shannon, L., Oki, L., and Murashige, T.,** Soybean agglutinin. A mitogen for soybean callus cells, *Exp. Cell Res.,* 107, 448, 1977.

127. **Ibrahim, R. K. and Edgar, D.,** Phenolic synthesis in *Perilla* cell suspension cultures, *Phytochemistry,* 15, 129, 1976.

128. **Ibrahim, R. K., Thakur, M. L., and Permanand, B.,** Formation of anthocyanins in callus tissue cultures, *Lloydia,* 34, 175, 1971.

129. Ikeda, T., Matsumoto, T., and Noguchi, M., Formation of ubiquinone by tobacco plant cells in suspension culture, *Phytochemistry*, 15, 568, 1976.

130. Ikeda, T., Matsumoto, T., Kato, K., and Noguchi, M., Isolation and identification of ubiquinone 10 from cultured cells of tobacco, *Agric. Biol. Chem.*, 38, 2297, 1974.

131. Ikuta, A., Syōno, K., and Furuya, T., Alkaloids of callus tissues and redifferentiated plantlets in the Papaveraceae, *Phytochemistry*, 13, 2175, 1974.

132. Ikuta, A., Syōno, K., and Furuya, T., Alkaloids in plants regenerated from *Coptis* callus cultures, *Phytochemistry*, 14, 1209, 1975.

133. Itokawa, H., Akasu, M., and Fujita, M., Several oxidized sterols isolated from callus tissue of *Stephania cepharantha*, *Chem. Pharm. Bull.*, 21, 1386, 1973.

134. Jain, S. C. and Jain, H. C., Glycoalkaloids from *Solanum* species *in vivo* and *in vitro*, in *All India Symp. 3rd Conf. Plant Tissue Culture*, The Maharaja Sayajirao University of Baroda, Baroda, 1978, 23.

135. Jain, S. C. and Khanna, P., Production of sterols from *Sesamum indicum* Linn. tissue cultures, *Indian J. Pharm.*, 35, 163, 1973.

136. Jain, S. C., Rosenberg, H., and Stohs, S. J., Steroidal constituents of *Trigonella occulta* tissue cultures, *Planta Med.*, 31, 109, 1977.

137. Jalal, M. A. F. and Collin, H. A., Polyphenols of mature plant, seedling and tissue cultures of *Theobroma cacao*, *Phytochemistry*, 16, 1377, 1977.

138. Jaspars, E.M.J. and Veldstra, H., An α-amylase from tobacco crown-gall tissue cultures. I. Purification and some properties of the enzyme. Pattern of α-amylase iso-enzymes in different tobacco tissues, *Physiol. Plant.*, 18, 604, 1965.

139. Jaspars, E. M. J. and Veldstra, H., An α-amylase from tobacco crown-gall tissue cultures. II. Measurements of the activity in media and tissues, *Physiol. Plant.*, 18, 626, 1965.

140. Jhang, J. J., Staba, E. J., and Kim, J. Y., American and Korean ginseng tissue cultures: growth, chemical analysis, and plantlet production, *In Vitro*, 9, 253, 1974.

141. Jindra, A. and Staba, E. J., *Datura* tissue cultures: arginase, transaminase and esterase activities, *Phytochemistry*, 7, 79, 1968.

142. Johnson, I. S. and Border, G. B., Metabolites from animal and plant cell culture, *Adv. Appl. Microbiol.*, 15, 215, 1972.

143. Johnson, I. S., Armstrong, J. G., Gorman, M., and Burnett, J. P., The *Vinca* alkaloids. A new class of oncolytic agents. Conference on Problems Basic to Cancer Chemotherapy, *Cancer Res.*, 23, 1390, 1963.

144. Jones, L. H., Plant cell culture and biochemistry. Studies for improved vegetable oil production, in *Industrial Aspects of Biochemistry*, Spencer, B., Ed., Federation of European Biochemical Societies, London, 1974, 813.

145. Jones, L. H., Propagation of clonal oil palms by tissue culture, *Oil Palm News*, 17, 1, 1974.

146. Kadkade, P. G. and Madrid, T. R., Glycoalkaloids in tissue cultures of *Solanum acculeatissimum*, *Naturwissenschaften*, 64, 147, 1977.

147. Kamimura, S. and Akutsu, M., Cultural conditions on growth of the cell culture of *Papaver bracteatum*, *Agric. Biol. Chem.*, 40, 899, 1976.

148. Kamimura, S. and Nishikawa, M., Growth and alkaloid production of the cultured cells of *Papaver bracteatum*, *Agric. Biol. Chem.*, 40, 907, 1976.

149. Kamimura, S., Akutsu, M., and Nishikawa, M., Formation of thebaine in the suspension culture of *Papaver bracteatum*, *Agric. Biol. Chem.*, 40, 913, 1976.

150. Kanamaru, K., Kato, K., and Noguchi, M., Isolation and identification of α-L-glutamyl-L-glutamic acid from tobacco cells in suspension culture, *Agric. Biol. Chem.*, 38, 2285, 1974.

151. Karstens, W.K. H. and de Meester-Manger Cats, V., The cultivation of plant tissues *in vitro* with starch as a source of carbon, *Acta Bot. Neerl.*, 9, 263, 1961.

152. Kato, K., Watanabe, F., and Eda, S., An arabinolgalactan from extracellular polysaccharides of suspension-cultured tobacco cells, *Agric. Biol. Chem.*, 41, 533, 1977.

153. Kato,K., Watanabe, F., and Eda, S., Interior chains of glucuronomannan from extracellular polysaccharides of suspension-cultured tobacco cells, *Agric. Biol. Chem.*, 41, 539, 1977.

154. Kaul, B. and Staba, E. J., Visnagin: biosynthesis and isolation from *Ammi visnaga* suspension cultures, *Science*, 150, 1731, 1965.

155. Kaul, B. and Staba, E. J., *Ammi visnaga* (L) Lam. tissue cultures. Multi-liter suspension growth and examination for furanochromones, *Planta Med.*, 15, 145, 1967.

156. Kaul, B., and Staba, E. J., *Dioscorea* tissue cultures. I. Biosynthesis and isolation of diosgenin from *Dioscorea deltoidea* callus and suspension cells, *Lloydia*, 31, 171, 1968.

157. Kaul, B., Stohs, S. J. and Staba, E. J., *Dioscorea* tissue cultures. III. Influence of various factors on diosgenin production by *Dioscorea deltoidea* callus and suspension cultures, *Lloydia*, 32, 347, 1969.

158. Kaul, B., Wells, P., and Staba, E. J., Production of cardio-active substances by plant tissue cultures and their screening for cardiovascular activity, *J. Pharm. Pharmacol.*, 19, 760, 1967.

159. **Keller, H., Wanner, H., and Baumann, T. W.,** Kaffein-synthese in Fruchten und Gewebekulturen von *Coffea arabica, Planta,* 108, 339, 1972.

160. **Khanna, P.,** Role of auxin, phytohormones and ascrobic acid on production of secondary metabolites from *in vitro* tissue cultures of different plant species, in *All India Symp. 3rd Conf. Plant Tissue Culture,* The Maharaja Sayajirao University of Baroda, Baroda, 1978, 17.

161. **Khanna, D.,** Effect of auxins, phytohormones and ascorbic acid on production of opium alkaloids in *in vitro* tissue cultures of *Papaver* species, in *All India Symp. 3rd Conf. Plant Tissue Culture,* The Maharaja Sayajirao University of Baroda, Baroda, 1978, 18.

162. **Khanna, P. and Jain, S. C.,** Effect of nicotinic acid on growth and production of trigonelline by *Trigonella foenum-graecum* L. tissue cultures, *Indian J. Exp. Biol.,* 10, 248, 1972.

163. **Khanna, P. and Jain, S. C.,** Diosgenin, gitogenin and tigogenin from *Trigonella foenum-graecum* tissue cultures, *Lloydia,* 36, 96, 1973.

164. **Khanna, P. and Mohan, S.,** Isolation and identification of diosgenin and sterols from fruits and *in vitro* cultures of *Momordica charantia* L., *Indian J. Exp. Biol.,* 11, 58, 1973.

165. **Khanna, P. and Nag, T. N.,** Production of amino acids *in vitro* tissue culture, *Indian J. Exp. Biol.,* 11, 310, 1973.

166. **Khanna, P. and Nag, T. N.,** Isolation, identification, and screening of phyllemblin from *Emblica officinals* Gaertn. tissue culture, *Indian J. Pharm.,* 35, 23, 1973.

167. **Khanna, P. and Staba, E. J.,** Antimicrobials from plant tissue cultures, *Lloydia,* 31, 180, 1968.

168. **Khanna, P., Mohan, S., and Nag, T. N.,** Antimicrobials from plant tissue cultures, *Lloydia,* 34, 168, 1971.

169. **Khanna, P., Sharma, G. L., and Uddin, A.,** Atropine from *Atropa belladonna* tissue cultures, *Indian J. Exp. Biol.,* 15, 323, 1977.

170. **Kirkland, D. F., Matsuo, M., and Underhill, E. W.,** Detection of glucosinolates and myrosinase in plant tissue cultures, *Lloydia,* 34, 195, 1971.

171. **Kita, K. and Sugii, M.,** Tissue culture studies on *Panax ginseng* C. A. Meyer. I. On the cultural requirements of callus, *Yakugaku Zasshi,* 39, 1474, 1969.

172. **Klein, R. M.,** Plant tissue cultures, a possible source of plant constituents, *Econ. Bot.,* 14, 286, 1960.

173. **Klein, R. M., Caputo, E. M., and Witterholt, B. A.,** The role of zinc in the growth of plant tissue cultures, *Am. J. Bot.,* 49, 323, 1962.

174. **Knobloch, K. H. and Hahlbrock, K.,** 4-coumarate: CoA ligase from cell suspension cultures of *Petroselinum hortense* Hoffm., *Arch. Biochem. Biophys.,* 184, 237, 1977.

175. **Kordan, H. A. and Morganstern, L.,** Flavonoid production by mature citrus fruit tissue proliferating *in vitro, Nature (London),* 195, 163, 1962.

176. **Kovacs, B. A., Wakkary, J. A., Goodfriend, L., and Rose, B.,** Isolation of an anti-histaminic principle resembling tomatine from crown gall tumors, *Science,* 144, 295, 1964.

177. **Kulkarni, D. D., Ghugale, D. D., and Narasimhan, K.,** Chemical investigations of plant tissues grown *in vitro:* isolation of β-sitosterol from *Morus alba* (mulberry) callus tissues, *Indian J. Exp. Biol.,* 8, 347, 1970.

178. **Kupchan, S. M., Komoda, Y., Thomas, G. J., and Hintz, H. P. J.,** Maytanprine and maytanbutine, new antileukaemic ansa macrolides from *Maytenus buchananii, J. Chem. Soc. Chem. Commun.,* 1065, 1972.

179. **Kupchan, S. M., Komoda, Y., Branfman, A. R., Dailey, R. G., and Zimmerly, V. A.,** Novel maytansinoids. Structural interrelations and requirements for antileukemic activity, *J. Am. Chem. Soc.,* 96, 3706, 1974.

180. **Kupchan, S. M., Uchida, I., Branfman, A. R., Dailey, R. G., and Fei, B. Y.,** Antileukemia principles isolated from Euphorbiaceae plants, *Science,* 191, 571, 1976.

181. **Kupchan, S. M., Komoda, Y., Court, W. A., Thomas, G. J., Smith, R. M., Karim, A., Gilmore, C. J., Haltiwanger, R. C., and Bryan, R. F.,** Maytansine, a novel antileukemic ansa macrolide from *Maytenus ovatus, J. Am. Chem. Soc.,* 95, 1354, 1972.

182. **Lacharme, J. and Netien, G.,** Acides amines et organiques des cultures de tissus, *Physiol. Veg.,* 7, 1, 1969.

183. **Lackmann, I.,** Wirkungsspektren der Anthocyansynthese in Gewebekulturen und Keimlingen von *Haplopappus gracilis, Planta,* 98, 258, 1971.

184. **Lamba, S. S. and Staba, E. J.,** Effect of various growth factors in solid media on *Digitalis lanata* Ehrh. and *Mentha spicata* L. cell suspensions, *Phyton (Argentina),* 20, 175, 1963.

185. **Lang, E. and Hörster, H.,** An Zuker gebundene regulare Monoterpene. II. Untersuchungen zur Olibildung und Akkumulation ätherischer Öle in *Ocimum basilicum* Zellkulturen, *Planta Med.,* 31, 112, 1977.

186. **Lee, J. D.,** Ginseng tissue cultures, *Yak-up Shinmun,* Nov. 4, 6, 1971.

187. **Lee, P. K., Carew, D. P., and Rosazza, J.,** *Apocynum cannabinum* tissue cultures. Growth and chemical analysis, *Lloydia,* 35, 110, 1972.

188. **Lee, T. T. and Starratt, A. N.**, Growth substance requirements and major lipid components of tissue cultures of *Euphorbia esula* and *E. cyparissias, Can. J. Bot.*, 50, 723, 1972.

189. **Leistner, E.**, Isolierung, Identifizierung und Biosynthese von Anthrachinonen in Zellsuspensionskulturen von *Morinda citrifolia, Planta Med.*, Suppl., 214, 1975.

190. **Lichtenthaler, H. K. and Straub, V.**, Die Bildung von Lipochinonen in Gewebekulturen, *Planta Med.*, Suppl., 198, 1975.

191. **Lin, A. and Mathes, M. C.**, The *in vitro* secretion of growth regulators by isolated callus tissues, *Am. J. Bot.*, 60, 34, 1973.

192. **Lin, M. and Staba, E. J.**, Peppermint and spearmint tissue cultures. I. Callus formation and submerged culture, *Lloydia*, 24, 139, 1961.

193. **Loewus, M. W. and Loewus, F.**, The isolation and characterization of D-glucose 6-phosphate cycloaldolase (NAD-dependent) from *Acer pseudoplatanus* L. cell cultures, *Plant Physiol.*, 48, 255, 1971.

194. **Mandels, M., Parrish, F. W., and Reese, E. T.**, β-(1 → 3) glucanases from plant callus cultures, *Phytochemistry*, 6, 1097, 1967.

195. **Mante, S. and Boll, W. G.**, Comparison of growth and extracellular polysaccharide of cotyledon cell suspension cultures of bush bean (*Phaseolus vulgaris* cv. Contender) grown in coconut-milk medium and synthetic medium, *Can. J. Bot.*, 53, 1542, 1975.

196. **Maretzki, A., dela Cruz, A., and Nickell, L. G.**, Extracellular hydrolysis of starch in sugarcane cell suspensions, *Plant Physiol.*, 48, 521, 1971.

197. **Marshall, J. G. and Staba, E. J.**, Hormonal effects on diosgenin biosynthesis and growth in *Dioscorea deltoidea* tissue cultures, *Phytochemistry*, 15, 53, 1976.

198. **Marshall, J. G. and Staba, E. J.**, Steroids and an artifact from *Dioscorea deltoidea* tissue cultures, *Lloydia*, 39, 84, 1976.

199. **Mathes, M. C.**, Antimicrobial substances from aspen tissue grown *in vitro, Science*, 140, 1101, 1963.

200. **Mathes, M. C.**, The secretion of antimicrobial materials by various isolated plant tissues, *Lloydia*, 30, 177, 1967.

201. **Medora, R. S., Tsao, D. P. N., and Albert, L. S.**, Tissue culture of *Digitalis mertonensis*. I. Effect of certain steroids on the callus growth and formation of Baljet positive substances in *D. mertonensis, J. Pharm. Sci.*, 56, 67, 1967.

202. **Mehta, A. R. and Staba, E. J.**, Presence of diosgenin in tissue cultures of *Dioscorea composita* Hemsl. and related species, *J. Pharm. Sci.*, 59, 864, 1970.

203. **Metz, H. and Lang, H.**, Verfahren zur Zuchtung von differenziertem Wurzelgewebe, German Patent, 1,216,009, 1966.

204. **Misawa, M., Samejima, H., and Kinoshita, S.**, Plant Cell Suspension Cultures for Production of Useful Substances, paper presented at Joint U.S.-Republic of China Seminar on Plant Cell and Tissue Culture, Taipei, Taiwan, May 14—22, 1974.

205. **Misawa, M., Tanaka, H., Chiyo, O., and Mukai, N.**, Production of a plasmin inhibitory substance by *Scopolia japonica* suspension cultures, *Biotechnol. Bioeng.*, 17, 308, 1975.

206. **Misawa, M., Hayashi, M., Tanaka, H., Koh, K., and Misato, T.**, Production of plant virus inhibitor by suspension culture of *Phytolacca americana, Biotechnol. Bioeng.*, 17, 1335, 1975.

207. **Mitra, G. C. and Kaul, K. N.**, *In vitro* culture of root and stem callus of *Rauvolfia serpentina* Benth. for reserpine, *Ind. J. Exp. Biol.*, 2, 49, 1964.

208. **Mizukami, H., Konoshima, M., and Tabata, M.**, Variation in pigment production in *Lithospermum erythrorhizon* callus cultures, *Phytochemistry*, 17, 95, 1978.

209. **Mizusaki, S., Tanabe, Y., Noguchi, M., and Tamaki, E.**, *p*-Coumaroylputrescine, caffeoylputrescine and feruloylputrescine from callus tissue culure of *Nicotiana tabacum, Phytochemistry*, 10, 1347, 1971.

210. **Morris, J. A.**, Sweet taste — basic research with practical applications, *Manuf. Confect.*, 52(7), 38, 1972.

211. **Nabeta, K., Kasai, T., and Sugisawa, H.**, Phytosterol from the callus of *Stevia rebaudiana* Bertoni, *Agric. Biol. Chem.*, 40, 2103, 1976.

212. **Naef, J. and Turian, G.**, Sur les carotenoides du tissu cambial de racine de carotte cultive *in vitro, Phytochemistry*, 2, 173, 1963.

213. **Nettleship, L. and Slaytor, M.**, Limitations of feeding experiments in studying alkaloid biosynthesis in *Peganum harmala* callus cultures, *Phytochemistry*, 13, 735, 1974.

214. **Nickell, L. G.**, The continuous submerged cultivation of plant tissue as single cells, *Proc. Natl. Acad. Sci. U.S.A.*, 42, 848, 1956.

215. **Nickell, L. G.**, Production of gibberellin-like substances by plant tissue cultures, *Science*, 128, 88, 1958.

216. **Nickell, L. G.**, Antimicrobial activity of vascular plants, *Econ. Bot.*, 13, 281, 1959.

217. **Nickell, L. G.**, Submerged growth of plant cells, *Adv. Appl. Microbiol.*, 4, 213, 1962.

218. **Nickell, L. G. and Brakke, M. K.**, Secretion of α-amylase by *Rumex* virus tumors *in vitro*. Biological studies, *Am. J. Bot.*, 41, 390, 1954.

219. **Nickell, L. G. and Maretzki, A.**, The utilization of sugars and starch as carbon sources by sugarcane cell suspension cultures, *Plant Cell Physiol.*, 11, 183, 1970.

220. **Nickell, L. G. and Tulecke, W. R.**, Growth substances and plant tissue cultures. In *Plant Growth Regulation*, Iowa State University Press, Ames, 1961, 675.

221. **Ogutuga, D. B. A. and Northcote, D. H.**, Biosynthesis of caffeine in tea callus tissue, *Biochem. J.*, 117, 715, 1970.

222. **Ogutuga, D. B. A. and Northcote, D. H.**, Caffeine formation in tea callus tissue, *J. Exp. Bot.*, 21, 258, 1970.

223. **Olson, A. C.**, Secreted polysaccharides and proteins from *Nicotiana tabacum* suspension cultures, *Colloq. Int. C.N.R.S.*, 193, 411, 1971.

224. **Otten, L. A. B. M., Vreugdenhil, D., and Schilperoort, R. A.**, Properties of D (+)-lysopine dehydrogenase from crown gall tumor tissue, *Biochim. Biophys. Acta*, 485, 268, 1977.

225. **Overton, K. H. and Roberts, F. M.**, Biosynthesis of trans, trans and cis, trans-farnesols by soluble enzymes from tissue cultures of *Andrographis paniculata*, *Biochem. J.*, 144, 585, 1974.

226. **Overton, K. H. and Roberts, F. M.**, Interconversion of trans, trans and cis, trans farnesol by enzymes from *Andrographis*, *Phytochemistry*, 13, 2741, 1974.

227. **Pandya, K. P., Mascarenhas, A. F., and Sayagaver, B. M.**, Ubiquinone (Coenzyme Q) of normal and crown gall tissue cultures of *Parthenocissus* sp., *Indian J. Biochem.*, 3, 127, 1966.

228. **Patterson, B. D. and Carew, D. P.**, Growth and alkaloid formation in *Catharanthus roseus* tissue cultures, *Lloydia*, 32, 131, 1969.

229. **Paupardin, C.**, Sur les variations de la teneur en acide gentisique des tissus de tubercules de topinambour (*Helianthus tuberosus* L. var. violet de rennes) cultives *in vitro* dans diverses conditions, *Colloq. Int. C.N.R.S.*, 193, 259, 1971.

230. **Persinos, G. J.**, Extraction of Stevioside from the Leaves of *Stevia rebaudiana*, U. S. Patent 3,723,410, 1973.

231. **Peterkova, I.**, Elektrophoretisches Bild der Peroxidase in verschiedenen Klonen einer Calusgewebekultur von *Nicotiana tabacum* L. var. Samsun, *Acta Fac. Rerum Nat. Univ. Comeianae Physiol. Plant.*, 4, 81, 1971.

232. **Peters, R. A., and Shorthouse, M.**, Formation of monofluorocarbon compounds by single cell cultures of *Glycine max* growing in inorganic fluoride, *Phytochemistry*, 11, 1339, 1972.

233. **Petiard, V., Demarly Y., and Paris, R. R.**, Mise en evidence d'heterosides cardiotoniques dans les cultures de tissus de *Digitalis purpurea*, *C. R. Acad. Sci.*, 272, 1365, 1971.

234. **Phillips, R. and Henshaw, G. G.**, The regulation of synthesis of phenolics in stationary phase cell cultures of *Acer psendoplatanus* L., *J. Exp. Bot.*, 28, 785, 1977.

235. **Pisetskaya, N. F.**, On the problem of the selection of suitable nutrient medium for the tissue culture of *Panax ginseng* C. A. Meyer., *Rastit. Resur.*, 6, 516, 1970.

236. **Puhaa, Z. and Martin, S. M.**, The industrial potential of plant cell culture, *Prog. Ind. Microbiol.*, 9, 13, 1971.

237. **Radwan, S. S., Spener, F., Mangold, H. K., and Staba, E. J.**, Lipids in plant tissue cultures. IV. The characteristic patterns of lipid classes in callus cultures and suspension cultures. *Chem. Phys. Lipids*, 14, 72, 1975.

238. **Ramawant, K. G. and Arya, H. C.**, Alkaloid contents in *Ephedra* species *in vitro* and *in vivo*, in *All India Symp. 3rd Conf. Plant Tissue Culture*, The Maharaja Sayajirao University of Baroda, Baroda, 1978, 24.

239. **Ranganathan, B., Mascarenhas, A. F., Sayagaver, B. M., and Jagannathan, V.**, Growth of *Papaver somniferum* L. tissue *in vitro*, in *Plant Tissue and Organ Culture — a Symposium*, Int. Soc. Plant Morphol., University of Delhi, India, 1963, 108.

240. **Rao, S. and Mehta, A. R.**, Tyrosine ammonium lyase in tissue cultures of *Arachis hypogaea* L., in *All India Symp. 3rd Conf. Plant Tissue Culture*, The Maharaja Sayajirao University of Baroda, Baroda, 1978, 21.

241. **Reichling, J. and Becker, H.**, Calluskulturen von *Matricaria chamomilla*. I. Mitteilung: Anlage und Wachstums verhalten der Calluskultur und erste phytochemische Untersuchungen, *Planta Med.*, 30, 258, 1976.

242. **Reinert, J. and White, P. R.**, The cultivation *in vitro* of tumor tissues and normal tissue of *Picea glauca*, *Physiol. Plant.*, 9, 177, 1956.

243. **Reinert, J., Clauss, H., and Ardenne, R. V.**, Anthocyanbildung in Gewebekulturen von *Haplopappus gracilis* in Licht verschiedener Qualitat, *Naturwissenschaften*, 51, 87, 1964.

244. **Reinert, J., Schraudolf, H., and Tazawa, M.**, Extrazellulare Enzyme und Auxinbedarf von Gewebkulturen, *Naturwissenschaften*, 44, 588, 1957.

245. **Reinhard, E., Boy, M., and Kaiser, F.**, Umwandlung von *Digitalis*-glycosiden durch Zellsuspensionskulturen, *Planta Med.*, Suppl., 163, 1975.

246. **Reinouts van Haga, P.**, Biosynthese von Alkaloiden in Sterilen Wurzelkulturen von *Atropa belladonna*, *Dtsch. Akad. Wiss. Berlin Kl. Chem. Geol. Biol.*, 7, 102, 1956.

247. **Remillard, S., Rebhun, L. I., Howie, G. A., and Kupchan, S. M.,** Antimitotic activity of the potent tumor inhibitor maytansine, *Science,* 189, 1002, 1975.

248. **Riker, A. J. and Hildebrandt, A. C.,** Plant tissue cultures open a botanical frontier, *Annu. Rev. Microbiol.,* 12, 469, 1958.

249. **Roddick, J. G. and Butcher, D. N.,** Isolation of tomatine from cultured excised roots and callus tissues of tomato, *Phytochemistry,* 11, 2019, 2, 1972.

250. **Roller, U.,** Selection of plants and plant tissue cultures of *Catharanthus roseus* with high content of serpentine and ajmalicine, in *Production of Natural Compounds by Cell Culture Methods,* Alfermann, A. W. and Reinhard, E., Eds., Proc. Int. Symp. Plant Cell Culture: BPT-Report 1/78, Gesellschaft fur Strahlen und Umweltforschung mbH, Munich, 1978, 95.

251. **Routien, J. B. and Nickell, L. G.,** Cultivation of Plant Tissue, U. S. Patent 2,747,334, 1956.

252. **Rucker, W. and Radola, B. J.,** Isoelectric patterns of peroxidase isoenzymes from tobacco tissue cultures, *Planta,* 99, 192, 1971.

253. **Saka, H. and Maeda, E.,** Characteristics and varietal differences of α-amylase isoenzymes in rice callus, *Nippon Sakumotsu Gakkai Kiji,* 42, 307, 1973.

254. **Sakato, K. and Misawa, M.,** Effects of chemical and physical conditions on growth of *Camptotheca acuminata* cell cultures, *Agric. Biol. Chem.,* 38, 491, 1974.

255. **Sakato, K., Tanaka, H., and Misawa, M.,** Broad-specificity proteinase inhibitors in *Scopolia japonica* (Solanaceae) cultured cells, *Eur. J. Biochem.,* 55, 211, 1975.

256. **Sakato, K., Tanaka, H., Mukai, N., and Misawa, M.,** Isolation and identification of camptothecin from cells of *Camptotheca acuminata* suspension cultures, *Agric. Biol. Chem.,* 38, 217, 1974.

257. **Saleh, N. A. M., Fritsch, H., Kreuzaler, G., and Grisebach, H.,** Flavanone synthase from cell suspension cultures of *Haplopappus gracilis* and comparison with the synthase from parsley, *Phytochemistry,* 17, 183, 1978.

258. **Sargent, J. A. and Skoog, F.,** Scopoletin glycosides in tobacco tissue, *Physiol. Plant.,* 14, 504, 1961.

259. **Scharlemann, W.,** Acridin-Alkaloide aus Kalluskulturen von *Ruta graveolens* L., *Z. Naturforsch.,* 27, 806, 1972.

260. **Schrall, R. and Becker, H.,** Produktion von Catechinen und oligomeren Proanthocyanidinen in Callus — und Suspensionskulturen von *Crataegus monogyna, C. oxyacantha* und *Ginkgo biloba, Planta Med.,* 32, 297, 1977.

261. **Schultz, W. D.,** Camptothecin, *Chem. Rev.,* 73, 385, 1973.

262. **Scott, R. W., Burris, R. H., and Riker, A. J.,** Nonvolatile organic acids of crown galls, crown gall tissue cultures and normal stem tissue, *Plant Physiol.,* 30, 355, 1955.

263. **Seidmann, J.,** New sweetening agents for foods, *Lebensm. Ind.,* 18, 407, 1971.

264. **Sekiya, J. and Yamada, Y.,** Partial characterization of RNA polymerase from cultured tobacco cells, *Agric. Biol. Chem.,* 38, 1101, 1974.

265. **Sethi, J. K. and Carew, D. P.,** Growth and betaine formation in *Medicago sativa* tissue cultures, *Phytochemistry,* 13, 321, 1974.

266. **Shafiee, A. and Staba, E. J.,** Allergens from short ragweed leaf tissue culture, *In Vitro,* 9, 19, 1973.

267. **Shafiee, A., Lalezari, I., and Yassa, N.,** Thebaine in tissue culture of *Papaver bracteatum* Lindl, population Arya II, *Lloydia,* 39, 380, 1976.

268. **Sharghi, N. and Lalezari, I.,** *Papaver bracteatum* Lindl., a high rich source of thebaine, *Nature (London,)* 213, 1244, 1967.

269. **Shiio, I. and Ohta, S.,** Nicotine production by tobacco callus tissues and effect of plant growth regulators, *Agric. Biol. Chem.,* 37, 1857, 1973.

270. **Shinshi, H. and Noguchi, M.,** Comparison of isoperoxidase patterns in tobacco cell cultures and in the intact plant, *Phytochemistry,* 15, 556, 1976.

271. **Shinshi, H., Miwa, M., Kato, K., Noguchi, M., Matsushima, T., and Sugimura, T.,** A novel phosphodiesterase from cultured tobacco cells, *Biochemistry,* 15, 2185, 1976.

272. **Shyr, S. E. and Staba, E. J.,** Examination of squill tissue cultures for bufadienolides and anthocyanins, *Planta Med.,* 30, 86, 1976.

273. **Simola, L. K.,** Changes in the activity of several enzymes during root differentiation in cultured cells of *Atropa belladonna, Z. Pflanzenphysiol.,* 68, 373, 1973.

274. **Sipply, K. J. and Friedrich, H.,** Alkaloide im Kallus von *Duboisia myoporoides, Planta Med., Suppl.,* 186, 1975.

275. **Slabecka-Szweykowska, A.,** Warunki tworzenia sie antocjanu w tkance *Vitis vinifera* hodowanej *in vitro, Acta. Soc. Bot. Pol.,* 21, 538, 1952.

276. **Slepyan, L. I.,** Pharmacological activity of callus tissues of ginseng grown under *in vitro* conditions, *Tr. Leningr. Khim.-Farm. Inst.,* 26, 236, 1968.

277. **Slepyan, L. I.,** Callus development in isolated ginseng root tissue culture, *Rastit. Resur.,* 7, 175, 1971.

278. **Slepyan, L. I., Brushwitzky, I. V., and Butenko, R. G.,** *Panax ginseng* C. A. Meyer as an object for introduction into tissue culture, *Probl. Pharmacog.,* 21, 198, 1967.

279. Song, M. and Tattrie, N., Lipid composition of morning glory (*Ipomoea* sp.) cells grown in suspension cultures, *Can. J. Bot.,* 51, 1893, 1973.

280. Speake, T., McCloskey, P., Smith, W. K., Scott, T. A., and Hussey, H., Isolation of nicotine from cell cultures of *Nicotiana tabacum, Nature (London),* 201, 614, 1964.

281. Spurr, H. W., Ascorbic acid oxidase and tyrosinase activities during crown-gall development on tomato, *Diss. Abstr.,* 22, 1790, 1961.

282. Spurr, H. W., Holcomb, G. E., Hildebrandt, A. C., and Riker, A. J., Influence of 2,4-dichloro-phenoxyacetic acid on growth and enzymatic activity of normal and crown-gall tissue cultures, *Plant Physiol.,* 37 (Suppl.), 731, 1962.

283. Spurr, H. W., Holcomb, G. E., Hildebrandt, A. C., and Riker, A. J., Distinguishing tissue of normal and pathological origin on complex media, *Phytopathology,* 54, 339, 1964.

284. Staba, E. J., Production of cardiac glycosides by plant tissue cultures. I. Nutritional requirements in tissue cultures of *Digitalis lanata* and *Digitalis purpurea, J. Pharm. Sci.,* 51, 249, 1962.

285. Staba, E. J., The biosynthetic potential of plant tissue cultures, *Rev. Ind. Microbiol.,* 4, 193, 1963.

286. Staba, E. J., Product Production from Plant Cell and Tissue Culture, paper presented at Joint U. S.-Republic of China Seminar on Plant Cell and Tissue Culture, Taipei, Taiwan, May 14—22, 1974.

287. Staba, E. J. and Kaul, B., Production of Diosgenin by Plant Tissue Culture Technique, U. S. Patent 3,628,287, 1971.

288. Staba, E. J. and Lamba, S. S., Production of cardiac glycosides by plant tissue cultures. II. Growth of *Digitalis lanata* and *Digitalis purpurea* in suspension culture, *Lloydia,* 26, 29, 1963.

289. Staba, E. J. and Shafiee, A., Production of allergens by plant tissue culture technique, U.S. Patent Application 346,074, 1973.

290. Staba, E. J., Shik Shin, B., and Mangold, H. K., Lipids in plant tissue cultures. I. The fatty acid composition of triglycerides in rape and turnip rape cultures, *Chem. Phys. Lipids,* 6, 291, 1971.

291. Stanko, S. A. and Bardinskaya, M. S., Anthocyanins of callus tissues in *Parthenocissus tricuspidata, Proc. Acad. Sci. USSR, Sect. Agrochem.,* 146, 956, 1962.

292. Stanko, S. A., and Bradinskaya, M. S., Authocyanins of callus tissue of *Parthenocissus tricuspidata,Proc. Acad. Sci. USSR, Sect. Agrochem.,* 146, 1152, 1962.

293. Steck, W. and Constabel, F., Biotransformation in plant cell cultures, *Lloydia,* 37, 185, 1974.

294. Steinhart, C. E., Tissue cultures of a cactus, *Science,* 137, 545, 1962.

295. Stobart, A. K., Weir, N. R., and Thomas, D. R., Phytol in tissue cultures of *Kalanchoe crenata, Phytochemistry,* 8, 1089, 1969.

296. Stohs, S. J., The metabolism of progesterone by plant microsomes, *Phytochemistry,* 8, 1215, 1969.

297. Stohs, S. J. and El-Olemy, M. M., Cholesterol metabolism by *Cheiranthus cheiri* leaf and tissue culture homogenates, *J. Steroid Biochem.,* 2, 293, 1971.

298. Stohs, S. J. and El-Olemy, M. M., Metabolsim of progesterone by *Dioscorea deltoidea* suspension cultures, *Phytochemistry,* 11, 1397, 1972.

299. Stohs, S. J. and Rosenberg, H., Steroids and steroid metabolism in plant tissue cultures, *Lloydia,* 38, 181, 1975.

300. Stohs, S. J. and Staba, E. J., Production of cardiac glycosides by plant tissue cultures. IV. Biotransformation of digitoxigenin and related substances, *J. Pharm. Sci.,* 54, 56, 1964.

301. Stohs, S. J., Kaul, B., and Staba, E. J., The metabolism of ^{14}C-cholesterol by *Dioscorea deltoidea* suspension cultures, *Phytochemistry,* 8, 1679, 1969.

302. Stohs, S. J., Rosenberg, H., and Billetts, S., Sterols of *Yucca glauca* tissue cultures and seeds, *Planta Med.,* 28, 257, 1975.

303. Stohs, S. J., Sabatka, J. J., Obrist, J. J., and Rosenberg, H., Sapogenins of *Yucca glauca* tissue cultures, *Lloydia,* 37, 504, 1974.

304. Stohs, S. J., Sabatka, J. J., and Rosenberg, H., Incorporation of 4-^{14}C-22,23-^{3}H-sitosterol into diosgenin by *Dioscorea deltoidea* tissue suspension cultures, *Phytochemistry,* 13, 2145, 1974.

305. Stohs, S. J., Wegner, C. L., and Rosenberg, H., Steroids and sapogenins in tissue cultures of *Dioscorea deltoidea, Planta Med.,* 28, 101, 1975.

306. Straus, J., Anthocyanin synthesis in corn endosperm tissue cultures. I. Identity of the pigments and general factors, *Plant Physiol.,* 34, 536, 1959.

307. Straus, J., Invertase in cell walls of plant tissue cultures, *Plant Physiol.,* 37, 342, 1962.

308. Straus, J. and Campbell, W. A., Release of enzymes by plant tissue cultures, *Life Sci.,* 1, 50, 1963.

309. Subbaiah, K. V. and Mehta, A. R., Hormonal effect on growth and polyphenol production in *Datura* cell suspension cultures grown *in vitro,* in *All India Symp. 3rd Conf. Plant Tissue Culture,* The Maharaja Sayajirao University of Baroda, Baroda, 1978, 19.

310. Sugano, N. and Hayashi, K., Possible scheme for the biosynthesis of anthocyanin and phenolic compounds in a carrot aggregen as indicated by tracer experiments. Studies on anthocyananins. LVIII. *Bot. Mag.,* 80, 481, 1967.

311. **Sugano, N., Miya, S., and Nishi, A.,** Carotenoid synthesis in a suspension culture of carrot cells, *Plant Cell Physiol.*, 12, 525, 1971.

312. **Sugisawa, H. and Ohnishi, Y.,** Isolation and identification of monoterpenes from cultured cells of *Perilla* plant, *Agric. Biol. Chem.*, 40, 231, 1976.

313. **Suhadolnik, R. J.,** Amaryllidaceace alkaloid formation by floral primordial tissue and callous tissue, *Lloydia*, 27, 315, 1964.

314. **Suhadolnik, R. J., Fischer, A. G., and Zulalian, J.,** Biogenesis of the Amaryllidaceae alkaloids. II. Studies with whole plants, floral primordia and cell free extracts, *Biochem. Biophys. Res. Commun.*, 11, 208, 1963.

315. **Suzuki, H., Ikeda, T., Matsumoto, T., and Noguchi, M.,** Isolation and identificatio of rutin from cultured cells of *Stevia rebaudiana* Bertoni, *Agric. Biol. Chem.*, 40, 819, 1976.

316. **Suzuki, H., Ikeda, T., Matsumoto, T., and Noguchi, M.,** Isolation and identification of hydrangenol and umbelliferone from cultured cells of Amacha (*Hydrangea macrophylla* Seringe var. *Thunbergii* Makino), *Agric. Biol. Chem.*, 41, 205, 1977.

317. **Tabata, M., Yamamoto, H., and Hiraoka, N.,** Alkaloid production in the tissue cultures of some solanaceous plants, *Colloq. Int. C.N.R.S.*, 193, 389, 1971.

318. **Tabata, M., Mizukami, H., Hiraoka, N., and Konishima, M.,** Pigment formation in callus cultures of *Lithospermum erythrorhizon*, *Phytochemistry*, 13, 927, 1974.

319. **Tabata, M., Yamamoto, H., Hiraoka, N., and Konoshima, M.,** Organization and alkaloid production in tissue cultures of *Scopolia parviflora*, *Phytochemistry*, 11, 949, 1972.

320. **Tabata, M., Hiraoka, N,. Ikenoue, M., Sano, Y., and Konoshima, M.,** The production of anthraquinones in callus cultures of *Cassia tora*, *Lloydia*, 38, 131, 1975.

321. **Tahara, A.,** Synthesis of sweeteners from pine resin, *Kagaku Kogyo*, 23, 398, 1972.

322. **Tahara, A.,** Diterpenoids. XXII. Hydrofluorene compound with strong sweetness, *Yakugaku Zasshi*, 93, 951, 1973.

323. **Takahashi, M. and Yamada, Y.,** Regulation of nicotine production by auxins in tobacco cultured cells *in vitro*, *Agric. Biol. Chem.*, 37, 1755, 1973.

324. **Tamaki, E., Morishita, I., Nishida, K., Kato, K., and Matsumoto, T.,** Process for preparing licorice extract-like material for tobacco flavoring, U. S. Patent 3,710,512, 1973.

325. **Tanaka, H., Machida, Y., Tanaka, H., Mukai, N., and Misawa, M.,** Accumulation of glutamine by suspension cultures of *Symphytum officinale*, *Agric. Biol. Chem.*, 38, 987, 1974.

326. **Tarng, C. S. and Stohs, S. J.,** A phytochemical investigation of *Corchorus olitorius* and *C. capsularis* tissue cultures, *Planta Med.*, 27, 77, 1975.

327. **Tattrie, N. H. and Veliky, I. A.,** Fatty acid composition of lipids in various plant cell cultures, *Can. J. Bot.*, 51, 513, 1973.

328. **Taylor, W. I. and Farnsworth, N. R.,** *The Catharanthus Alkaloids. Botany, Chemistry, Pharmacology, and Clinical Uses,* Marcel Dekker, New York, 1975, 324.

329. **Teuscher, E.,** Problems der Produktion sekundarer Pflanzenstoffe mit Hilfe von Zellkulture, *Pharmazie*, 28, 6, 1973.

330. **Thorpe, T. A., Maier, V. P., and Hasegawa, S.,** Phenylalanine ammonium-lyase activity in citrus fruit tissue cultured *in vitro*, *Phytochemistry*, 10, 711, 1971.

331. **Tomita, Y. and Seo, S.,** Biosynthesis of the terpenes, maslinic acid and 3-epimaslinic acid in tissue cultures of *Isodon japonicus* Hara, *J. Chem. Soc. Chem. Commun.*, 1973, 707, 1973.

332. **Tomita, Y. and Uomori, A.,** Structure and biosynthesis of protokoronin in tissue cultures of *Dioscorea tokoro*, *Phytochemistry*, 13, 729, 1974.

333. **Tomita, Y., Uomori, A., and Minato, H.,** Sesquiterpenes and phytosterols in the tissue cultures of *Lindera strychnifolia*, *Phytochemistry*, 8, 2249, 1969.

334. **Tomita, Y., Uomori, A., and Minato, H.,** Steroidal sapogenins and sterols in tissue cultures of *Dioscorea tokoro*, *Phytochemistry*, 9, 111, 1970.

335. **Tulecke, W. and Nickell, L. G.,** Production of large amounts of plant tissue by submerged culture, *Science*, 130, 863, 1959.

336. **Tulecke, W. and Nickell, L. G.,** Methods, problems and results of growing plant cells under submerged conditions, *Trans. N. Y. Acad. Sci.*, 22, 196, 1960.

337. **Turner, T. D.,** Pharmaceutical applications of plant tissue cultures, *Pharm. J.*, 1971, 341, 1971.

338. **Uddin, A.,** Production of amino acids in *Ephedra foliata* suspension cultures, *Curr. Sci.*, 46, 825, 1977.

339. **Ukita, M., Furuya, A., Tanaka, H., and Misawa, M.,** 5′ — phosphodiesterase formation by cultured plant cells, *Agric. Biol. Chem.*, 37, 2849, 1973.

340. **Vagujfalvi, D., Maroti, M., and Tetenyi, P.,** Presence of diosgenin and absence of solasodine in tissue cultures of *Solanum laciniatum*, *Phytochemistry*, 10, 1389, 1971.

341. **van de Voort, F. and Townsley, P. M.,** A comparison of the unsaponifiable lipids isolated from coffee cell cultures and from green coffee beans. *J. Can. Inst. Food Sci. Technol.*, 8, 199, 1975.

342. **van der Wel, H.**, Isolation and characterization of the sweet principle from *Dioscoreophyllum cumminsii, Fed. Eur. Biochem. Soc. Lett.,* 21, 88, 1962.

343. **van der Wel, H. and Loeve, K.**, Isolation and characterization of thaumatin I and II, the sweet-tasting proteins from *Thaumatococcus danielli, Eur. J. Biochem.,* 31, 221, 1972.

344. **van Huystee, R. B. and Turcon, G.**, Rapid release of peroxidase by peanut cells in suspension culture, *Can. J. Bot.,* 51, 1169, 1973.

345. **Vasil, I. K. and Hildebrandt, A. C.**, Growth and chlorophyll production in plant callus tissues grown *in vitro, Planta,* 68, 69, 1966.

346. **Veliky, I. A.**, Synthesis of carboline alkaloids by plant cell cultures, *Phytochemistry,* 11, 1405, 1972.

347. **Veliky, I. A. and Barker, K. M.**, Biotransformation of tryptophan by *Phaseolus vulgaris* suspension cultures, *Lloydia,* 38, 125, 1975.

348. **Veliky, I. A. and Genest, K.**, Growth and metabolites of *Cannabis sativa* cell suspension cultures, *Lloydia,* 35, 450, 1972.

349. **Veliky, I., Sandkrist, A., and Martin, S. M.**, Physiology of, and enzyme production by, plant cell cultures, *Biotechnol. Bioeng.,* 11, 1247, 1969.

350. **Verma, D. D. S. and van Huystee, R. B.**, Cellular differentiation and peroxidase enzymes in cell culture of peanut cotyledons, *Can. J. Bot.,* 48, 429, 1970.

351. **Volk, R., Harel, E., Mayer, A. M., and Gan-Zvi, E.**, Catechol oxidase in tissue culture of apple fruit, *J. Exp. Bot.,* 28, 820, 1977.

352. **Wall, M. E., Wani, M. C., Cook, C. E., Palmer, K. H., McPhail, A. T., and Sim, G. A.**, Plant antitumor agents. I. The isolation and structure of camptothecin, a novel alkaloidal leukemia and tumor inhibitor from *Camptotheca acuminata, J. Am. Chem. Soc.,* 88, 3888, 1966.

353. **Wang, C. and Staba, E. J.**, Peppermint and spearmint tissue culture. II. Dual carboy culture of spearmint tissues, *J. Pharm. Sci.,* 52, 1058, 1963.

354. **Warick, R. P. and Hildebrandt, A. C.**, Free amino acid contents of stem and *Phylloxera* gall tissue cultures of grape, *Plant Physiol.,* 41, 573, 1966.

355. **Washitani, I. and Sato, S.**, Studies on the formation of proplastids in the metabolism of *in vitro* cultured tobacco cells. I. Localization of nitrite reductase and NADP — dependent glutamate dehydrogenase, *Plant Cell Physiol.,* 18, 117, 1977.

356. **Washitani, I. and Sato, S.**, Studies on the formation of proplastids in the metabolism of *in vitro* cultured tobacco cells. II. Glutamine synthetase/glutamate synthetase pathway, *Plant Cell Physiol.,* 18, 505, 1977.

357. **Washitani, I. and Sato, S.**, Studies on the formation of proplastids in the metabolism of *in vitro* cultured tobacco cells. III. Source of reducing power for amino acid synthesis from nitrite, *Plant Cell Physiol.,* 18, 1235, 1977.

358. **Washitani, I. and Sato, S.**, Studies on the formation of proplastids in the metabolism of *in vitro* cultured tobacco cells. IV. Gluconeogenetic pathway, *Plant Cell Physiol.,* 18, 1243, 1977.

359. **Weber, N.**, 3-Ketosteroide in soja-suspensionskulturen, *Phytochemistry,* 16, 1849, 1977.

360. **Weinstein, L. H., Nickell, L. G., Larencot, H. J., and Tulecke, W.**, Biochemical and physiological studies of tissue cultures and the plant parts from which they are derived. I. *Agave toumeyana* Trel., *Contrib. Boyce Thompson Inst.,* 20, 239, 1959.

361. **Weinstein, L. H., Tulecke, W., Nickell, L. G., and Larencot, H. J.**, Biochemical and physiological studies of tissue cultures and the plant parts from which they are derived. III. Paul's Scarlet Rose. *Contrib. Boyce Thompson Inst.,* 21, 371, 1962.

362. **West, F. R. and Mika, E. S.**, Synthesis of atropine by isolated roots and root-callus cultures of belladonna, *Bot. Gaz.,* 119, 50, 1957.

363. **Wickremasinghe, R. L., Swain, T., and Goldstein, J. L.**, Accumulation of amino-acids in plant cell tissue cultures, *Nature (London),* 199, 1302, 1963.

364. **Widholm, J. M.**, Control of tryptophan biosynthesis in plant tissue cultures: lack of repression of anthranilate and tryptophan synthetases by tryptophan, *Physiol. Plant.,* 25, 75, 1971.

365. **Widholm, J. M.**, Tryptophan biosynthesis in *Nicotiana tabacum* and *Daucus carota* cell cultures: site of action of inhibitory tryptophan analogs, *Biochem. Biophys. Acta,* 261, 44, 1972.

366. **Widholm, J. M.**, Control of aromatic amino acid biosynthesis in cultured plant tissues: effect of intermediates and aromatic amino acids on free levels, *Physiol. Plant.,* 30, 13, 1974.

367. **Widholm, J. M.**, Relation between auxin autotrophy and tryptophan accumulation in cultured plant cells, *Planta,* 134, 103, 1977.

368. **Williams, B. L. and Goodwin, T. W.**, The terpenoids of tissue cultures of Paul's Scarlet Rose, *Phytochemistry,* 4, 81, 1965.

369. **Wilson, G.**, The application of the chemostat technique to the study of growth and anthraquinone synthesis by *Galium mollugo* cells, in *Production of Natural Products by Cell Culture Methods,* Alfermann, A. W. and Reinhard, E., Eds., Proc. Int. Symp. Plant Cell Culture: BPT-Rep. 1/78, Gesellschaft für Strahlen und Umweltforschung mbH, Munich, 1978, 147.

370. **Wu, C. H., Zabawa, E. M., and Townsley, P. M.,** The single cell suspension culture of the licorice plant, *Glycyrrhiza glabra, Can. J. Food Sci. Technol.,* 7, 105, 1974.

371. **Wu, W. L., Staba, E. J., and Blumenthal, M. N.,** Multiliter production and immunochemical cross-reactivity of plant tissue culture antigens, *J. Pharm. Sci.,* 65, 102, 1976.

372. **Yaklich, R. W. and Gentner, W. A.,** Anthocyanin pigments and thebaine of *Papaver bracteatum, Physiol. Plant.,* 31, 326, 1974.

373. **Yanagawa, H., Kato, T., Kitahara, Y., and Kato, Y.,** Chemical components of callus tissues of rice, *Phytochemistry,* 11, 1893, 1972.

374. **Yanagawa, H., Kato, T., Kitahara, Y., Kameya, T., and Takahashi, N.,** Chemical components of callus tissues of pumpkins, *Phytochemistry,* 10, 2775, 1971.

375. **Yu, P. L. C., el-Olemy, M. M., and Stohs, S. J.,** A phytochemical investigation of *Withania somnifera* tissue cultures, *Lloydia,* 37, 593, 1974.

376. **Zenk, M. H., El-Shagi, H., and Schulte, U.,** Anthraquinone production by cell suspension cultures of *Morinda citrifolia, Planta Med.,* Suppl., 79, 1975.

377. **Zenk, M.H., El-Shagi, H., and Ulbrich, B.,** Production of rosmarinic acid by cell-suspension cultures of *Coleus blumei, Naturwissenschaften,* 64, 585, 1977.

378. **Zenk, M. H., El-Shagi, H., Arens, H., Stöckigt, J., Wesler, E. W., and Deus, B.,** Formation of the indole alkaloids serpentine and ajmalicine in cell suspension cultures of *Catharanthus roseus,* in *Proceedings in Life Sciences: Plant Tissue Culture and its Bio-technological Application,* Barz, W., Reinhard, E., and Zenk, M. H., Eds., Springer-Verlag, Berlin, 1977, 27.

379. **Zheng, G. Z. and Zheng, L.,** Studies on tissue culture of medicinal plants. I. Callus cultures of *Scopolia acutangula* for the production of hyoscyamine and scopolamine, *Acta Bot. Sinica,* 18, 163, 1976.

380. **Zheng, G. Z. and Zheng, L.,** Studies on tissue culture of medicinal plants. II. Chemical control of callus growth and synthesis of hysocyamine and scopolamine by *Scopolia acutangula* callus, *Acta Bot. Sinica,* 19, 209, 1977.

N

W

X

Y

Z